Paediatric Problems in General Practice

THIRD EDITION

Oxford General Practice Series • 36

MICHAEL MODELL
Professor of Primary Health Care,
University College London Medical School

ZULF MUGHAL
Consultant Paediatrician,
St Mary's Hospital, Manchester
and
Honorary Senior Lecturer in Child Health,
University of Manchester

and

ROBERT BOYD
Professor of Paediatrics,
University of Manchester

OXFORD NEW YORK TORONTO
OXFORD UNIVERSITY PRESS
1996

Oxford University Press, Walton Street, Oxford OX2 6DP
Oxford New York
Athens Auckland Bangkok Bombay
Calcutta Cape Town Dar es Salaam Delhi
Florence Hong Kong Istanbul Karachi
Kuala Lumpur Madras Madrid Melbourne
Mexico City Nairobi Paris Singapore
Taipei Tokyo Toronto
and associated companies in
Berlin Ibadan

Oxford is a trade mark of Oxford University Press

Published in the United States
by Oxford University Press Inc., New York

A catalogue record for this book is available from the British Library

Library of Congress Cataloging in Publication Data

Modell, Michael, 1937–
Paediatric problems in general practice / Michael Modell,
Zulf Mughal, Robert Boyd. — 3rd ed.
p. cm. — (Oxford medical publications) (Oxford general practice series ; 36)
Includes index.
ISBN 0-19-262512-8 (pbk)
1. Pediatrics. 2. Family medicine. I. Mughal, Zulf. II. Boyd, Robert (Robert David Hugh)
III. Title. IV. Series. V. Series: Oxford general practice series ; no. 36.
[DNLM: 1. Pediatrics. 2. Family Practice. W1 OX55 no. 36 1996 / WS 200 M689p 1996]
RJ45.M554 1996
618.92—dc20
DNLM/DLC
for Library of Congress 96–13499 CIP

Typeset by
Advance Typesetting Ltd, Oxfordshire

Printed in Great Britain by Biddles Ltd, Guildford

Preface to third edition

Encouraged by the response to earlier editions, we have again based this book firmly on the practical realities of delivering child care in primary care, and have expanded the authorship to maintain this and widen our perspective.

The book has been radically revised and about a third has been rewritten to include those changes in paediatric diagnosis and treatment that appear genuine improvements. We have also tried to reflect and respond to deeper trends: rising patient and family expectations and their empowerment through greater knowledge; the increasing autonomy of adolescents; doctor accountability through more open note-keeping; the revolution of applied genetics driven by DNA technology and antenatal imaging; the new immigrants, more refugees from Africa and Europe but fewer economic migrants; the decline of developmental surveillance contrasting with the GP contract-driven desire for greater health promotion; the greater integration of disabled children into general education; the continued increase in the skill and profile of members of the primary care team; the rapid advance in applied information technology, the slower move to base health care decisions on reliable evidence; the worrying increase in childhood poverty, family instability, and the expanding number of neighbourhoods which fail to give a safe and secure environment.

Readers will note that we have usually used the male person or pronoun. We considered avoiding gender pronouns altogether, being impersonal or labelling the doctor as she and patient as he, but eventually decided as male authors that this would be a distraction. No insult is intended.

Alec Anson, Frank Bamford, Jon Couriel, Stephen D'Souza, Amra Darr, Peter Davenport, Tim David, Caroline Doig, Pam George, Elena Garralda, Simon Gowers, Stuart Handyside, Jonathan Jagger, Roy McGregor, Ian McKinley, Bernadette Modell, Tariq Mohammed, David Morris, Patricia Morris-Jones, Tahra Mughal, Richard Newton, Valerie Newton, Roger Palmer, Bob Poslethwaite, Wendy Rankin, Jill Roland, Helen Roper, Dick Stevens, Karen Mee, and Adrian Thomas have commented on sections of this or the last edition. Gill Yudkin read several chapters and commented most usefully from the perspective of a GP heavily involved in the care of families. We are most grateful to them for the mistakes they prevented us making and ask them to forgive us for occasions when we have failed to follow their advice. We also thank Zeenat Mughal for her secretarial support.

London and Manchester
April 1996

M.M.
Z.M.
R.D.H.B.

Contents

1 Communication

Until recently, hospital consultants formed a more powerful and prestigious part of the medical establishment in the UK than GPs, but this is changing. General practitioners are closer to the 'consumers' than hospital doctors, and their patterns of referral for secondary care can have a more direct influence on which services are provided by which hospital or other provider. Their opinion is being sought and they are being wooed by other sections of the health service in an unprecedented manner. In turn, decision-making and power are also being shared with nurses, pharmacists, and other health professionals, who are being given prescription rights, formalized advisory roles and direct access to patients. Registers of practitioners of complementary medicine are being established; managerial power and numbers are increasing. The advent of fund-holding practices means that, for the first time in almost 50 years, there is a significant financial component to the doctor–patient interaction. Even without fund-holding there may be a perception by patients that treatment is being withheld because of cost. The new arrangements present an opportunity for closer liaison between primary and secondary care, and for GPs to negotiate contracts for paediatric services (especially for non-emergencies) which emphasize quality and relevance as well as cost. It remains to be seen whether the changes will lead to a better, more cost-effective, or an increasingly fragmented service.

Within the practice the GP's responsibilities remain:

1. To provide 24-hour care for children who are sick; referring when necessary.
2. To promote health and prevent avoidable illness; to support parents and help them improve their expertise.
3. To co-operate with other health and non-health professionals in the care of children, especially those with chronic disorders or disabling conditions.

THE CHILD-FRIENDLY PRACTICE

Services should be provided in a cheerful, safe environment containing picture-books and toys. There should be easy access for prams, pushchairs and wheelchairs including somewhere where these can be protected from bad weather. For the child health clinic, a play area, appropriate toilets, and a fridge to store vaccines are all important. Equipment and drugs must be readily available for the occasional paediatric emergency—nebulizers, a resuscitation box including drugs for managing anaphylaxis and meningococcal septicaemia, airways and ambu bags for face mask ventilation of infants and children. All drugs need to be locked in a cabinet away from the inquisitive fingers of wandering toddlers.

Doctors should not leave their sharps boxes or open medical bags in empty, unlocked consulting-rooms.

Many practices make special arrangements to ensure that sick children are promptly assessed, with a few appointments for them left unbooked during each surgery session. Quick access to the doctor is especially important for the sick infant (p. 10). Parents are often willing to save the GP a home visit and bring an unwell child to the practice if they can be promised a prompt consultation. If the child cannot be brought into the surgery, a request for a home visit to a vomiting feverish baby should be treated more urgently than one to an adult with an infected varicose ulcer. Sick infants may change rapidly after the initial consultation. The GP may need to alert the colleague who is on duty in the evening, to the possibility of further contact by the family if the child's condition deteriorates. More forcefully, early follow-up by phone or visit may sometimes need to be agreed at the initial consultation.

Child-friendly receptionists are the key to the child-friendly practice. Their initial training programme should include instructions on why ill babies and children need to be seen promptly. Doctors and receptionists are not the only staff involved. With special training practice nurses may be able to help identify those children who need urgent medical attention.

CHILD-CENTRED CONSULTATIONS

The consultation is the key role of the GP, even though this central task sometimes appears to be overtaken by a plethora of administrative duties.

A number of books (required reading for the MRCGP) describe different models of the consultation (Pendleton *et al.* 1984; Neighbour 1987). The models generally identify fundamentally similar elements of a successful interaction between doctor and patient. These include a relaxed atmosphere in which the parents (or patient) is able to describe why she has consulted at that particular time, and is given the opportunity to express her own ideas of the nature of the problem.

Balint (1957), coming from a psychoanalytic tradition, had an important influence. He emphasized that patients often present with physical manifestations of psychological problems and that the doctor's emotional reaction during the consultation can be of considerable diagnostic importance. If he feels angry, depressed or 'put upon', this may reflect the effect the patient has on other people in their lives. The doctor's emotions may also reflect how the patient is actually feeling.

Many consultations do not just deal with acute illnesses. If time permits, there may be the possibility of opportunistic health promotion or of following-up unresolved issues raised on a previous occasion.

Mrs Hunt came to tell the doctor about the breakdown of her marriage. She did not think her depressed mood was having much effect on her intelligent four-and-a-half-year-old daughter. The GP gently reminded her that when Louise had been asked to 'draw mummy' at her pre-school check a few weeks earlier the following picture had been produced.

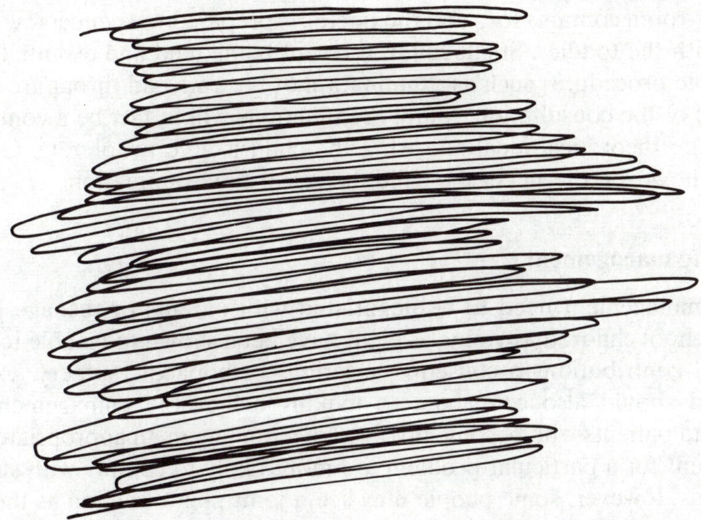

'Do sit down ...', 'How can I help you?' are useful opening remarks to give parents and adolescents a broad opportunity to express their real concerns. The former are usually acute observers of their children's behaviour and are able to give an accurate description of the problem. The doctor needs to listen carefully as valuable diagnostic clues to the cause of the problem may almost incidentally emerge; for example, 'the colds go to her chest' (asthma).

The doctor should also focus on the young person concerned, observing an infant whilst the parent is giving the history or smiling in an encouraging way at the toddler who wishes to explore the room. He needs to know the patient's name, however young, and use it. It can be worrying and irritating for older children to be discussed as if they were absent. Many older children can give a good account of their symptoms and should be encouraged to do so. Parents can usually be persuaded politely not to interrupt by making it clear that the doctor's attention is selectively focused on the child. Even younger children may make helpful contributions, especially if they feel secure, for example, by sitting on their mother's lap. Siblings who are brought into the room should not be ignored. 'What is your baby's name ...,' 'I like your jumper ...'.

Examination

An unhurried approach is essential. The infant will be more relaxed and less inclined to cry if in physical contact with the mother, and if the doctor starts by a brief pretend examination of the parent or of the child's doll or teddy bear. He will also be more at ease if allowed to play with the stethoscope before it is placed on his chest. The toddler may allow the examination to proceed only if the doctor does not insist on the vest being removed An opportunistic examination is necessary in this age group—do what you can when you can. This is often easier if the consulting-room contains toys and the doctor is prepared to spend a few minutes playing with the toddler. Small children resent being held and essential but uncomfortable procedures such as examination of the ears and throat are best left to the end of the consultation. Many examinations will in fact be a compromise between the theoretical ideal and what the child is able to tolerate. Generally speaking, however, the sicker the child the easier the examination.

Negotiating management

Plans of management need to be negotiated with parents or teenage patients. Primary school children as young as eight have been shown to be able to make a thoughtful contribution to consent for serious orthopaedic surgery (Alderson 1993), and should also contribute to making achievable management plans. Parents and patients who become involved in agreeing on an appropriate plan of management for a particular problem are more likely to comply with suggested treatments. However, some people may see a joint plan of action as the doctor abdicating responsibility or prefer a parent–child relationship with their GP. Such attitudes are only changed slowly over time. Sometimes the issues are clear cut. For example, the child with suspected acute appendicitis or meningococcal septicaemia obviously requires prompt admission to hospital. Much more frequently a dogmatic approach is inappropriate and the parents' or child's view may be the deciding factor. Should the infant with a prolonged cold be prescribed penicillin? Is it necessary to postpone a foreign trip because the infant is feverish? Would medicine or tablets be preferred for a urinary tract infection?

Education of parents and children plays an important role. For example, a review of seven controlled trials of asthma education for children (Clark 1989) showed improved outcomes, including an approximately one-third reduction in emergency attendances and admission days (Lewis *et al.* 1984) compared to controls.

Well-written leaflets are a useful adjunct to verbal instructions and can be taken home and read at leisure. These are, however, no substitute for clear verbal instructions at the end of a consultation, for example, when to stop dioralyte in an infant with gastro-enteritis, or re-contact the doctor if the fever does not subside.

GPS AND PAEDIATRICIANS

Doctors may communicate with each other, by electronic mail, more usually by fax, telephone, letter, or face-to-face; the latter sometimes in paediatric clinics held in practice premises or health centres. Postgraduate activities present another opportunity for contact, especially as the didactic lecture is slowly being replaced by seminars and workshops.

A practice is likely to have a considerable amount of contact with the local paediatric department. Communication will be enhanced if the GP and consultant know and respect each other. The initiative for this needs to come from a young principal or registrar when he or she joins the practice. Visiting patients in hospital, sitting in out-patient sessions, dialogue at postgraduate courses, and invitations to attend the practice lunchtime meetings to discuss a relevant topic are all useful methods of building up a relationship with a hospital department. The GP registrar may have already worked as an SHO in the local hospital.

These efforts may be time-consuming initially, but not in the long run if smooth communication leads to trouble-free admissions and discharges, and a welcoming response from the paediatric team to a request for an urgent hospital referral or telephone advice. Some hospitals have regular weekday paediatric emergency clinics where GPs can get an urgent opinion. These are very useful, but should not be used for children with minor or non-urgent problems. If they are not available it is reasonable for the GP to expect to be able to get an urgent out-patient consultation within 24–48 hours of the request.

The telephone

Telephone conversations are the commonest form of spoken communication between a consultant and a GP. Both may need considerable chasing around until contact is made, though this is easier if practices have the mobile phone or direct-line number of the local paediatricians. General practitioners should usually be prepared to be interrupted during a consultation, as should consultants during ward rounds and out-patient clinics, when requested to speak urgently to a colleague. Many practices have developed a system for ensuring that hospital doctors are able to speak to the relevant GP out-of-hours if urgent information is needed.

The commonest reasons for telephone contact are: for discussion of a possible referral or admission; for provision of additional information about delicate social problems that the GP does not wish to mention in a letter, and to confer

Table 1.1 Communication between GPs and hospital consultants

Referral letter
Degree of urgency
Main problems
Findings on examination
GP's diagnostic opinion
Medication so far
Important past history
(including history of immunization and prenatal history when relevant)
Important social and family history
Information given to patients
Reason for referral (diagnosis, reassurance for the doctor or the patient, or management advice)
Preferred follow-up arrangements

(The last two points are very important if the GP is to receive an appropriate response.)

Consultant's reply
Diagnosis, reason for making it and any doubts about it
Available results of relevant investigations and those still outstanding
Management
Prognosis
Information given to family
Follow-up arrangement
Answer specific questions of GP
(re-read referral letter before dictating reply)

(Separate copies may need to be sent, if the parent agrees, to a health visitor if not practice-attached.)

about diagnostic or therapeutic possibilities before they are mentioned to the child's parents. Telephone calls are an important interim means of communication before the discharge letter arrives at the practice—vital if an early home visit by the health visitor or GP is needed, or if the child has died, or the family has been given devastating news.

Letters

Table 1.1 sets out the key items of information to be included in letters or faxes to and from hospital. Ideally, a patient should be referred to a named doctor, but not if it is important that the child is rapidly seen by the first available consultant. However, the quality of a letter is likely to be higher when the GP knows who is going to read it.

Various issues may need to be clearly negotiated between the consultant and the GP. These include: (1) shared care arrangements. For example, a child with severe asthma may be best served by surveillance by the practice, coupled with six-monthly visits to out-patients and easy access to casualty in the event of a severe attack. The hospital department may employ specialist nurses (e.g. in diabetes or asthma) who may visit the child at home and be on call for advice; (2) deciding who has the responsibility for prescribing and monitoring complex and expensive drug regimes, such as erythropoietin or growth hormone.

Patients now have the right to read their own medical records (and presumably those of their young children) unless the information contained may cause serious physical or mental harm to the patient or a third party. The days have gone when doctors could carelessly write of 'stupid mothers' or 'aggressive fathers'. In addition, it is sometimes helpful for the GP to go through a consultant's letter with parents to ensure that everything is understood and to reassure them that there are no secrets kept from the family. It is a challenge to ensure that this openness does not lead to vacuous, unhelpful correspondence.

Paediatric clinics in practice premises

This increasingly common development has many potential benefits. These can include: improved hospital–practice communication; useful education for all the health professionals concerned, including the paediatricians; consultations with families who would be reluctant to go to the hospital; good public relations for the paediatric department concerned. Joint consultations increase parents' confidence in the practice personnel when they see GP, health visitor, and paediatrician conferring together, respecting each other's expertise and agreeing on how best the problem should be managed. Some fund-holding practices request these clinics as a means of improving the quality of care provided. However, some practices have been hosting these outreach clinics for many years.

The benefits will only be realized if real communication occurs (Modell and Boyd 1984), and this is disappointingly rare (Bailey *et al.* 1994). The ideal is for the GP and/or health visitor to join the consultation, or, at a minimum, to discuss the problem with the consultant after he has seen the family, perhaps at a practice meeting. Otherwise the child may as well be sent to hospital. Similarly the consultant should bring feed-back of practice patients admitted or seen in out-patients since the previous clinic. The consultant may learn a lot about the family from the practice team, especially when the discussion includes contributions from health visitors, counsellors and others, and will then be able to contribute more effectively to a management plan especially for the socially disadvantaged. In short, education is a two-way process.

There are some drawbacks to these clinics. If the session occurs once a month, it is difficult for the GP who sees a child with an urgent problem to wait until the consultant's next visit. Whilst blood and urine can be taken for tests in the practice, more elaborate investigations will mean that the child is not saved a hospital visit. Finally, the practice, or group of practices, has to generate enough useful consultations to make it worth the paediatrician spending half a day away from the hospital.

Computers

In some practices computers are mainly used for housekeeping functions, such as maintaining an age–sex register, issuing repeat prescriptions, recall reminders, lists of appointments, and facilitation of claims for fees and allowances. Databases usually contain only sparse medical histories, but the practice needs to be aware that the method of storing information and obtaining access must conform to the Data Protection Act. In many practices target groups who need regular surveillance can be easily identified electronically. These include children with chronic conditions, such as asthma, glue ear with deafness, recurrent urinary tract infection or failure to thrive. The quality of the output will depend entirely on the quality of the original material. Whatever system is used needs to integrate records produced by different members of the primary care team, health visitors and practice nurses as well as GPs.

More and more practices are making much more comprehensive use of their computers and some are already paperless. Computers are becoming more user-friendly and a more valuable tool for clinical care, audit and research. At the moment, entering data during a consultation is a laborious and time-consuming activity which often detracts from doctor–patient interaction. Links are being set up with local hospitals for direct booking of appointments and admission dates for surgery and quick access to X-rays and pathological results. Referrals and consultants' responses will soon be sent by electronic mail. Screening and immunization records of community units or trusts and the Health Authority will be easily accessible, as will Medline searches. GPs visiting a patient at home can sometimes access information from the surgery database via a modem link to their laptop computer. An electronic link to the outside world of computer software means vast amounts of medical information will become available to members of the primary care team (and patients) via the internet. At the moment, computers present clinical data, leaving the user to decide on the best course of action. Some systems include templates which act as an 'aide-memoire' for patients who are seen with a particular problem, such as asthma or diabetes. The next step is a computerized decision-support system which presents the user with patient-specific advice. Such a system is being developed for the management of asthma in primary care. It will electronically compare information obtained at the presenting consultation with that acquired at previous encounters between the patient and the primary care team. It aims to aid diagnosis in atypical patients, suggest a management plan in accordance with the agreed guidelines and help in monitoring the patient's progress.

Other computer advances on the horizon are interactive software which provide patients with enough information to enable them to make an informed choice about the most appropriate treatment and receive tailored health advice, and 'smart cards' which enable doctors to have instant access to an individual's medical history—particularly important for a mobile population. Continue to watch this space.

Bibliography

Alderson, P. (1993). *Children's consent to surgery*. Open University Press, Milton Keynes, Buckingham.

Bailey, J. J., Black, M. E., and Wilkin, D. (1994). Specialist outreach clinics in general practice. *British Medical Journal*, **308**, 1083–6.

Balint, M. (1957). *The doctor, his patient and the illness*. Pitman Press, Tunbridge Wells.

Clark, N. M. (1989). Asthma self management education. *Chest*, **95**, 1110–13.

Lewis, C. E., Rachelefsky, G., Lewis, M. A., De La Sota, A., and Kaplan, M. (1984). A randomised trial of asthma care training for kids. *Pediatrics*, **74**, 478–86.

Modell, M. and Boyd, R. D. H. (1984). A consultant in a health centre. *The Practitioner*, **228**, 968–71.

Neighbour, R. (1987). *The inner consultation*. MPT Press, Lancaster.

Pendleton, D., Schofield, T., Tate, P., and Havelock, P. (1984). *The consultation: an approach to learning and teaching*. Oxford University Press.

2 Catastrophes and potential catastrophes in infants

Avoidable death and avoidable brain damage haunt any doctor treating babies and children. Disabilities are discussed in Chapter 8 and we are concerned in this chapter mainly with sudden infant death and with symptoms in babies that may mean life-threatening illness. However, many potentially fatal conditions can also lead to disabilities if the child survives. One of the challenges of general practice is to be able to pick out the child who has a major life-threatening disease from the majority, who have relatively minor self-limiting conditions.

Worldwide, most deaths in infancy and childhood result from the interaction of infectious disease with poor nutritional status. Today, in Britain, while many deaths are the results of accidents, often contributed to by social problems, most of the rest come at the end of a long period of illness following malformation *in utero*, genetic disorder, poor antenatal growth, premature delivery or malignant disease. Sometimes, however, death or near death comes out of a clear sky without much warning, the topic of the present chapter.

THE ACUTELY ILL YOUNG BABY—WARNING SIGNS AND SYMPTOMS

It may be difficult to spot serious disease early in babies. All of us have sent infants home from the surgery or from hospital only for them to be admitted a few hours later, seriously ill from acute conditions that we have missed. Perhaps doctors treating a sick baby should ask themselves at the end of the consultation: 'If this child is found dead tonight will I be justified in feeling that I made an adequate assessment?' A positive answer requires a sound clinical approach, summarized in Table 2.1.

Infants are especially vulnerable to systemic infection in the first few weeks of life and may deteriorate within hours and become fatally ill. The GP must treat neonatal infections with great respect and have a low threshold for sending the sick neonate into hospital. Although infection is the commonest danger, metabolic disorders such as hypoglycaemia, renal failure, an acute abdomen, gross anaemia, adverse effects of drugs, and intracranial haemorrhage from

Table 2.1 The acutely ill young baby—key points

History	Has the baby lost interest in feeds? Is he vomiting; is it persistent or bile stained? Is there profuse watery diarrhoea or blood in the stools? Is there persistent moaning or a high-pitched cry; can the parents console him? Does the mother say she cannot wake him up properly, or that he is persistently drowsy or has lost interest in his surroundings?
Observation	Look at the way the baby is lying; is tone reduced? Can the baby (after three or four weeks of age) make sustained eye contact ? Is he febrile (check resting temperature if doubtful), tachypnoeic, or wheezy?
Once undressed	Is he dehydrated; sunken fontanelle, reduced skin turgor, tachycardia? Is the fontanelle over full? Is there marked intercostal or subcostal recession ? Is there jaundice, pallor or a purpuric or petechial rash? Is there an obstructed, incarcerated, or strangulated inguinal hernia; or a tender abdomen? Is there an inactive or deformed limb? Can you console his crying even briefly, or is he worse when lifted?

non-accidental injury may all present non-specifically in an acutely ill baby, as may many other rare conditions.

The most striking features of acute illnesses in infancy are listlessness, floppiness, and anorexia. It is almost safe to say that, with the sole exception of dehydration, a baby who has just taken a good feed is not acutely ill. The ill baby's muscle tone is reduced and skin blood flow is impaired. He therefore lies pale and inactive. The knees are less bent than usual and the baby looks as though he has been 'poured out' on to the cot mattress. His temperature may be raised, normal or subnormal. The following specific signs and symptoms may or may not be found superimposed on the general picture of acute illness.

Vomiting

Vomiting, though common in gastro-enteritis, is also a non-specific feature of acute infection in babies. Repeated vomiting in a sick baby may be a symptom of meningitis or encephalitis. Green, bile-stained vomit is often important as it may mean intestinal obstruction. Persistent vomiting can also, in infancy, be a presenting symptom of a urinary tract infection; the baby may appear well. More rarely, it may indicate a metabolic problem, for example galactosaemia. Commoner than all this are small vomits, 'possetting', in an otherwise healthy infant.

Dehydration causing acute loss of weight

Loss of 250–500 g over 24–48 hours, unless there has been an error in weighing, can only mean dehydration, usually from diarrhoea and vomiting. Dehydration (p. 209) is fairly easily spotted if lowered fontanelle tension, a dry mouth, sunken eyes and reduced skin turgor are looked for. Very rarely, an ill baby with severe gastro-enteritis, who may have been fed too much salt, may show weight loss without a reduced tissue turgor being obvious.

Breathlessness and cyanosis

A sustained tachypnoea is the most useful single sign of pneumonia or of heart-failure in a baby. Normal young babies often have a very odd pattern of respiration compared with adults. They have periods of fast respiration, several seconds when they do not breathe at all, and odd sighs and quivers. Respiratory rates of up to 50 per minute are acceptable, especially in a baby with fever. Persistent breathing above 50 per minute, when the baby is not crying or excited, is definitely abnormal. The baby is having to work extra hard to ventilate the lungs and this is shown by use of the sternomastoids, and—an important sign—by in-drawing of the intercostal spaces with each inspiration and by subcostal recession.

If rhinorrhoea, a cough, and, perhaps, a fever are associated with tachypnoea, pneumonia or bronchiolitis are likely. It is sometimes difficult to differentiate between them, although a hyperinflated chest and expiratory wheeze is more prominent in the latter. Breathlessness, with a liver enlarged 3 cm or more below the costal margin and an easily palpable heart-beat is more likely to mean heart-failure. Occasionally tachypnoea is seen as a ventilatory response to acidosis in dehydration, in some inborn errors of metabolism, in renal failure, or after excess salicylate ingestion from teething gels.

The best test of exercise tolerance in a baby is his ability to take a feed, so it is useful to ask the mother whether he is too breathless to suck properly. However, it is important to exclude simple nasal obstruction as a cause of this. In heart-failure he may manage a few sucks but tires easily. Added sounds on auscultation are often transmitted from the upper airways, but high-pitched sounds, either fine inspiratory crackles or a persistent high-pitched expiratory wheeze, are more likely to mean pneumonia, bronchiolitis, or heart-failure.

Blue hands and feet are seen in any chilly baby, whereas central cyanosis is always pathological. It may be difficult to be sure that central cyanosis is a real finding. It helps to compare the tongue's colour with the examiner's finger. A sick blue baby probably has a respiratory infection; a well blue one, cyanotic heart disease.

Irritability and unresponsiveness—is it meningitis?

The possibility that a child's symptoms may be caused by bacterial meningitis is a source of anxiety for most GPs as the avoidance of brain damage, and, indeed, the very survival of the baby may depend on early diagnosis and appropriate antibiotic therapy. If meningitis is not recognized, but antibiotics have already been given for one reason or another, then the signs of meningitic inflammation may be less obvious.

Irritability is a difficult symptom to assess; the inconsolable screaming of 'three-month colic' (p. 70) can be alarming to parent and doctor, but the condition is physically harmless. So is the screaming reported by fraught parents requesting a late evening visit to a well baby who has got into a state. Nevertheless, prolonged crying may be the clue to a number of important diagnoses, in addition to meningitis or other intracranial disease. The commonest is perhaps otitis media.

An infant with meningitis is an unhappy baby who probably has a headache, though he cannot complain of it specifically. Most babies will stop crying, if only briefly, when comforted by the mother, whereas the baby with meningeal inflammation will often continue to be uncomfortable, unhappy, and 'whingeing' even when the mother cuddles him and may even be made worse by cuddling. In the young baby, under about three months, neck stiffness is a pretty useless sign because it is usually absent, except at a late stage of meningitis. A better sign in young infants is increased tension of the anterior fontanelle, often slight, but sometimes so extreme that a visible lump is present. Unfortunately, even the fontanelle pressure may be normal in some infants with meningitis, especially if they are dehydrated. Reliance has to be placed on the more intangible sign of the baby's level of consciousness. Is the baby 'on the ball' in terms of eye-to-eye contact and alertness? Does his attention tend to fade away as soon as contact has been made? Dopiness linked to irritability means meningitis should remain on the agenda. As the baby gets older, a stiff neck gradually becomes a more reliable indicator of meningeal irritation. The irritable, angry infant who throws his head back when approached by the doctor may be difficult to assess. A period of observation, which can last 5 or 10 minutes before the laying-on of hands, may demonstrate the definite absence of any neck stiffness at all. If the infant is seen to smile or if the baby sitting on his mother's lap is alert enough to flex the head voluntarily to look at the bunch of keys rattled in front of his tummy, meningitis is very unlikely.

Clouding of consciousness, fits, or excessive vomiting suggest meningitis but can also be a feature of certain fulminating encephalopathies of early childhood, such as Reye's syndrome, in which liver failure with hypoglycaemia, hyperammonaemia, and clotting defects are associated with brain swelling, and haemorrhagic shock encephalopathy (HSE), a clinically somewhat similar encephalopathy. An epidemiological association between the use of aspirin in febrile toddlers and the onset of Reye's syndrome is the reason why this drug is not used for simple childhood fever. Mortality in either of these conditions is of the order of 50 per cent.

Skin lesions

Examining the skin may provide the vital clue to the diagnosis of a sick baby. For example, pustules and paronychia may indicate a staphylococcal septicaemia.

Almost any rash can occur in meningococcal septicaemia. It can vary from a few petechiae to confluent purpura covering much of the body surface. More confusing, only a maculo-papular rash may be apparent. All GPs must be aware of the potentially serious significance of a haemorrhagic rash in a sick, febrile child; it may be due to a meningococcal septicaemia until proved otherwise. If there is any suspicion of this diagnosis, the infant under one year should be given a parenteral antibiotic, e.g. benzylpenicillin 300 mg i.m. into the lateral aspect of the thigh before transferring to hospital. Older children are given 600 mg.

Purpuric or petechial lesions may also be seen in ill babies with other septicaemias, in those who are suffering the effects of intrauterine viral infections, notably rubella, in those who have themselves, or whose mothers have, idiopathic thrombocytopenic purpura (ITP), or in those who have acute clotting defects, perhaps with associated melaena. Bruises, cigarette burns, and purpuric lesions may be the only outward sign of non-accidental injury in a child who has had an intracranial haemorrhage after a blow on the head. An erythematous rash is a feature of Kawasaki syndrome (fever >40 °C for at least 5 days, conjunctivitis, sore mouth, desquamatous erythema and lymphadenopathy and coronary aneurysms).

Convulsions

Convulsions are often difficult to recognize in young infants as they may consist only of short-lived twitching of the side of the face, of shaking of a limb in a baby who is otherwise quiet, or of brief eye-rolling, perhaps with momentary stiffness or cyanosis. They are usually repetitive. Causes of fits in the first few days of life include maldevelopment of the brain, birth injury presenting within a day or two after a difficult delivery, metabolic causes—notably hypoglycaemia (in small-for-dates babies or infants of diabetic mothers), hypocalcaemia (in mothers with osteomalacia), or withdrawal from intrauterine exposure to, for example, tranquillizers or opiates—and meningitis or encephalopathy. Any neonate with a suspected convulsion should be immediately referred to hospital. Simple febrile convulsions are very uncommon until the age of six months. Indeed, most patients under one year who have a supposedly febrile convulsion need a lumbar puncture to exclude the possibility of meningitis. About 30 per cent of babies with meningitis have a convulsion. Infantile spasms (Salaam fits) are often overlooked in young babies. These are repetitive flexion spasms with brief loss of concentration which can even be mistaken for unusually emphatic hiccups. They are seen in a baby who has stopped making developmental progress and the long-term prognosis for development is poor. Urgent referral for EEG diagnosis is important, as early steroid treatment conceivably improves the prognosis.

Paralysis

A sudden complaint that a baby is failing to move a limb or part of a limb is occasionally the mother's first observation of a long-standing neurological lesion, such as cerebral palsy. Occasionally, there is a true acute neurogenic paralysis. The most common reason is pseudo-paralysis from either osteomyelitis (p. 291), septic arthritis, or injury, accidental or deliberate, sometimes with an underlying fracture. The limb will be painful and the baby or toddler may scream rather than quieten when cuddled.

Choking

'Choking' can mean almost anything from the concerns of an anxious granny to an inhaled foreign body, a brief convulsion, dyspnoea, a sore throat, a cold, gastro-oesophageal reflux, or the paroxysms of whooping cough. It is a frequent, but not always unimportant, complaint, whose cause can usually be sorted out by eliciting a detailed account of exactly what happened. Was the baby feeding or sucking a toy when he choked, did his eyes roll, does he have a runny nose? Was it really an apnoeic attack?

Jaundice

In the first week of life

The main danger with early jaundice is of an unconjugated plasma bilirubin concentration sufficiently high to cause irreversible damage to the basal ganglia—kernicterus. Most yellow neonates, especially those of low-birth-weight, have physiological jaundice, but this should not be accepted as the diagnosis without further investigation if it is present before 24 hours of age. At that stage it may then be an early sign of haemolysis from rhesus or other blood group incompatibility between baby and mother and indicates a need for immediate hospital investigation. The GP should have a low threshold for requesting an urgent bilirubin estimation throughout the first week to exclude levels dangerous to the brain (over 300 μmol/L; less in very sick or low-birth-weight infants, or during the first two or three days of life, when levels may rise rapidly higher). Deep jaundice in the first week of life can also be a sign of infection. In black babies visual assessment of bilirubin is obviously difficult, and in them several cases of kernicterus have been reported in which severity of jaundice had been underestimated.

After the first week

Deepening jaundice after seven days, or jaundice that persists at all after two weeks, is not usually dangerous in itself but is nevertheless sometimes the sign of serious disorder. The jaundice may be pre-hepatic with excess haemolysis, usually at this stage from an inherited defect of red blood cells, such as glucose-6-phosphate dehydrogenase deficiency, or hepato-cellular or obstructive jaundice. In hepato-cellular jaundice there is difficulty in bilirubin conjugation in the liver cells. It is this group that is likely to give the GP difficulty in diagnosis. Most such babies have a normal sized liver and normal coloured stools. They often appear quite well even in the presence of serious disease. Serious causes of poor conjugation include hypothyroidism, hopefully picked up by neonatal screening programmes before symptoms develop, even in the absence of slow feeding, hoarse cry, umbilical hernia, and coarse facies typical of thyroid deficiency; septicaemia, which makes the baby look ill, or an *E.coli* urinary infection; certain rare enzyme defects, such as galactosaemia.

Very much commoner than any of these is jaundice induced by breast-milk. The cause of breast-milk jaundice remains obscure but it is quite harmless. It presents something of a management dilemma for the clinician. How is one to avoid missing important disease which may cause prolonged jaundice while allowing a mother and her jaundiced baby to continue breast-feeding? If the well, breast-fed baby is only moderately jaundiced (bilirubin concentration under 200 μmol/L, of which >90 per cent is unconjugated), is passing yellow–green pigmented stools and has a normal urine culture and a normal thyroid screening test, the GP is unlikely to make a serious mis-diagnosis, even though there are some unusual presentations, with jaundice, of rare disorders, such as the very occasional case of cystic fibrosis or of alpha 1-antitrypsin deficiency that may be diagnosed late with a low-key approach.

The hallmarks of obstructive jaundice from biliary atresia, are pale stools and yellow-stained urine. If diagnosed early and treated by twelve weeks, but not later, about half the cases can be given long-term palliation through surgery. Neonatal hepatitis (a different condition from hepatitis in later childhood) also causes a similar obstructive picture. These conditions are difficult to differentiate without laparoscopy and liver biopsy following hospital referral.

SUDDEN DEATH IN INFANCY SYNDROME (SIDS, COT DEATHS)

Approximately one in 1500 babies in the UK is found unexpectedly dead during the first year of life. In 10% a plausible cause of death is found (Gilbert *et al.* 1990)—a congenital malformation, a metabolic defect, or a potentially treatable condition, such as meningitis or pneumonia. In the remainder no cause has been found to explain the death, even after a thorough post-mortem with full virological and bacteriological studies. These deaths make up the 'sudden infant death syndrome' (SIDS or 'cot death') and are a leading 'cause' of death in the first year. Despite much research the reason for death in a given child remains elusive. Suggested mechanisms include apnoea, especially when lying in the prone position, perhaps from an abnormality of the respiratory control system, or a sudden cardiac arrhythmia.

Only the first three or perhaps four items listed in Table 2.2 provide realistic opportunities for prevention. The death rate for cot death has fallen for some years. There is recent evidence that breast-feeding has a protective effect (Ford *et al.* 1993) and the death rate has more than halved since general advice to sleep babies face upwards. This advice was based on some 20 retrospective case-control studies which indicated that sleeping face down is associated with an incidence of SIDS between 3 and 8-fold higher than face up. There is also a 2–3-fold

Table 2.2 Factors affecting the likelihood of SIDS

If the baby sleeps face down
If the mother smoked antenatally or household members smoke
If there are too many bed clothes
Following recent symptoms of excessive crying, diarrhoea, unusual drowsiness or upper respiratory tract infection
Between one and four months of age and in winter
Between midnight and 9 a.m.
In boys
In large sibships
Following twin or multiple pregnancy
After low-birth-weight
In social classes 4 or 5
With young mothers

Adapted from Department of Health (1993).

increase in the risk of SIDS associated with antenatal maternal and postnatal parental cigarette smoking. Hyperthermia brought on by over-wrapping and over-heating during mild illnesses increases the risk of SIDS. The *Back to sleep* campaign leaflet from the UK Health Departments suggests that:

babies should be kept warm but they must not be allowed to get too warm. Keep the temperature in your baby's room so that you feel comfortable in it. Use lightweight blankets which you can add to or take away according to the room temperature. Do not use a duvet or baby nest which can be too warm and can easily cover a baby's head. Feverish babies should have few or even no blankets.

Most cot deaths occur at home. After the devastating discovery of their dead or dying child the majority of parents will dial 999 or go straight to the local hospital. However, the GP is often, but not always, involved either by a telephone call from the hospital or perhaps directly by the parents.

The GP was rung up late one morning from the local casualty department. Elaine, aged five months, has been brought in dead an hour before. Mrs Bryant was about to go home and the casualty medical officer felt that the GP ought to know what had happened. He went round to visit the family a few hours later. Mrs Bryant's first husband had died previously and she had been living for some years with the father of Elaine. She explained in a numb, flat way how she had found the baby dead in the cot that morning. The father sat in the sitting room unable to say very much and their 3-year-old daughter was behaving as if nothing very extraordinary had happened. Whilst the doctor was attempting to comfort the family, the Coroner's Officer arrived to take a statement, telling them about the post-mortem that was going to be performed the next day.

The GP may have to discuss the post-mortem findings with the parents and provide explanation about SIDS, not only to them but also to older siblings and to grandparents. Leaflets providing information are available from the Foundation for the Study of Infant Deaths, 14 Halkin Street, London SW1.

Because there have been occasional reports of twin siblings dying cot deaths in quick succession, the GP will naturally be anxious about a surviving twin. In our view admission and careful observation for a day or two in the local paediatric department is sensible.

It is, of course, important to cancel all appointments inviting the dead child for immunizations or to any other clinics and to suppress lactation if the mother has been breast-feeding (bromocriptine 2.5 mg daily for three days and then twice daily for 14 days).

The devastating and unexpected nature of SIDS and any lack of explanation may lead to difficulties with grieving and with accepting the death. The parents should be given ample time to express their own ideas and fears. It is worth warning them that they may find their emotions disturbed for several months and that they may have vivid fantasies about the continuing existence of the child and violent positive or negative emotional feelings towards other members of the family. As time passes they need help in rebuilding their confidence in the handling and rearing of their other children, with repeated reassurance and easy access to the doctor. All the ground may have to be gone over repeatedly. There has to be a particularly sympathetic and careful approach to the next pregnancy, which is easier if the obstetrician and midwife are told the history. Parents are often edgy when the new baby approaches the age at which its predecessor died, and they may expect the GP to be aware of this without being told the reason.

Very occasionally, in families with a history of multiple incidences of SIDS, infanticide, usually by suffocation, may be the explanation (Emery 1985), but in the great majority of cases parents are not to blame in any way, and any hint that they are can be disastrously demoralizing for a family who are already coping with police investigation and with their own natural feelings of guilt. The GP can help the family to cope with the tragedy by emphasizing how well the child was cared for and how the parents are not to blame.

Near-miss cot deaths (acute life-threatening episodes)

Parents sometimes rush an infant to the doctor, believing the baby has been briefly lifeless—pale and not breathing. Sometimes parents are anxiously misinterpreting normal irregularity of breathing. At other times there may indeed be a genuine problem: a convulsion, inhaled food, the start of an acute illness (see above), or acid reflux into the lungs from a hiatus hernia. We generally take a careful history for both therapeutic and diagnostic reasons and then under-react unless the history suggests one of the above causes, or the baby appears unusually vulnerable, having been markedly premature, had a sibling die perhaps a cot death, or comes from a very socially disorganized family; occasionally the described episode is an oblique confession of parental violence towards the baby. A brief admission for observation and reassurance is sometimes useful.

It has become common practice for babies who have had a 'near-miss' or who have a history of cot death in a sibling to be issued with an apnoea alarm, but more than 99% in either group will not die a cot death without an alarm and it is not clear that the alarm can prevent death in the remainder. Unfortunately, the alarms often go off with normal ventilatory irregularity and, conversely, may not alarm in the presence of true apnoea. Some babies have died while attached to an alarm. No controlled trial has demonstrated their value, but an enormous one would be needed because of the low incidence of death. Nevertheless, parents who have had previous cot deaths sometimes say that the alarm gives them enough confidence to go to bed instead of spending the night watching the baby. An alarm is often used as a placebo. If the doctor is really serious about using it the parents need to learn what to do if it bleeps and the baby looks dead. This means teaching them how to give mouth-to-mouth respiration and external cardiac massage correctly; babies have been injured by incompetent resuscitation. We do not ourselves recommend alarms in this situation, but do not refuse their use if the parents are very keen.

Bibliography

Department of Health. (1993). *Report of the Chief Medical Officer's Expert Group on the Sleeping Position of Infants in Cot Death*. HMSO, London.

Emery, J. L. (1985). Annotation, infanticide, filicide, and cot death. *Archives of Disease in Childhood*, **60**, 505–7.

Ford, R. P., Taylor, B. J., Mitchell, E. A., Enright, S. A., Stewart, A.W., Becroft, D. M., *et al.* (1993). Breastfeeding and the risk of sudden infant death syndrome. *International Journal of Epidemiology*, **22**, 885–90.

Gilbert, R. E., Fleming, P. J. Berry, J., and Rudd, P. T. (1990). Signs of illness preceding sudden and unexpected death in infants. *British Medical Journal*, **301**, 45–6.

3 Practising prevention

The aims of health promotion are to abolish avoidable child death and disease, to manage disability and resultant handicap, to mitigate the effects of deprivation and poor parenting, and to encourage healthy habits for children to take into adult life. Its aims do not include an over-dependence on medication or an exaggerated concept of what medicine can solve. They do include a positive attitude to life and the ability to make the most of one's resources and opportunities.

If we can discourage young teenagers from starting to smoke, more will be achieved for the health of the community than is accomplished by hundreds of specialists treating the end result of damage caused by cigarettes.

Health promotion means giving families the confidence to manage minor childhood ailments themselves; and informing them how they can make best use of the services the practice offers. Most health promotion by the doctor occurs opportunistically. There is a chance during most consultations to offer advice about preventive care and the natural history of disease. This may enable the parents to cope with a recurrence of the same problem. Much more health promotion is the remit of the health visitor.

The ideal health care system for children is a partnership between the family and the practice team, with parents becoming aware of the importance of measures to promote healthy living, of how to get most benefit from the services the practice offers, and of the early signs of potentially serious disease. The family is the front line and, although a consultation about a child with a minor self-limiting illness may be worthwhile, leading on to a discussion of other important issues, it is more appropriate if the same minor problem does not lead to repeated consultations. An important part of the doctor's role is thus to increase parents' knowledge and self-confidence in the management of their child's health. Hand outs may have some value and Pike (1980) showed that parents who were given a booklet on aspects of child care showed some improvement in their knowledge two or three weeks later. The biggest improvement occurred in social classes 4 and 5, and amongst unemployed parents. Some excellent literature is available, an example being *Birth to five: a guide to the first five years of being a parent* (Health Education Authority 1989).

Health promotional services are provided partly by the practice team, partly by community trusts and partly by schools. Unless clear communications are established, these divisions lead either to duplication, or to tasks not being carried out because each organization considers them another's responsibility. Many family doctors, recognize that they are 'Community Physicians' for their registered population and the structure and organization of practices have been adapted to enable selected groups to be easily and quickly identified. These may include individuals at particular risk, for example children who have had a parent die young from premature coronary artery disease, or migrants at risk from tuberculosis (TB).

THE HEALTH VISITOR

There are many facets to the work of a health visitor. These include: health promotion and education; prevention of physical and emotional ill health; developmental assessment and the early detection of health problems; and the surveillance and support of the child and family with medical and parental difficulties. For example, following a child protection case conference the health visitor may be identified as the designated key worker with the family. Health visitors mainly work with parents and their young children. However, families with a chronically sick or disabled child will benefit from their support over many years.

THE PRACTICE NURSE

In many practices nurses play a central role in the care of children and adolescents. They are seen about minor injuries, before foreign travel and for childhood immunizations and blood tests. Parents and, indeed, young people themselves may ask the nurse for advice when they are either too embarrassed to talk to the GP or worried that their symptoms are too trivial to 'bother the doctor with'. Teenage girls may initially prefer to consult a nurse about contraception or the possibility of a pregnancy. Many of these consultations provide excellent opportunities for health promotion.

Nurses are increasingly involved in the care of asthmatic patients. They are often better than GPs in following management guidelines and more careful to select the correct inhaler device, spending more time teaching the child how to use it. A parent may take a sick child with a rash, fever, cough, earache or sore throat directly to the nurse, particularly if it is difficult to get immediate access to their doctor.

Practices should not be afraid of extending the role of their nurses. However, it is important to make sure that appropriate training has been given (for example, to assess an unwell child) and that boundaries of responsibilities are understood. It is a waste of their talents if their work is limited to traditional nursing tasks only, or to jobs the doctor finds tedious or difficult.

The allocation of tasks within primary care, especially those concerned with surveillance, health promotion and the management of chronic disease is evolving rapidly at the interface between practice nurse, health visitor, specialist nurse, doctor and other health professional. Tasks that used to be the preserve of the doctor are now being undertaken more appropriately by other health professionals.

THE CHILD HEALTH CLINIC IN THE PRACTICE

The most recent review of child health surveillance (Hall 1996) concluded that many of the routine screening tests in common usage were unreliable and should be scrapped. There is now greater emphasis on targeting services on families with problems, and parental involvement in monitoring a child's progress.

At present, child health surveillance is partly provided by general practices and partly by clinics organized by community trusts. Though some community-based clinics provide a high standard of care, the system leads to duplication of services. Ideally, child health surveillance should be carried out by an enthusiastic, appropriately trained primary care team. Its members provide comprehensive care for the family, have access to medical records, can prescribe, and carry out pathological investigations without referral to a consultant. The expertise of more experienced CMOs could be used more effectively in co-operation with the primary care team. The advantages of health visitor attachment to the practice, namely ease of communication between health professionals leading to a more comprehensive and often earlier identification of problems needing health visitors' help, appear to us overwhelming. Arrangements have to be made to cover the patients of practices too small to justify their own full-time health visitor, and for families who are not registered at all. In some inner city areas special health visitor support is needed for homeless young families placed temporarily in 'bed and breakfast' accommodation. Under the 1990 contract, GPs can apply to join the under-five child health surveillance list of their local FHSA. If they are approved (and criteria vary) they get paid a small annual fee for each child they look after.

A practice with three principals will need to hold a weekly half-day child health clinic, the usual setting for the detection of unreported disease or disability in the preschool child. There are many unresolved questions. How useful do young mothers find them? How much screening should the GP do and how much should be left to the health visitor? Clinics seem to be best conducted by health visitors with suitably trained GPs, not the reverse. Time should be set aside at the end of each session for a discussion of the families seen in the clinic. There should be no ambiguity about which member of staff is responsible for following-up the problems identified.

Parent-held records help to involve parents in monitoring their child's progress. Assuming health visitors and doctors actively promote their use, they are likely to be available wherever and whenever the child is seen, and can provide immediate information to a GP who has not yet received a new family's medical records. They also contain useful health information and are an aide-memoire, reminding the parent to bring the child for a routine check or immunization. On the other hand, it is not always easy to find one's way around the booklet; it requires doctor discipline to use it. GP and health visitor still tend to use their own clinic records in addition.

Although the extensive use that young mothers make of these clinics is evidence of their popularity, the most vulnerable members of the community, as in most screening programmes, tend to be least likely to avail themselves of the service. To counteract this, such families need to be easily identified and contacted, for example following a computer prompt. The clinic organization and timing needs to be flexible, giving working mothers the opportunity to attend outside conventional hours. This is easier in large group practices, where several health visitors and doctors can hold clinics throughout the day.

GPs must work with health visitors in the surveillance of young families who will not come to the clinic. This means a greater readiness to assess children at home, which goes against the present tendency for fewer home visits by GPs. The notification of births provides the information health visitors need to carry out the first visit to mothers and children, and to discuss with them the advantages of attendance at the child health clinic. They carry out many of the assessments and may already have made contact with the mother before the birth, if there has been appropriate communication from the GP antenatal clinic and the midwife.

There are several different activities at the child health clinic, and the clinic's value cannot be assessed by considering only the role of the health visitor and the GP. We must look at the total picture:

1. *Mutual support*—According to conventional clinical criteria about ten per cent of mothers are depressed within three months of giving birth (Hall 1996). Their isolation and that of other mothers may be reduced by having opportunities to meet. Discussion groups run by health visitors, centring around the difficulties of bringing up small children, may be helpful in sharing common problems.

2. *Surveillance*—of general health, nutrition, growth, vision, hearing and physical development, including head circumference. Children should sometimes be weighed and their length entered on a centile chart, especially during their first year. The height of older children should also be recorded occasionally; this requires a Raven Minimeter height measuring tape or its equivalent (p. 91). Lengths of younger babies can also be useful in the assessment of failure to thrive, but to be accurate an infant measuring table with a fixed headpiece and sliding footpiece is required. An accurate length or height measurement above the 99.6 centile or below the 0.4 centile, is an indication for referral (Hall 1996).

3. *Health promotion*—Mothers, particularly with their first baby, are not only a semi-captive population, but also probably receptive to advice. In the clinic, the

health visitor can work with the doctor in her central role of health promotion, helped by posters in appropriate languages, exhibitions, leaflets, video displays and, in the future, patient-activated computer programs.

Topics appropriate for educational airing include not only those dealing directly with infant care (feeding, weaning, sensible dietary habits, immunization, general handling and safety, and the early recognition of symptoms of disease), but also how to integrate the baby into family life and stimulate him to play and to enjoy him. Other useful issues include women's health generally, contraception, cervical screening, the needs of older siblings, prevention of accidents and the hazards of pets. 'Passive' smoking is detrimental to the health of a child. Parents may find a discussion of the local neighbourhood aids to child rearing helpful: mutual support systems, the social services, playgroups, and nursery schools. In addition, the special needs of ethnic minorities can be picked up: language classes, health precautions for children on returning to their country of origin, and how to get interpreter and advocacy services. For most mothers advice from peers and relatives has more influence, though this is not always positive.

4. *Immunization*—(see p. 33)

5. *Early diagnosis of social disorganization and maternal depression*—(see Chapter 5)

6. *Positive reinforcement from professionals that in most respects parents are doing a good job*

In the rest of the chapter we describe the stages of development and their routine assessment at some length. This is not because we feel the routine surveillance of the low-risk child is very important in itself, but because the GP involved in routine surveillance becomes gradually conversant with the normal range of development since he continues to see many healthy, normal children of all shapes, sizes, and colours in the clinic. His really productive screening will be done during the normal surgery consultations or when he visits the sick child at home. If he is confident in his assessment of the normal child he will be alert to incidental problems of development or to the unreported disability that he sees in a child brought in for another reason. It may be appropriate for many of these children to be referred by the GP to himself to be assessed at leisure in the child health clinic.

Physical development

Some head control develops early and a 12-week infant can lift his head above the plane of the rest of his body; by 20–24 weeks there is no head lag when the baby is pulled up. He sits when he is aged about 28 weeks, is able to stand well a few months later, and then walks unsteadily on a wide base, gradually becoming more sure-footed as the months go by. The infant becomes adept at using his fingers and hands several months before he stands and walks.

The initial generalized mass response of infants is replaced with time by a much more specific approach to objects. Thus a 20-week infant has an ataxic, bidextrous approach to a brick placed in front of him. By the time he is aged 40 weeks he can accurately and quickly touch an object with one finger or pick up a small object between his finger and thumb. The younger baby shows his pleasure and excitement by moving several parts of his body, whereas the older child may just smile or laugh while keeping quite still.

In each of the four main areas of development—locomotive, manipulative, linguistic and social—there is an order in which individual skills are mastered. For example, motor development proceeds in a cephalo-caudal direction. However, the speed of maturation in one area does not necessarily equal that in another, so that the child who is not yet able to sit without support may be relatively dextrous with his fingers and pick up objects with one hand, readily transferring them to the other. Gross disparity between the various areas of development is likely to be of significance.

The primitive reflexes, such as the Moro reflex, although of great theoretical interest, are of little importance in developmental screening. Their orderly suppression, a feature of normal development, is disturbed in cerebral palsy in which they are abnormally persistent. But cerebral palsy will usually present more definitely with delay in maturation of locomotor or manipulative skills, seen most obviously in failure to use one or other hand. It is important to note whether all four limbs are moving normally and the Moro reflex is a useful way to check if both arms move symmetrically in the young infant.

All parents are concerned that their child should be normal, and any anxiety that this is not the case is likely to be more acute if there has been some real or imagined abnormality in the pregnancy or delivery. One of the main benefits of the consultation will be lost unless parents tell the doctor of their worries about a viral infection in pregnancy or a difficult delivery by Caesarean section and receive appropriate reassurance. In the case of severely disabled children, the history will often provide pointers to the cause of the disability. With less obvious abnormalities it may provide an early clue to the presence of a problem; thus a history of difficulties in feeding may be the first sign of slow development, and if the mother feels her baby is not hearing properly, she may well be right.

The doctor's assessment of the baby's general behaviour is the central issue and is vital. How alert is he? How intently is he interested in what is going on? How long will he concentrate on his little tasks before he gets bored? An interested, alert, socially responsive infant who is fun to examine is not going to turn out to have a severe learning difficulty, even if he is somewhat slow in his developmental milestones. Early diagnosis of a disabling disorder, especially before the mother becomes pregnant again, may be important; female carriers of fragile X (an important cause of mental retardation) can be identified by DNA studies (p. 298) and offered prenatal diagnosis. Also parents of children with specific syndromes may be able to accept the situation more easily if given a diagnostic label.

However, considerable anxiety may be caused by false alarms leading to hospital referral. Examples are the large child with a normally big head who is considered for a time to be possibly hydrocephalic, or the 7-month-old baby who does not turn to sounds, because he is not quite mature enough or is bored or is involved with what is going on in front of him, and is therefore considered to be possibly deaf. Generally, the rule must be: if in doubt, wait and see; re-examine the child after a suitable interval. But it is difficult to get the balance between over- and under-anxiety precisely correct. Perhaps the answer is: (i) parents worried and GP or health visitor uncertain; mothers are often right—refer? (ii) GP or health visitor uncertain, mother unconcerned; wait and re-examine.

Timing and content of routine visits

We discuss 'checks' during the first week, 6 weeks, 15–18 months, 2–2½ years, and 3½–4 years, although at least one of the last three can be dropped unless the child is at risk or the parents are worried about some specific aspect of development. Much monitoring of a child's progress is carried out by health visitors. However, it is important that the GP does not lose his expertise, partly because he is likely to be asked to assess children the health visitor is unsure about (and vice versa). We include the neonatal examination as routine. It is a weakness of some practices that the GP does not get to grips with a new baby's problems until the infant is brought in for his six weeks' check. By this stage the period of highest risk to physical health is already over. He will also have missed a good opportunity to reinforce relationships with the family. However, advice about the need to ensure adequate domestic support from family and friends and, if possible, a long period off work post-partum, needs to have been given earlier, during the mother's pregnancy. Health visitors and community midwives are the ideal personnel to discuss these issues.

Each examination should involve charting the weight (and height for the last check) and reacting if it is falling off; watching general alertness and health, confidence, and cuddliness with the mother and her response; identifying important malformations at some stage in infancy, preferably at the first examination; making a rough assessment of physical development; noting disorders of vision or hearing early, and referring children with communication problems before school starts and often as early as three years.

Bearing these general principles in mind, we now mention some specific points to be looked out for at each visit. Details of hearing and sight testing are discussed separately.

First week

The aims of the neonatal examination are fourfold. First, to examine for problems of adjustment to extra-uterine life; in particular, whether the baby's lungs and cardiovascular system are working normally and whether he has a good urinary stream and normal bowel motions. Secondly, are there problems with feeding; is breast-feeding becoming established satisfactorily, and are there any obvious difficulties of bonding which require intensive work by the health visitor? Thirdly, are there any important defects, including dislocation of the hips and malformations of the back, mouth, or eyes, which are easily missed? Finally, does the baby fall into a high-risk group that requires extra attention; was he born prematurely or small for dates; did his mother take drugs or drink excessively; has he failed to regain his birth weight by early in the second week? Is there any persistent jaundice?

Six to eight weeks

Even if the GP has done the first-week examination, a full check for malformations is needed including an assessment of hip stability. The presence of more than one significant malformation is an indication for a genetic assessment. Has the infant got the normal red reflex when a light is shone on the pupils? Is he floppy when lifted? Is the Moro reflex symmetrical? Are both testes descended? Is the skin of normal colour? Has the baby got evidence of a severe congenital heart defect—tachypnoea even at rest, a large liver, a murmur (not invariably present) and perhaps cyanosis? Are the femoral pulses palpable? Is the head circumference crossing the centile lines? Most infants with a big head will have inherited it from their parents. Does the child look unusually odd? Dysmorphic features may be associated with defects of vision and hearing. Does he fix on his mother's face and smile? Most congenital abnormalities will be of minor significance and will be pointed out to the doctor by the mother. Weight gain and nutrition are particularly important at six weeks. This is an appropriate time for the doctor to discuss contraception (unless he has already done so during the mother's post-natal examination) and check the baby is fit to start the course of immunizations two weeks later.

Seven to eight months

This is an important age for checking development in terms of alertness, co-ordination, sitting and the use of all limbs. Can either hand be used to grasp and release objects? Are fallen toys looked for? Does the baby vocalize and has he passed his hearing test? This visit and the next present a good opportunity to discuss nutrition, sleeping pattern, prevention of accidents in the home, use of safety harnesses in cars, dental care and the avoidance of sunburn. Many of these items can most appropriately be reviewed with the health visitor. In a healthy child, physical examination can be restricted to weighing and testing for hip stability, listening to the heart and confirming testicular descent.

Fifteen to eighteen months

This is a crucial home visit for the health visitor who wishes to review a poor and under-stimulating home situation. Should the social services department be involved in some sort of intervention? Should the baby and mother both be attending a day nursery? Time is running out for successful initiatives on behalf of the child from a severely deprived environment. Most 18-month-old infants are able to walk, say a few words with meaning and understand many more.

Two to two-and-a-half years
This is another assessment which is often carried out by the health visitor in the child's home. Is he walking and talking normally? Children whose speech delay causes concern should be referred to a specialist clinic for hearing testing. It is not too early to refer the poor speaker to a speech therapist after the examiner has satisfied himself the child has normal hearing and has not got an anatomical or neurological problem and that there is no significant mental handicap. Children of this age are at an increased risk of iron deficiency, particularly if their diet is made up of foods with inadequate amounts of iron. An Hb concentration of less than 11 g/dL in the absence of thalassaemia trait (p. 253), makes iron deficiency likely.

Three-and-a-half to four years
Check whether all the immunizations have been given and discuss with the parents any particular concerns they may have about the child's progress, hearing or sight. Observe the relationship between child and parent; does he cling to the mother's skirt or feel confident enough to play with toys in another part of the room? By this age speech should be quite complex, with sentences containing a subject, verb and object. Assuming hearing is normal, if speech is unintelligible to the parents or causing concern for some other reason, the GP should consider whether social problems or developmental delays are likely before referring to a speech therapist. It is not difficult to make a reasonable assessment of sight and hearing of a four-year-old child; and the ability of the child to co-operate gives a good indication of his intelligence and general togetherness. Fine motor co-ordination can be tested by asking the child to copy a circle (by three years) or a cross (by four years). Alternatively, most older children can draw a picture of their mother which includes a head, body, facial features and limbs (although not always emerging from the anatomically correct positions).

Physical examination is often pretty cursory; especially as many young children do not like to undress completely. However, the routine visit provides an opportunity to discuss organic as well as psychosocial causes of previous recurrent ill-health, slow toilet training or poor growth. Topics for health promotion include avoidance of road traffic accidents and how the child should respond when approached by strange adults. Children should have hearing and vision tests by the school nurse shortly after starting school.

VISION AND HEARING TESTING

The validity of most of these tests depends on a suitable environment and the skill of the examiner, who in the future may not always be the GP or health visitor. The sensitivity and specificity of many of the tests is low, especially if done under pressure by a non-expert. Perhaps a community-based orthoptist may be most adept at identifying treatable visual problems. However, early diagnosis of squint and profound deafness do seem to meet the criteria for worthwhile screening, in that early treatment is possible and leads to better results than late treatment. In addition, a child who starts nursery or primary school with an unrecognized sensory defect is at a disadvantage. Testing of children between two and four should perhaps be restricted to those who are considered to be 'at risk' for one reason or another, or if there is parental concern.

Vision

A baby on the first day of life can fix with his eyes and the retina should look red when examined through the ophthalmoscope—best seen from 20 cm using a + lens—the red reflex. By six weeks or earlier, most infants make eye-to-eye contact on feeding and are able to follow a bright object over a range of at least 90 degrees. If they do not the parents may correctly suspect seriously impaired vision. Roving nystagmus can be an important presenting sign of visual defect. So obviously are silhouettes against the red reflex (cataracts) or eyes of markedly different size, which may indicate congenital glaucoma. Infants who need more careful examination include: those born after infection in pregnancy or very preterm (especially if they had a stormy neonatal course), those who are small for date, are neurologically impaired, have a malformation syndrome or a family history of severe errors of refraction. A fixed squint at any age is abnormal, and an intermittent squint, especially persisting after 6 months, is also important.

The visual acuity of a three-month-old baby is probably about 6/60 and improves to 6/9—6/6 by the age of three to four years. In children between six months and two years, visual acuity can be roughly tested as follows: the infant sits on his parent's knee and watches the examiner rolling a tiny white plastic ball a few feet away or picks up a tiny pellet from the table in front of him. The 15-month-old toddler will frequently run and pick up objects two or three metres away, particularly if shown how to do so by the parent. By 2½ years, matching toys is a useful technique. The examiner picks up a large toy and asks the child to pick out the same object from a collection put in front of him. As soon as the child has got the idea, the examiner walks to the other side of the room and, showing the child a small version, asks him to match it with toys in front of him. Unfortunately, many children of this age are impossible in the surgery; the test may be done more profitably at home by the health visitor.

Over the age of about three years, the toy test can be replaced by more formal letter recognition. Naming letters on an optician's chart is beyond most preschool children, but a child's ability to match pairs of objects can again be made use of. The child is given a card with a number of letters printed on it. The examiner has a booklet of letters of different size, one to each page, or better still grouped in a row (this will detect astigmatism). He shows these in turn from a distance of three metres while the child points out which letter on his card matches the letter on display. The Sonksen-Silver test of visual acuity incorporates a row of test letters and meets the Snellen standards of specification. If the child will not allow each eye to be tested separately, another attempt will be made a few

Table 3.1 Hints for parents to defect deafness

Can your baby hear you?

Here is a checklist of some of the general signs you can look for in your baby's first year:

Shortly after birth—Your baby should be startled by a sudden loud noise such as a hand clap or a door slamming and should blink or open his/her eyes widely to such sounds.

By 1 month—He/she should be beginning to notice sudden prolonged sounds like the noise of the vacuum cleaner and should pause and listen to them when they start up.

By 4 months—He/she should quieten or smile to the sound of your voice even when he cannot see you. He may also turn his head or eyes towards you if you come up from behind and speak to him from the side.

By 7 months—He/she should turn immediately to your voice across the room or to very quiet noises made on each side if he is not too occupied with other things.

By 9 months —He/she should listen attentively to familiar everyday sounds and search for very quiet sounds made out of sight. He should also show pleasure in babbling loudly and tunefully.

Based on McCormick, in Polnay and Hull (1993), p. 327.

months later. Children with visual acuity of 3/6 or worse in either or both eyes need to be referred. As well as testing visual acuity, the way the child copes with the test helps to show whether he can organize his intellectual activities in a way appropriate for his age. A child may not co-operate if he find the test too simple and boring. School-aged children can cope with a formal Snellen's chart at six metres.

Hearing

Those babies at special risk of deafness include those with a positive family history, those of markedly low-birth-weight or who have had severe birth asphyxia or neonatal jaundice, meningitis, rubella, or cytomegalovirus *in utero* and those who have malformations of the face or ears or a white forelock of hair (Waardenburg syndrome). Hearing problems in older children are more likely if the parent suspects deafness, or if there was delayed speech, cerebral palsy or a cleft palate. Neonatal hearing tests are complicated, and not yet universally available or fully validated. Tests include assessing the baby's reaction to noise (acoustic cradle), or measuring the effect of sound on the brain's electrical activity (auditory brain stem evoked response). At risk neonates with apparently normal hearing, should be tested some months later to make sure that a hearing problem has not developed. According to Polnay and Hull (1993), about 1 in 1000 children will have severe sensorineural deafness, and 1 in 500 will be moderately affected and the problem may not be detected until later childhood. Milder, often fluctuating conductive deafness is seen in children with glue ear. A checklist to detect deafness (Table 3.1) can help parents decide whether their child may have a problem with hearing.

The often inadequately performed distraction tests of hearing, in which the baby turns to a quiet sound are particularly difficult until the child is about seven months old.

Most babies are routinely tested in a sound-proof room in community screening programmes. If it is necessary to test in the practice, the baby sits on his mother's knee with the examiner standing behind in such a way that there is no question of his reflection being seen (an important cause of really deaf children being thought to have normal hearing). A third adult positions herself a few feet in front of the child with a mildly interesting silent toy. The examiner produces quiet, short sounds three feet away from each ear, at about ear level and a few inches behind the child. A mixture of verbal and non-verbal noises, perhaps a low-frequency hum, a hiss, a short shake of a high-frequency rattle (Manchester rattle—6000 Hertz) and stroking the inside of a cup with a spoon give a reasonable range. The baby should turn towards the sound, but even a small prompt deviation of the eyes towards the stimulus noticed by the assistant is satisfactory.

Many **two-year-olds** will have a vocabulary of 50–200 words and be speaking in two word phrases. However, quite a few will not be saying much that is intelligible, except perhaps to their doting parents. Comprehension and hearing can be tested by showing a co-operative two-year-old five or six toys (for example, cup, spoon, brush, ball, and car) one at a time and then placing them in front of him. The examiner then asks the child to point out each toy in turn and, if all goes well, repeats the request in a soft voice a few feet away. These toys can be used to test comprehension by seeing if the toddler understands simple little commands (e.g., 'put the spoon in the cup', 'brush the baby's hair'). Indications for referral for assessment include a vocabulary with few recognizable words and a dismal performance from a co-operative child in the test described above. An alternative test is to ask children, softly from two or three metres away, to point to parts of their own or their mother's body or clothing. As with the toy test, children must be shown what to do first.

At **three-years-plus**, the 7-paired toy test is a useful method of assessing hearing. The examiner makes sure the child knows what the name of each toy is and puts them on a table in front of the child. He then retreats about three feet, covers his mouth, and asks the child to show a named toy. Ideally, a sound meter should be used to confirm a softly spoken voice of 40 dB. The items can be asked for in any order, but the child should correctly identify the paired objects, for example:

plane/plate	tree/key
man/lamb	duck/cup
horse/fork	shoe/spoon
house/cow	

If the child fails a few items, a test can be repeated a couple of months later. Anything worse than that, or an unintelligible vocabulary, are indications for referral. A simpler but less reliable test is to use a card with pictures of standard words such as seat, fish, ship, bike, cup, face, and car, which can be easily confused because of hearing loss. Again the child needs to be shown what to do. Ideally, each ear should be tested separately, but many children may object. Hall (1996) recommends that the two years plus hearing tests should not be done routinely on low-risk children. Pure tone audiometry gives precise information and is worth trying to achieve from about 3½ years of age onwards. A loss of more than 20 decibels at more than one frequency is significant.

Most babies who have failed screening tests for hearing or vision were too distracted, too tired or hot, miserable or bored, or the examiner was. The initial action, unless the failure is gross, is obviously to retest at a future date. An interpreter/advocate may help at the assessment of children from homes where English is not spoken. The paired toy test is obviously not appropriate in these cases.

ACTIVE IMMUNIZATION

The handbook *Immunization against infectious diseases* (1992) is an essential resource for health visitors, doctors and practice nurses involved in immunization.

A live attenuated vaccine (measles/mumps/rubella [MMR], poliomyelitis [OPV], BCG) causes a mild infection. A killed or inactivated vaccine is derived from virulent organisms (pertussis). A toxoid is an inactivated toxin (diphtheria, tetanus). Inactivated vaccines and toxoids may contain adjuvants which enhance their ability to stimulate antibody production (pneumovac). Some vaccines are produced from part of the pathogen, such as the polysaccharide coat. The body's response can then be enhanced by conjugation with another antigen, such as diphtheria or tetanus toxoid (*Haemophilus influenzae*—HiB).

The childhood immunization rate is now about 90 per cent for children under two years. The national pressure to achieve near 100 per cent immunization (including financial incentives for doctors) must be balanced, by avoiding coercing parents who are adamantly opposed.

A mild cold or runny nose is not a contra-indication to routine immunization, but the injection is best postponed if there is a significant febrile illness. Live vaccines are generally very effective but may be lethal in children with inadequate immunity due to anti-cancer therapy, lymphoma or leukaemia, or who are hypogammaglobulinaemic or on large doses of steroids. HIV positive children can be given all the routine immunizations except for BCG, and inactivated polio vaccine may be preferable. If more than one live vaccine need to be given together, different sites should be used (unless a standard combined preparation is used).

A list of false contra-indications is given in Table 3.2. Telephone advice lines and immunization advisory clinics have been established in some areas for health professionals and patients who are unsure whether a child is eligible for a specific vaccine. If the health visitor or doctor is uneasy, this is usually because there is a close family history of neurological disease or some sort of reaction to a previous immunization. Each edition of the immunization guidelines list fewer and fewer

Table 3.2 False contra-indications to childhood immunization

1. Personal or family history of:
   allergy (unless personal history of anaphylaxis—see p. 172)
   asthma
   hayfever
2. Family history of convulsions or of any adverse reaction following immunizations
3. Current treatment with antibiotics or topical or inhaled steroids
4. Breast-fed baby or baby's mother being pregnant
5. Jaundice after birth; do not postpone immunization because of prematurity
6. Previous history of pertussis, rubella, measles, or mumps
7. Stable neurological conditions, such as Down syndrome or cerebral palsy
8. Older age than usual at presentation for immunization
9. Contact with infectious disease in Britain

Questions before immunization is given

1. Was your baby born on time and was he or she well after delivery?
2. Has your baby had any fits or convulsions?
3. Is your baby well at the moment?
4. Did your baby have any reaction after the last immunization?

Questions 1–3 are asked before the first immunization, and 3–4 before each subsequent immunization.

Modified from *Immunisation against infectious disease* (1992).

contra-indications to routine immunization—the advice will nearly always be to go ahead. The four questions listed in the table are a quick and useful screening test.

Infants may be uncomfortable and have a mild febrile reaction to the DTP. If bothersome, one or two doses of paracetamol (60 mg) will lead to a more cheerful baby.

Immunization schedules

The DTP immunization schedule in the United Kingdom was changed from three, five, and nine months to two, three, and four months in 1990 in order to improve compliance and protect young babies against whooping cough. Vaccination against *Haemophilus influenzae* type b was added in October 1992. This schedule appears to produce adequate protection but antibody levels are probably not as high as with the old schedule (Booy *et al*. 1992).

Pertussis and DTP vaccine

Protection of babies from whooping cough in the first few months (the most vulnerable age) depends mainly on the state of immunity of their siblings, but vaccination at two months helps to protect them. Whooping cough is a serious

Table 3.3 Immunization schedules

Vaccine	Age	Notes
DTP and polio	1st dose 2 months	Primary course
Hib	2nd dose 3 months	
	3rd dose 4 months	
Measles/mumps/rubella (MMR)	12–18 months	Can be given at any age over 12 months
Booster DT and polio		
MMR if not previously given	4–5 years	
Rubella	10–14 years	Girls who have not had MMR
BCG	10–14 years or infancy	If tuberculin negative
Booster tetanus and polio	5–18 years	

Source: *Immunisation against infectious diseases* (1992).

disease in babies and vaccination appears to lessen its severity. Miller and Fletcher (1976) studied 1-to-2-year-olds with whooping cough, and found that only three per cent of 459 vaccinated cases were in the 'admitted to hospital' or 'severe illness treated at home' groups compared with 21 per cent of 575 unvaccinated children.

Like other vaccines prepared from killed bacteria (for example, parenteral typhoid vaccine and cholera vaccine) whooping cough vaccines are not as effective as toxoids or live vaccines. The vaccine also causes more reactions. Most severe triple immunization reactions are due to the pertussis component. A red, swollen injection site with a fever and a fretful baby is classified as a 'minor' reaction and is not a contra-indication to continuing the course. As with any intramuscular injection the child may be left with a hard nodule for a while, even if the pertussis component is omitted.

The central question is whether side-effects are ever associated with permanent damage to the brain. Evidence suggests that they may be, but extremely rarely. A report on the National Childhood Encephalopathy Study by Miller *et al.* (1981), compared encephalitic admissions to paediatric units with control cases. The increased risk of serious neurological reactions occurring within one week of immunization with DTP vaccine was 1 per 110 000 injections. In 1 in 310 000 the neurological disability was still present one year later (approximately 1 case per 4000 doctor years in practice). In some of these cases the standard contra-indications to vaccination had not been observed. Diphtheria and tetanus vaccination was not associated with a significant risk. A report from the Committee of the Institute of Medicine of the Washington National Academy of

Sciences (Howson and Fineberg 1992) concluded that there was no causal relationship between the DTP vaccine and SIDS, and insufficient evidence to decide whether the vaccine could lead to chronic neurological damage. The committee reached the following figures for the excess risks per 100 000 immunizations: acute encephalopathy 1, for anaphylaxis 6, shock and 'unusual shock like state' up to 300. Inconsolable persistent crying occurred in 0.1 to 6 per cent of children given a DTP injection.

Thus, while vaccination against pertussis should be encouraged, the contra-indications should be strictly observed. Babies with 'fever equal to or more than 39.5 ºC within 48 hours of vaccine; anaphylaxis; bronchospasm; laryngeal oedema; generalized collapse; prolonged unresponsiveness; prolonged inconsolable or high-pitched screaming for more than four hours; convulsions or encephalopathy occurring within 72 hours, should not be given another pertussis injection. The same applies to babies who develop an extensive indurated redness and swelling involving most of the antero-lateral surface of the thigh or a major part of the circumference of the upper arm. Specialist advice is recommended before immunizing children with a history of convulsions or cerebral damage in the neonatal period because it is difficult, to decide if any neurological disorder is 'stable or progressive' when the child is only a few months old.

A past history of febrile fits or a close family history of idiopathic epilepsy are no longer considered contra-indications. However, advice on reducing post-immunization fever is especially important in this group.

Diphtheria

Active immunization with absorbed diphtheria toxoid is highly effective and the disease has virtually disappeared from the United Kingdom. Reactions after immunization in children under 10 are usually mild. Sometimes there is a slight temperature and malaise, and there may be some swelling and redness at the injection site. There is a risk of a severe reaction if the standard vaccine is given to an older child or adult who is already immune. They should be given the low-dose preparation. Non-immune child contacts of a case of diphtheria should be given a course of erythromycin in addition to three injections of the standard diphtheria vaccine. Again the low-dose vaccine is recommended for those aged 10 years or over.

Tetanus (for use after injury, see p. 51)

If the preschool tetanus vaccination schedule has been completed, a booster is only needed every 10 years. More frequent injections may lead to severe local reactions but should nevertheless be given if there is a serious doubt as to the child's immunity. Local reactions may last for several days following vaccination; but a general reaction is unusual. Children who had a severe reaction to a previous dose should not be reimmunized.

Poliomyelitis

Oral polio vaccine (OPV) consists of a mixture of attenuated strains of each of the three types of polio virus. The response to one type may interfere with the response to another or be affected by other enteric infections; this is why two or three doses of the vaccine are needed to produce immunity to all three types, and why gastro-enteritis is a contra-indication to vaccination. Breast-feeding does not appear to inhibit development of antibodies, so vaccination need not be delayed until breast-feeding has been discontinued. The baby will excrete the virus for up to six weeks; a potential risk to the immunosuppressed or to non-immune contacts. It is perhaps sensible to advise parents and carers to wash their hands after nappy changing especially thoroughly during this period. If there are immunosuppressed individuals in the household, the baby should be vaccinated with killed polio vaccine rather than live OPV. Even though the vaccine may contain traces of penicillin, only a history of extreme hypersensitivity to penicillin is considered a contra-indication.

MMR vaccine

This live attenuated vaccine should be given to pre-school children from the age of about one year. It can be given with the DTP or DT and Polio vaccine. It results in protection against the three viruses in probably 95 per cent of cases. Parents should be warned that their immunized child may develop a fever lasting two or three days, possibly a rash about a week after the injection and cervical lymphadenopathy in the second week, and, rarely, a parotid swelling in the third. Affected children are not infectious and paracetamol is sufficient to reduce the fever. Miller *et al.* (1993) estimated that the risk of viral meningitis two to five weeks after the MMR was about 1 in about 11 000 injections. Most affected children usually presented with a febrile convulsion, usually accompanied by vomiting, drowsiness or irritability. Meningeal irritation is presumably due to the mumps component of the vaccine. Neurological complications following a wild mumps infection are four times more likely. Febrile convulsions caused by the measles component occur in 0.1% one to two weeks after immunization. The Joint Committee do not consider a personal or close family history of convulsions to be a contra-indication to the MMR, but if these fits were febrile the parents should be told to give paracetamol if fever develops a week or so later. If there is a history of anaphylactic reaction to egg-containing food, paediatric advice should be sought before immunization.

One sometimes feels that the benefits of immunization against common, usually not very severe, diseases are only marginal, but this is not always the case.

One morning, when she was well on the road to recovery, I was sitting on her bed showing her how to fashion little animals out of coloured pipe cleaners, and when it came to her turn to make one herself, I noticed that her fingers and her mind were not working together and she couldn't do anything. 'Are you feeling alright?' I asked her. 'I feel all sleepy,' she said. In an hour, she was unconscious. In 12 hours she was dead. The measles had turned into a terrible thing called measles encephalitis and there was nothing the doctors could do to save her [R. Dahl describing his daughter's death (*British Medical Journal* 1986)]

Haemophilus influenzae b

Conjugated Hib vaccine is over 90 per cent effective against the virulent b group strains of *H. influenzae* responsible for some cases of meningitis, epiglottitis, pneumonia and septicaemia. The incidence of these infections dropped by 80 per cent in the year after introduction of the vaccine in the UK. Side-effects are usually limited to local redness and a mild fever. Young infants are most vulnerable to these infections, but one dose of the vaccine is still recommended for children age 13–48 months who missed the primary course. It can be given at the same time as the MMR. Children under four years who have been in close contact with a case of virulent Hib disease should be immunized as well as being given rifampicin prophylaxis.

Rubella

Rubella vaccination is unique in being given to protect a potential fetus (see p. 157). The vaccine is a live attenuated virus which is given to girls aged 10–14 years who have not had the MMR or MR. Prospective studies have shown that rubella antibody levels are well maintained for 20 years. It is still uncertain whether immunity following vaccination in childhood will persist till the end of the reproductive years. Women must be screened for rubella antibody early in every pregnancy because the vaccine does not take in a few cases (<5 per cent), and a few women lose previously acquired immunity. The vaccine can cause a mild fever, rash, and lymphadenopathy; in adults arthralgia and arthritis may occur. Symptoms occur usually one to three weeks after vaccination. Pregnancy is considered a contra-indication to rubella vaccination and conception should be avoided for four weeks afterwards. It is reassuring, however, that the vaccine does not appear to be teratogenic.

BCG

In 1988 there were 294 newly diagnosed cases of tuberculosis in children under 15 years, a reduction of 60 per cent in 10 years. The rate for white children was 1.5/100 000, and 26/100 000 for children born in the UK whose parents originated from the Indian subcontinent (MRC 1994).

The freeze-dried, live, attenuated strain of *Mycobacterium tuberculosis* is over 70 per cent effective. Protection lasts some 15 years. It has been debated for some time whether routine BCG administration should be continued. At present, immunization is recommended for children aged 10–13 years, and for younger children when the parents request a BCG. A preliminary tuberculin skin test is essential; only those with a negative test are immunized. A strongly positive result may indicate active TB and should be investigated. BCG is also recommended for immigrants and neonatal immunization for their children. A preliminary tuberculin skin test is not necessary before immunizing neonates, but particular care should be taken with intradermal technique (p. 324). Most Authorities follow this general approach, but a minority still offer immunization of all neonates and this may produce a worthwhile reduction in the incidence of tuberculosis in childhood (Curtis *et al.* 1984).

A small papule develops two to six weeks after vaccination. This slowly increases in size for a further two to three weeks and may ulcerate and discharge. Any dressing used should be non-waterproof. Lymphadenopathy may develop, and the lesion heals over after about two months, leaving a small scar. The most frequent cause of severe injection site reactions is faulty injection technique. The vaccinator needs to be skilled in giving intradermal injections. The contraindications to live vaccines should be strictly adhered to, and BCG should be avoided in HIV positive children. Another live vaccine can be given with BCG, but otherwise there should be at least a gap of three weeks between the BCG and other live vaccines. There is no need to delay the primary immunization course following a neonatal BCG—but inject in a different limb. Newborn babies with a parent who has active TB should be given prophylactic isoniazid.

Other vaccines

Influenza vaccine given annually in the autumn is usually reserved for children with cystic fibrosis, sickle cell disease and HIV infection, or other severe chronic lung or heart disorders, or who live in a residential home. The split virion vaccine is recommended for younger children. In the event of an epidemic, unvaccinated high-risk children can alternatively be immunized at the onset of exposure and given amantadine for two weeks until an immune response has had time to develop. It should not be given to children who are very allergic to eggs, as egg protein is present in the vaccine.

Hepatitis B vaccine is recommended for infants born to carriers, or to mothers infected during pregnancy. One dose is given as soon after birth as possible, the second a month later, and the third when the infant is six months of age. These babies also need simultaneous passive immunization with hepatitis B immunoglobulin (HBIG) with the first dose of the vaccine. Antenatal screening for hepatitis B should be offered to all pregnant women. Vaccination may also be necessary for teenagers planning to enter certain occupations (for example, medicine).

Multivalent pneumococcal vaccine is useful in reducing the risk of pneumococcal pneumonia and septicaemia in patients who have impaired splenic function, as in sickle cell anaemia, or who have had a splenectomy, or the nephrotic syndrome. Protection is not complete. It is recommended that the vaccine should be given only after two years of age as antibody response is poor before that age, though some paediatricians advise that infants with sickle cell disease should be vaccinated at six months of age. It should also be given before a splenectomy. Reactions to repeated doses may be severe and the British National Formulary 1994 suggests 'revaccination after 3–5 years (not sooner) for children at highest risk'.

PASSIVE IMMUNIZATION

Human immunoglobulin (Ig) contains antibodies to various infectious organisms. The preparations used consist mainly of IgG antibodies, quantitatively the most important component of the body's serological defence. IgG has a mean plasma half-life of 25 days. Human Normal IgG (HNIG) is produced from a pool of human plasma from normal donors, whereas specific IgG contains an increased amount of a specified antibody. Systemic reactions are rare if IgG is given intramuscularly, but may occur if it is given intravenously by mistake. In general, IgG has been used for travellers to areas where there has been a high incidence of hepatitis, and for post-exposure prophylaxis. Since the protective effect falls off sharply as the days pass after exposure to an infection, immunoglobulin should be given before, or as early as possible after, contact. HNIG may interfere with the antibody response to live vaccine, and ideally these should be given either three weeks before, or three months after an injection of HNIG. That gap may not be feasible for travellers needing a booster dose of a polio vaccine. There is no evidence that the AIDS virus has been transmitted by batches of immunoglobulin available in the UK.

Measles

HNIG can be used to prevent or attenuate measles in immunocompromised contacts. It can also be given to babies under a year, particularly if they have had a recent serious illness, to be followed by MMR after a gap of at least three months.

Rubella

HNIG does not prevent infection, but may mask the signs and symptoms of 'German measles'. The Joint Committee consider it may 'possibly reduce the risks to the fetus' and may thus be considered for a non-immune pregnant rubella contact who would not consider termination of pregnancy.

Infectious hepatitis A

HNIG should be offered to household contacts of a case of hepatitis A and to the infrequent traveller just before leaving for an endemic area. The frequent traveller should be offered hepatitis A vaccine which produces, after two doses, a more than 50-fold higher antibody level than HNIG.

Hepatitis B (see p. 163)

Chickenpox

Human varicella-zoster immunoglobulin (VZIG) should be given to children at high risk. These include immunosuppressed children and those who have recently been on steroids. For perinatal infections, see p. 155.

Mumps

HNIG does not appear to work, and mumps-specific immunoglobulin is not made any more.

Immunoglobulin deficiency

A number of rare immunoglobulin deficiencies can be fairly successfully treated with repeated intramuscular injections of HNIG.

FOREIGN TRAVEL

Advice to families intending to travel, particularly to tropical or subtropical countries, needs to contain more than a list of recommended injections. Do they know how to protect against sunburn, how to avoid contaminated food and water (freshly cooked food is safer than salads, soft fruit, or ice-cream)? Is malarial prophylaxis needed? Are they also aware of the financial hazards of illness or accidents abroad? The United Kingdom has reciprocal medical arrangements with a number of countries, including those in the European Union, but families will need private insurance to cover medical costs elsewhere, and even for EU countries to avoid bureaucratic delays in treatment. The Department of Health issues a useful booklet, *Health advice for travellers*, on health protection for people intending to travel abroad. It includes a table of vaccinations recommended for most countries, and information on health insurance and reciprocal arrangements.

Diarrhoea is common and parents of infants may need reminding that fluid and electrolyte replacement is the mainstay of treatment (take along some sachets of Dioralyte or Rehidrat). The management of diarrhoea on return from abroad is discussed in Chapter 13.

Vaccinations for travel

Updating routine vaccinations—in particular against polio, tetanus, and diphtheria—is as important as any extra ones, such as cholera or typhoid. Most travellers even to the more exotic countries, will only need two visits, separated by four to six weeks for the necessary immunization. Even a single does of most live vaccines will give worthwhile protection.

Cholera vaccine is not recommended for infants under one year. It usually gives only about 50 per cent protection lasting three to six months, and the main reason for giving it is to satisfy officials at the frontiers of some countries. A certificate with evidence of one recent injection is usually sufficient.

Typhoid monovalent whole cell vaccine protects 70–80 per cent of recipients. It is not advised for babies under one year, and ideally the primary course should be given as two injections separated by four weeks. Booster injections are needed only every three years. A capsular polysaccharide typhoid vaccine has recently been introduced. A single dose also appears to give 70–80 per cent protection for three years and adverse reactions tend to be less severe than after a whole cell vaccine. An oral live attenuated vaccine is also available, but is not recommended for children under six years.

Hepatitis occurs particularly where sanitation is poor. Immunoglobulin given just before departure is satisfactory for the very occasional visitor abroad; more regular travellers or wandering school-leavers should be actively immunized against hepatitis A and hepatitis B.

BCG for a tuberculin negative child may be advisable a few months before an extended visit to rural areas of Asia, Africa or South America.

Yellow fever, a viral infection transmitted by a variety of mosquitoes, occurs in parts of South America.

Meningococcal vaccine does not protect against *Neisseria meningitidis* Group B, the commonest pathogen in the UK. Children over the age of two months, who have been or may be in contact with Group A or Group C meningitis in parts of Africa or Saudi Arabia, for example, should be given the vaccine in addition to chemoprophylaxis. One dose of the vaccine protects for ten years.

Rabies is a possibility following a bite or scratch by a potentially infected animal, and immunization is recommended for backpacking adolescents travelling to remote parts of the world. Unfortunately they will have to pay for the vaccine.

Diarrhoea in travellers

This almost inevitable accompaniment of a holiday in the tropics is due to a variety of organisms, including *E.coli*, viruses, shigella, salmonella, giardia and *E.histolytica*. Food may be the culprit or water, perhaps from swimming pools or the sea. The patient should know that fluid replacement is the mainstay of treatment, ideally using a glucose–electrolyte mixture (vital for infants and young children) or by drinking soups containing some extra salt, fruit juices, and eating boiled rice or bread and bananas (potassium). The role of antibiotics is controversial. They are indicated for toxic children with severe diarrhoea.

Co-trimoxazole, trimethoprim or ciprofloxacin may reduce the length and severity of the illness. Prophylactic antibiotics may work (Farthing 1993) but are not usually indicated in children.

BREAST-FEEDING

Breast-milk production is stimulated by prolactin secretion from the anterior pituitary gland in response to the infant sucking; frequent breast feeds on demand induce higher levels of prolactin and produce better lactation than a 'four-hourly' regimen. Breast-feeding may be better established by putting the infant on the breast as early as possible after birth (oxytocin secretion will also encourage contraction of the uterus after birth). Successful breast-feeding also depends on a positive and relaxed atmosphere, a mother who is healthy, well nourished, and drinking adequately and an infant who is healthy and has a vigorous suck. Co-administration of dextrose, water or formula feeds should be avoided if possible as this may jeopardize lactation.

If there is a problem, watching a breast-feed may identify the cause. Difficulties result from faulty technique such as trying to feed in a position uncomfortable to the mother or child, carrying on a feed after the nipples get sore, or failure to alternate the side of starting. Sore or cracked nipples can usually be prevented if the nipple goes well into the baby's mouth and is not chewed at the tip; it is easier if the mother sits in a comfortable chair leaning slightly forward to feed, as gravity assists in this. An established cracked nipple can be very painful. The baby should be fed from the good side first to allow the 'let down' of the milk in both breasts, so that feeding is then easier from the cracked side. If very bad the breast can be expressed manually or using a pump. If the cracked nipple is due to monilial infection, both the mother and the infant should be treated. A warm, red, tender, lumpy segment of breast in a toxic patient implies mastitis, or a blocked duct if there is less toxicity. The keystone of treatment is thorough emptying of the breast with each feed, together with flucloxacillin if there is toxicity. Breast-feeding should continue in order to reduce the risk of a breast abscess. Similarly, expression, either manually or with a breast pump, is necessary for the painful breasts of engorgement; the pain may be eased with a hot or cold compress.

Failure to thrive because of insufficient breast-milk is more likely if the mother is over-tired or over-anxious. The baby may be constipated or produce more frequent, small, slightly greenish "hunger" stools and gain weight poorly. Although undernourished, some appear to be satisfied and sleepy after a feed, although others cry hungrily and do not settle well. The infant may suck vigorously at the breast, but test-weighing (difference in infant's body weight before and immediately after a feed without change of clothing) shows inadequate intake of breast-milk. Regular test-weighing itself can be stressful enough to reduce milk production. If there is an insufficient supply of milk it is important to make sure that the mother has emptied both breasts by the end of the feed, if necessary by manual expression. Expressed milk can be refrigerated for use later in the day. Even with the best will in the world it is sometimes impossible for the mother to produce enough milk for the baby to thrive, and complementary or total bottle feeding is necessary. Mothers who are unhappy breast-feeding or who do not produce enough milk should not be made to feel guilty.

Breast-fed babies have fewer serious gastro-intestinal and respiratory infections. They are less likely than bottle-fed babies to become obese. Breast-feeding encourages the development of a close physical relationship between the mother and baby. It is probably not true that potentially allergic infants are protected by breast-feeding and it is no longer felt that a marked family history of atopy is a special indication for prolonged breast-feeding, with the late introduction of solids. In any case, breast-feeding does not completely exclude dietary antigens which may be absorbed by the mother's intestine and enter breast milk. There are certain disadvantages to breast-feeding, apart from the relatively minor ones of not knowing how much the infant is taking, and of dealing with the loose stools of the fully breast-fed baby. Only the mother can feed the baby and she is less able to spend time away from the house, although after some months if breast-feeding is well established, the baby can take a bottle by day and merely have a breast-feed night and morning.

The combined oestrogen–progesterone contraceptive pill is not usually suitable for women who are breast-feeding because it may lessen the supply of milk. A reasonable alternative is the progesterone-only pill, but this is not quite so effective a contraceptive and must be taken at the same time every day. The loss of efficacy is counterbalanced by the contraceptive effect of breast-feeding. Breast-milk jaundice resulting in peak unconjugated bilirubin levels of around 250 μmol/L in the second week of life in a term infant is a major nuisance, since it often results in an otherwise healthy and thriving infant being investigated for rarer causes of prolonged jaundice, such as hypothyroidism. Breast-milk is low in vitamin K. Thus, exclusively breast-fed infants who have not received intramuscular vitamin K shortly after birth (because of an, as yet unproven, association between an increased risk of childhood malignancies and intramuscular vitamin K administration in the neonatal period) are at risk of developing haemorrhagic disease of the newborn. It is current practice to give them oral vitamin K. In an HIV positive mother there is potential for transmitting the virus via breast milk.

ARTIFICIAL FEEDING

Formulae are prepared from cows' milk by reducing of the protein and mineral content and by substituting of vegetable for butter fat, to simulate the composition of human milk. They are fortified with iron and vitamins. Babies usually thrive provided that the feeds are prepared in accordance with manufacturers' instructions. Unmodified cows' milk is not recommended until the child is about 12 months old, because it may contribute to hypernatraemic dehydration and be less digestible. When used, it need not be boiled provided it is pasteurized and kept refrigerated. More recently, follow-on formulae have been introduced which contain higher protein, salt, vitamin and iron concentrations than standard formulae. These are rarely necessary, except for the occasional infant over six months of age who refuses all solids. Soya protein based formulae are free of cows' milk protein and lactose and are often used for infants with cows' milk allergy (often incorrectly diagnosed because of symptoms such as 'colic'). Many infants with true cows' milk allergy are also allergic to soya protein. These formulae are suitable for short-term management of transient milk protein–lactose intolerance after gastro-enteritis (p. 212).

A number of special artificial formulae are produced for babies intolerant of sugars, suffering from a metabolic disorder or allergic to cows' milk protein. These formulae, described in the section of the BNF on 'Foods for special diets', and soya based formulae, are available on prescription. Occasionally a mother has alleged dependence on soya formulae in order to obtain free milk.

Vitamin supplements are advisable for infants fed on a specialized formula not supplemented with vitamins (most are), low-birth-weight infants, and those solely breast-fed over the age of six months. Babies with limited exposure to ultra-violet light (usually Asians) also require vitamin D supplementation which should be continued through childhood. It is important to note that a marked excessive vitamin D intake may lead to pathological hypercalcaemia with vomiting, constipation, and failure to thrive.

HEALTHY EATING

All children need an adequate intake of food with the necessary vitamins and trace minerals such as iron. This is not achieved in many parts of the world. It is hoped that current dietary advice to parents of healthy children may reduce the incidence of obesity, coronary artery disease, hypertension, cancer and gastrointestinal disorders in the next generation, as early nutrition may be an important factor in the development of these complex diseases. Evidence for atherosclerosis beginning in childhood comes from post-mortems of young adults killed in wars. It would seem sensible to reduce dietary intake of saturated fats, though there is as yet no proof that this will prevent later coronary heart disease. It is recommended that in adults and children over the age of five years, no more than 30–35 per cent of daily calories should be derived from fats, with 12–15 per cent derived from saturated fats. Fat is an important source of energy and zealous dietary restriction is not advisable for infants and toddlers. Thus, full-fat-milk should be given to children under two years, with gradual change to semi-skimmed milk after this age, and the intake of carbohydrates should be increased to meet the resultant shortfall of calories. The addition of salt to infants' food, which may be dictated by parental taste, is not recommended. Excessive milk drinking or frequent snacks of high-calorie, high-fat crisps or biscuits frequently leads to a complaint that a one-or-two-year old 'is not eating anything'.

Meals for older children and teenagers should contain less fat in total, but a rise in the polyunsaturated–saturated fat ratio, less sugar and salt and more fibre. This means eating more wholemeal bread, wholemeal breakfast cereals, peas, beans, lentils, fruit and vegetables, less jams and marmalades and salt in cooking, fewer sweets, chocolates, cakes, and biscuits. Skimmed or semi-skimmed milk is better for drinks and cereals than full-cream milk, and polyunsaturated margarine should be spread thinly on toast rather than thickly spread butter. Grilling is better than frying and vegetable oils high in polyunsaturated fats (for example, sunflower, corn, and soya oils) are better than butter or lard. Chicken and fish have little fat, unlike sausages and mince. Low-fat fast foods include jacket potatoes and baked beans. Regular exercise will help to maintain a body-weight in accordance with height.

Any recommended dietary changes need to take into account the family's present eating habits as well as their income, which may only permit intake of high-calorie (but affordable) foods, such as custard, biscuits, sausages, and chips. It is only possible to alter what children eat by influencing the diet of the whole family, and even then fads and fancies may prevail. Knowledge of the best childhood diet is evolving, and in the future advice may become more specifically related to the disease patterns of individual families. Where there is not convincing data, health visitors and doctors should avoid a 'nanny knows best' attitude. Dietary advice should also be appropriate to the different cultures in our society.

LOW-BIRTH-WEIGHT BABIES

Increasing numbers of very low-birth-weight babies are surviving. Some may be as much as 16 weeks premature with a birth weight of 1 kg or less. Most achieve developmental milestones at roughly the usual time, once allowance is made for the number of weeks of prematurity. The lower the birth-weight, the greater the degree of prematurity, and the more severe the illness and complications of the neonatal period, the more likely is mental handicap and cerebral palsy.

Post-discharge care

By the time of discharge most babies are being fed four to six hourly and taking some 180–200 ml/kg per day. Some do not settle well on milk feeds, and early weaning with, for example, baby rice, appears to be satisfactory, even if started as early as two weeks after the expected date of delivery. Others seem quite happy with milk only for another three or four months. A preterm baby's nutritional stores are much impaired, as many nutrients cross the placenta predominantly in the last six weeks of gestation. Most babies born before 35 weeks will be kept on folic acid (2.5 mg), iron (5 mg) daily and vitamin drops such as Abidec (0.6 ml) daily until completely weaned. Immunizations are often begun at two months from the actual date of birth, provided that the baby is clinically well by this stage. Pertussis is usually avoided if the baby was thought to be neurologically abnormal while in the neonatal unit, or if ultrasound scans showed large haemorrhages in the ventricles or any haemorrhage into the brain, or ischaemic damage to the brain. Smaller haemorrhages just into the sub-ependymal region or into the ventricle are usually ignored. Many preterm babies by the time of discharge, are below the second centile, and they should be expected to continue parallel to this, or to move towards it over the ensuing months. Failure to do so is an indication to reassess the baby. Increasing numbers of babies surviving with severe bronchopulmonary dysplasia (a chronic lung disorder caused by damage to lungs brought about by oxygen toxicity and high-pressure ventilation) require long term domiciliary oxygen. All low-birth-weight infants need to be carefully monitored in the child health clinic, even though they are also likely to be followed up by hospital or community paediatricians. Babies who have been ventilated in the neonatal period more commonly suffer from chest infections in infancy.

DENTAL HEALTH

Dental caries and periodontal disease (disease of the gums and tooth-supporting structures) are the commonest chronic diseases in children, and doctors tend to be lamentably ignorant about them. However, there has been a significant decrease in dental decay in the last 20 years, at least partly due to the measures discussed below. Many parents do not realize that the first molar that appears when the child is about six years old is a permanent tooth. It is prone to decay and there is no replacement tooth behind it.

Dental caries is a bacterial disease. The susceptibility of the child is influenced by many factors, including his genes, age, diet, oral hygiene, fluoride content of the water, and general state of health. Micro-organisms collect upon the surface of the tooth. In the presence of saliva and food debris they form a strong adherent film—dental plaque. This almost invisible deposit will form rapidly in places which are not smooth and self-cleansing, such as fissures and interdental spaces. Fermentable carbohydrates, particularly sucrose, are the main substrate for the production of acids which first decalcify the enamel, then erode the underlying dentine, which becomes demineralized. If left untreated a pulpitis may develop and eventually the pulp of the tooth becomes necrotic and the bacteria may pass through the opening at the end of the root and cause an abscess. This in turn may cause a gum boil or a facial swelling.

Antibiotics may be necessary to control the infection and abscesses can be treated by a root-canal filling or by removing the tooth. They can sometimes be drained by drilling a hole in the occlusal surface of the tooth.

The GP's examination and advice can help to reduce dental decay and periodontal diseases in children. Tooth enamel which has incorporated the fluoride ion into its crystalline structure is more resistant to destruction by acid than enamel which is fluoride free. The presence of fluoride to a level of one part per million in the public water supply would probably reduce dental caries by about a half. Fluoride tablets are only advised, from the age of six months, if the water contains less than 0.3 mg of fluoride/litre (see BNF for dose). Excess use may discolour the teeth. The daily use of toothpaste containing fluoride and the topical application of fluoride gel to the teeth by dentists can also reduce caries.

On examining the child's throat it may be more important to look at the teeth and gums. Large, carious cavities are easy to spot and so is gingivitis, with sore gums which bleed easily. Children with these need referral to a dentist. By the age of 12–18 months toddlers should have enough teeth to have them cleaned with a small, soft toothbrush with a small amount of children's fluoride-containing toothpaste. Teeth should be cleaned regularly. The child of two to two-and-a-half should pay his first six-monthly visit to the dentist.

Most infants can be educated to eat non-sweetened rather than to sweetened food. Sugary substances between meals are more damaging than sugar ingested at meal times, when saliva and other foods tend to neutralize the tooth-destroying acid. Comforters made of dummies dipped in syrup or a mini-feeder containing a sugary liquid can cause rampant dental caries in the young child. The upper primary incisor teeth are the first affected, followed by the maxillary posterior teeth; the lower anterior teeth are less severely affected. We disagree with each other on how far sweets should be restricted altogether; is this really 'a middle-class puritanical fad'? Iatrogenic caries is common in children on long-term medication with sugar-containing formulations, though several have been changed to remove sugar; they are labelled 'sugar free' in the BNF. If sugar medicines cannot be avoided they should be at least followed by a tooth cleaning session, especially last thing at night. Tablets are better if the child will tolerate them. These strictures especially apply if medicines are needed for months at a time.

Orthodontic treatment. Over-crowded and crooked teeth are commonplace but can usually be straightened by an orthodontic programme. This involves about two years of treatment with stainless steel attachments bonded to the teeth. Treatment is best between the ages of 10 and 14. The benefits are mainly cosmetic, but are no less important because of this. Orthodontic treatment has doubtful effects on the incidence of dental caries.

Emergency dental care is needed for subluxated or fractured teeth. Teeth that are knocked out should, if possible, be immediately replaced. If this is not feasible they should be kept moist, preferably in saline, and child plus tooth should be immediately dispatched to the dentist. Reimplanted teeth usually remain firmly fixed at least a few years, allowing the jaw to grow normally during childhood. Likewise, a dislocated tooth should be quickly splinted back in position.

HEART MURMURS

Most systolic murmurs heard during a febrile illness in a previously well child are unimportant flow murmurs that will be gone when the child is re-examined. A positive diagnosis of the commonly heard benign murmur, can usually be made from the examination. It is limited to systole and is usually relatively short and of mild intensity. It starts after a clearly heard first sound and is usually confined to the left of the lower sternum. If only heard high up and to the left an atrial septal defect is a possibility, especially if there is fixed splitting of the second sound. A benign murmur is never harsh or accompanied by a thrill or by a heaving cardiac impulse. The murmur may lessen or disappear when the child breathes in. The child with a benign murmur will be otherwise well, not abnormally short of breath on exercise or subject to more than the usual share of chest infections, and will be growing normally. Before reassuring parents that the murmur is benign (if it is decided to mention it at all) cyanosis must be looked for, and the precordium examined to be certain that the heart is not enlarged. Make sure that the femoral pulses are present.

Another benign sound is the venous hum which extends though systole and diastole, and can be confused with the murmur of a patent ductus arteriosus. It is heard most easily when the child sits up, and may disappear when he lies down or alters the position of his head. It is more often heard below the clavicles and in the neck. The murmur disappears on compression of the jugular vein, a useful diagnostic manoeuvre. It has no pathological significance.

If the doubtful GP decides to refer the child with a murmur, it saves time if referral is made to a department able to offer echocardiography. This is non-invasive and allows the exclusion of most childhood cardiac lesions, on an out-patient basis.

Bibliography

Bantock, H. and Modell, M. (1992). Child health surveillance—surveillance of the child under 5. In *Clinical guidelines—report of a local initiative*, (ed. A. Haines and B. Hurwitz). Royal College of General Practitioners, London.

Booy, R., Aitken, S. J. M., Taylor, S., Tudor-Williams, G., Macfarlane, J. A., Moxon, E. R. *et al.* (1992). Immunogenicity of combined diphtheria, tetanus and pertussis vaccine given at 2, 3, and 4 months versus 3, 5, and 9 months of age. *Lancet,* **339**, 507–10.

Bradshaw, C. L. (1985). Dental problems in children. In *Progress in child health,* Vol 2, (ed. J MacFarlane).

Cartwright, K. A. (1992). Vaccination against Haemophilus influenzae B disease. *British Medical Journal,* **305**, 485–6.

Court, S. D. M. (1976). *Fit for the future*—Report of the Committee on Child Health Services. HMSO, London.

Curtis, H. M., Leck, I., and Bamford, F. W. (1984). Incidence of childhood tuberculosis after neonatal BCG examination. *Lancet,* **i**, 145–8.

Farthing, M. J. G. (1993). Travellers' diarrhoea. *British Medical Journal*, **306**, 1425–6.

Hall, D. (ed.) (1996). *Health for all children,* Report of the third Joint Working Party on Child Health Surveillance, (3rd edn). Oxford University Press.

Hart, C. and Bain, J. (1989). *Child care in general practice*, (3rd edn). Churchill Livingstone, London.

Health Education Authority (1989). *Birth to Five: a guide to the first five years of being a parent.*

Houston, W. J. B. (1986). Current trends in orthodontic treatment. *Archives of Disease in Childhood,* **61**, 536–7.

Howson, C. P. and Fineberg, H. V. (1992). Ricochet of magic bullets. Summary of the Institute of Medicine Report—Adverse effects of pertussis and rubella vaccines. *Pediatrics,* **89**, 318–23.

Immunisation against infectious diseases (1992). HMSO, London.

Kinder, J., Louise, T., Rao, M., Bridgman, G., and Kurian, A. (1992). False contra-indications to childhood immunisation. *British Journal of General Practice*, **42**, 160–1.

Lancet. (1992). Hepatitis A: a vaccine at last. *Lancet*, **339**, 1198–9.

Medical Research Council Cardiothoracic Epidemiology Group. (1994). Tuberculosis in children: a national survey of notifications in England and Wales in 1988. *Archives of Disease in Childhood*, **70**, 497–500.

Miller, C. L. and Fletcher, W. B. (1976). Severity of notified whooping cough. *British Medical Journal,* **1**, 117–19.

Miller, C. L., Ross, E. M., Alderslade, R. *et al.* (1981). Pertussis immunisation and serious acute neurological illness in children. *British Medical Journal*, **1**, 1595–9.

Miller, E., Goldacre, M., Pugh, S., Colville, A., Farrington, P., Flower, A. *et al.* (1993). Risk of aseptic meningitis after measles, mumps and rubella vaccine in UK children. *Lancet,* **341**, 979–82.

Pike, L. A. (1980). Teaching parents about child health using a practice booklet. *J. Roy. Coll. Gen. Pract.,* **30**, 517–19.

Polnay, L. and Hull, D. (1993). *Community Paediatrics*, (2nd edn). Churchill Livingstone, London.

Steim, E. R. (1979). Standard and special human immune serum globulins as therapeutic agents. *Pediatrics,* **63**, 301–19.

4 Accidents and poisonings

Childhood accidents are the commonest cause of death between the ages of 1 and 15. It has been estimated that 20 per cent of all paediatric admissions to hospital are due to accidents, and one out of six children will attend an Accident and Emergency Department each year (Polnay and Hull 1993). The risk of accidents in different environments varies according to age: toddlers and preschool children are at greater risk at home, while school age children are more likely to be injured at school during games and sports, and, more importantly, on the roads as pedestrians. Boys outnumber girls by a ratio of 3:2. Children from economically deprived backgrounds have a higher death rate from accidents. Poor housing, such as high rise flats, poor access to nearby parks or play areas, overcrowding and lack of money to buy safety equipment (such as fire guards) contribute, as do more intangible social factors. Stressful situations such as parental depression, marital discord, or family illness increase the risk of childhood accidents. The various preventive measures appear to be having an effect as the rate of accidental death is declining.

Morton and Phillips's (1992) book on Accidents and emergencies in children (Oxford University Press) provides useful advice to the GP (2nd edition in press).

ROAD TRAFFIC ACCIDENTS

Boys between the ages of five and eight are most likely to be knocked down by a car. Two-thirds of deaths occur between 3 and 9 p.m. The majority of the deaths are due to serious head injuries. Young male drivers are a considerable danger to children. Without children of their own, they perhaps have difficulty in remembering that a small child does not have the ability to assess the risks of crossing the road, or the self-control to wait until a car has gone safely by; this group of drivers appears to show a similar childlike rashness.

DROWNING

About 80 children are drowned each year. Mouth-to-mouth resuscitation should continue until the ambulance arrives on the scene. In children hypothermic from drowning, the definition of death should be failure to respond to resuscitation after warming of the body. It is common sense to point out to parents the real hazards of leaving a toddler alone in the bath, or in a garden with a pond or water tub for even a few moments. These kill far more children of this age group than ingestion of tablets. Unfenced canals and swimming pools are also a danger which may need to be brought to the attention of local authorities. Kemp *et al.* (1994) found evidence suggestive of abuse in 10 out of 44 cases of children who suffered drowning or near-drowning in the domestic bathtub. Teenagers who drown tend to be boaters or swimmers who underestimate the dangers.

CUTS

Most cuts can be satisfactorily treated in the surgery without stitching, using adhesive strips such as Steristrip. Suturing is indicated for large wounds, or if the edges of the cut cannot be neatly brought together, or for cuts over a moving part, such as a joint. Before using adhesive strips, the cut is cleaned and dried and several strips are then applied. Gaps should be left between the strips, which can remain *in situ* for 7–10 days before being removed. A visit to the Accident and Emergency Department for an X-ray may still be necessary following small wounds to exclude the presence of fragments of glass, although only some types are radio-opaque. Non-adhering dressings such as Melolin next to the skin are easier to remove than sterile gauze swabs, but are not advisable if the wound is infected. Dressings on clean wounds can be left for several days before being changed. If the child has been immunized against tetanus no further prophylaxis is needed, unless the course was more than ten years ago (five years if the wound is very dirty or the course was incomplete). Human tetanus immunoglobulin is only indicated for the non-immune child with a dirty wound or one with a lot of tissue damage, particularly if it is more than six hours old.

BURNS AND SCALDS

Many burns occur in toddlers who have just started getting about but who have not yet got enough sense to avoid danger. Sometimes child abuse is the cause.

Burns can be divided into superficial, when there is partial skin loss, or deep, involving loss of the full thickness of the epidermis. The first will heal in two or three weeks but the second will only epithelialize following slow granulation. Grafting may be necessary to hurry the process and to reduce development of contractures and scarring, which may be appallingly disfiguring. The depth of a burn can sometimes be assessed by its appearance: a superficial burn will present as an area of redness, with or without blistering. The blister may have burst revealing a wet, painful, sensitive, pink area with deep red spots. Deep burns appear blanched and dry, and are later covered with exudate. Early appearances can be very misleading. Some burns that initially seem to be partial thickness are the precursor of a lifetime of deformity and vice versa. If there is uncertainty, refer. Early recognition of deep burns and early referral for surgical treatment improves eventual results.

The simplest initial treatment in the home is to place the burn instantly in cold water until pain is reduced, subsequently covering it with a clean tea-towel or handkerchief. In the surgery, the burnt area may be gently cleaned with cold water or isotonic saline solution. Loose skin may be removed but intact blebs and blisters are best left untouched. Sometimes it is difficult to put an effective dressing over a large intact blister, but to trim it may make the episode more painful as well as increasing the likelihood of infection. The area should be covered with non-adherent paraffin gauze or chlorhexidine impregnated dressing (for example, Bactigras) overlaid with sterile gauze and a thick layer of padding to absorb oozing. Finally, a crepe bandage will retain it all in place. This dressing is left undisturbed, if possible for several days, unless the outer surface becomes moist with exudate, increasing the likelihood of infection. A mild analgesic will be necessary at first to control the pain.

Indications for hospital referral include all full thickness burns, unless they are tiny, and partial thickness burns of over five per cent (half of the surface of an arm or an eighth of the trunk), burns on the face, especially near the eye, or if there is any question that smoke or steam have been inhaled, perhaps indicated by a burned mouth. Burns on the fingers or palms, which may lead to lasting disability, and electrical burns, which frequently cause deep tissue damage, should also be referred. Cigarette burns, perineal burns, or scalds from a too-hot bath are often a sign of child abuse. The management of any burnt child will depend on the social circumstances of the family and the nursing facilities of the practice, as well as upon the amount of tissue injured. A rare but life-threatening complication of burns is the toxic shock syndrome (headache, fever, scarlatiniform rash, conjunctivitis, vomiting, watery diarrhoea, and a rapid pulse), caused by exotoxin produced by certain strains of *Staphylococcus aureus* secondarily infecting the burned or scalded area.

FALLS AND HEAD INJURIES

The GP is liable to get an enquiry every two or three weeks about a child who has fallen and perhaps hurt his head. The vast majority sustain no serious injury. Those who do badly, if they do not die at once, most frequently remain unconscious from the time of the accident, they may occasionally recover, even after several weeks of coma. Such a child will often show residual motor handicap, behavioural disturbance, and sometimes epilepsy. A tiny but important group with intracranial, especially extradural, bleeding will be all right, or nearly all right immediately after the fall, but then begin to develop signs of raised intracranial pressure hours or even days later. Vomiting, drowsiness, and bradycardia proceed to coma, hemiplegic signs, squint, unequal pupils and, in the infant, a full fontanelle. Such lives will be lost without appropriate neurosurgery. The problem is to avoid missing these few, most, but not all, of whom will have been knocked out by the initial blow. Some paediatricians admit for observation all head injuries sufficiently severe to cause unconsciousness at the time of injury.

If the child has not had an obviously trivial injury, he will need to be seen by the GP, or, if appropriate, directed straight to the hospital. Knowledge of the circumstances of the accident is of some help in reaching a decision whether to refer or not. How severe was the impact? Did he fall on soft ground or on hard concrete? Was he involved in a road traffic accident? Was he quiet for a prolonged period before crying? Often a young child who is upset following a fall will vomit once or twice and then may want to go to sleep without there being any evidence of intracranial haemorrhage. It is important to ascertain the child's condition before the accident, as some children fall because they are unwell and the post-accident symptoms of irritability or fever can be due to preceding acute otitis media or tonsillitis. Much less commonly than in adults, an unexplained fall when a child is standing is caused by a fit, a cardiac arrhythmia or, in teenagers, a vasovagal attack (chapter 18).

As well as feeling the pulse, checking for associated infectious disease and making a brief neurological examination, the GP should look for injuries elsewhere. Is there any guarding or tenderness in the abdomen? Does the child wince when his thorax is squeezed? Do the limbs all move normally; is there any obvious deformity? Are all pulses present? Examination of the head includes inspection of the scalp for haematomas, lacerations or evidence of bony deformity which may indicate a depressed fracture, and of the face for local deformity or tenderness. Bruising behind the ears (Battle's sign) is a sign of fracture of the base of the skull, as are bilateral periorbital haematomas.. There may be bleeding or a CSF leak (like a watery runny nose or ear, though the discharge may be blood-stained) or neurological signs of intracranial bleeding. A displaced, fractured nose should be straightened within the first three weeks after injury but not until after the swelling has subsided. The only indication for urgent action is the uncommon haematoma of the nasal septum which will cause obstruction to airflow. X-rays are not of assistance in the diagnosis of a fractured nose; it is a clinical diagnosis.

If it is decided to keep the child with a head injury at home the parents may need to be asked to contact the doctor again or take him to hospital if any of the following occur:

1. The child becomes irritable, disorientated or abnormally drowsy—difficult to assess at bed-time. The parents should perhaps awaken the child once during the night, about two hours after he has gone to bed to make sure that he is all right.
2. The child has a convulsion.
3. He continues to vomit.

Table 4.1 Accidents and violent deaths under 15 years of age in England and Wales (1991)

	Male	Female
Motor vehicles	181	91
Falls—accidental	29	8
Possible accident or homicide	39	38
Poisoning	9	9
Fire	47	35
Some other causes		
Congenital anomalies	329	303
Asthma	12	8
Malignant neoplasms	208	157

From *Mortality statistics* (1992).

4. He complains of increasing headache in spite of paracetamol.
5. He becomes ataxic or develops a squint or weakness of a limb.

Social problems may present as imaginary head injuries. Parents whose angry feelings towards their children rightly alarm them may concoct a story of having dropped the baby. Some babies with brain damage from intracranial bleeding have sustained this as a result of parental violence, having either been thrown down or uncontrollably shaken. Indeed, in one study from the United States, of 84 children under one admitted to hospital with a head injury, 35 per cent of the total and 95 per cent of the severe ones were attributed to non-accidental injury (Billmire and Myers 1985). As with any accident, a fall on the head will also sometimes be symptomatic of poor supervision, as when extra stress within a family has diverted adult attention away from the toddler.

POISONING

Accidental ingestion of drugs and poisons by children is frequent. Fortunately, death is rare (Table 4.1). In recent years, tricyclic antidepressants have been the commonest fatal poison.

The GP is often contacted about a child who is feared to have taken a potential poison, either a drug, some household product, or unknown berries. Toddler overdoses are so common that GPs should warn parents of this danger when prescribing potentially dangerous drugs to a member of a household containing children. The occasion provides a good opportunity for parents to describe the arrangements they have made for keeping potentially poisonous substances in a safe place.

If the doctor is uncertain about the toxic effects of a substance, a phone call will usually provide the answer (for example, to the National Poisons Information Service, London, tel. 0171 635 9191). Unless it is clear that the amount of a substance ingested is safe, and it is often very difficult to be certain how much a toddler has swallowed, it is traditionally recommended that the stomach needs to be emptied, perhaps by the use of an emetic such as syrup of ipecacuanha (age 1–7: 15 mL; 30 mL for older child), followed by a large glass of water. A second dose may be necessary if the child has not vomited by half an hour. Although ipecacuanha is an effective emetic, it seems doubtful whether its use often prevents significant absorption (Vale *et al.* 1986). In any case, the syrup is contraindicated for semi-conscious or unconscious patients, or after the ingestion of corrosive agents or paraffins and similar hydrocarbons because of further damage to the oesophagus or to the lungs if inhaled. The whole lamentable business is often most conveniently delegated, without delay, to the Accident and Emergency Department, especially if the GP thinks a substantial overdose of a serious poison has been ingested. The parents should be reminded to take the container of tablets or fluid with them.

Tricyclics (cardiac arrhythmias), Lomotil (coma, respiratory depression; may be delayed), salicylates (tachypnoea, delayed effects), iron (shock, haemorrhagic necrosis of the gut, and CNS depression), co-proxamol (coma and respiratory depression), paracetamol (liver damage) are all potentially very dangerous, and require urgent hospital management if more than a definitely trivial overdose has been taken. There may be a latent period before symptoms occur, particularly likely if the child has swallowed sustained-release preparations or enteric-coated preparations (e.g. Nu-Seals aspirin), or iron, or paracetamol, or after the very poisonous amanita toadstools. Hallucinogenic fungi (magic mushrooms) are also sometimes taken by older children for their supposedly pleasurable properties. They are not very dangerous and the effects wear off after about six hours. However, children should not be left alone while they are hallucinated.

Many household chemicals are harmless (see Table 4.2). The dangerous offenders are paraffins (delayed pulmonary damage), caustics (oesophageal stricture), anti-freeze (blindness and renal failure), and paraquat weed-killer (delayed pulmonary fibrosis).

An ill child with bizarre symptoms may have taken a poison, as may a child who is unconscious. One striking form of child abuse, especially in the families of paramedical personnel, is the inappropriate administration of drugs (Meadow 1985). Occasionally it can be diagnostic to analyse a urine specimen for drugs in a child with obscure recurrent symptoms.

Table 4.2 Toxicity of domestic products

Non-toxic	**Potentially toxic**	**Toxic**
Pencils	Detergents	Anti-freeze
Crayons	Bleaches	Oven cleaners
Inks	Disinfectants	Dish-washing powder
Chalk	Wrights vapourizing fluid	Battery acid
Water-based glues	Disc or button batteries	Paraquat, herbicides and insecticides
Water-colour paint	Nail varnish remover	Petroleum distillates
Paints	Lavatory deodorizing blocks	Solvents
Putty		
'Blu-tak'		
Deodorants		
Suntan lotions		
Bath oils		
Lipstick		
Action		
Reassure and buy some more	Hospital referral is sometimes needed after consultation with Poisons Information Service	Refer to hospital promptly

Modified from Volans and Byatt (1985).

PREVENTION OF CHILD ACCIDENTS AND POISONING

Legislative and environmental solutions such as wearing of seat belts, fewer open fires, change to fire retardant foam in furniture and the use of child-resistant containers for medicines have resulted in a fall in childhood death due to accidents and poisoning. While there is little convincing evidence that health education campaigns, such as the Green Cross Code, have led to a reduction in accident rates in children (Grayson 1981, Colver *et al.* 1982) found that advice given by health visitors led to families installing safety equipment at home. Thus, the GP and health visitor have an important role in prevention of accidents and poisoning as part of child health surveillance, or opportunistically during a surgery consultation or home visit. The checklist in Table 4.4 is based on Sibert (1991).

Table 4.3 Some drug-induced symptoms

Coma	Alcohol (hypoglycaemia is a danger), barbiturates, tranquillizers and sedatives, phenytoin, diphenoxylate/atropine (Lomotil), antihistamines, co-proxamol (Distalgesic), severe aspirin overdose (causes over-breathing), tricyclics, lithium
Confusion, ataxia, excitement, or hallucination	Alcohol, tricyclics, anti-epileptics, antihistamines, phenothiazines, diphenoxylate/atropine, salbutamol, lithium, dexamphetamine, glue sniffing, LSD
Convulsions	Tricyclics, dexamphetamine, theophylline, alcohol, lithium, co-proxamol
Extra-pyramidal symptoms and/or dystonia (e.g. head retraction)	Tricyclics, phenothiazines including Stemetil, metoclopramide, antihistamines
Bradycardia, tachycardia, or cardiac arrhythmias	Digoxin, alcohol, salbutamol, dexamphetamine, tricyclics, theophylline, co-proxamol

FOREIGN BODIES

Children are liable to get small objects stuck in parts of their anatomy. The GP will be able to remove some of them in surgery without causing the child a lot of distress.

The nose

Unless the patient has pushed objects up both nostrils he will present with a unilateral nasal discharge which is often very offensive, smelling of blue cheese.

William was admitted to the ward from paediatric outpatients for investigation of an unusual odour. Diagnosis—presumed metabolic disorder. Sister pointed out that the odour was coming out of one nostril and a complete cure was achieved by removing the foreign body.

The discharge may have been going on for days or weeks before the child is seen. Very occasionally, the object can be manoeuvred out of the nose by applying pressure above it. An older child should be able to blow the nose while the opposite nostril is occluded. If these measures fail it may be possible to get

Table 4.4 Hints on preventing childhood accidents and poisoning

To prevent road traffic accidents
1. Encourage parents of children 8 years or less to take them to school
2. Encourage use of defined play areas for children
3. Encourage use of car safety seats for children
4. Encourage the use of bicycle safety helmets
5. Encourage parents to let their children attend bicycle riding instructions and to maintain bicycles adequately

To prevent domestic injury
1. Advise the use of stair guards to families with toddlers
2. Only use baby walkers when the child is closely watched
3. Check window and balcony design for child safety. Advise catches if necessary
4. Advise the use of safety glass

To prevent burns and scalds
1. Encourage use of smoke alarms
2. Encourage disposal of dangerous foam furniture
3. Discourage open fires—if they have to be used, use fireguards
4. Use coiled flex electric kettles
5. Emphasize dangers of hot liquids
6. Fit a cooker guard
7. Encourage safe use of fireworks
8. Set domestic water to a modest temperature

To prevent drowning
1. Advise parents of young children about the danger of baths, garden ponds and other open water
2. Teach children to swim
3. Fence, grid, or remove garden ponds and open water even if shallow
4. Supervise swimming in public pools
5. Fence private pools and drain them in winter
6. Use of life jackets for children in boats

To prevent accidental poisoning
1. Encourage use of child resistant containers by pharmacists (now standard)
2. Encourage storage of medicines and household products away from children

Adapted from Sibert (1991).

a bent ring probe along the septum and behind the object, but if there is any difficulty, or the child is young and frightened, he should be referred to an ENT surgeon.

The ear

Gentle syringing may remove the object in the older child. This should not be attempted if the whole meatus is blocked or the obstruction is of vegetable matter which could swell when soaked with water. Any difficult object should be removed under direct vision because of the risk of damaging the middle ear. It is said that insects in the ear can be drowned and washed out using olive oil, although we have never done so.

The larynx

A foreign body in the larynx is an emergency. The child may be blue and asphyxiating or have stridor and be coughing, spluttering, and choking. He should first be held with his head lower than his trunk and his back firmly slapped and then the lower chest squeezed suddenly. If this fails and the foreign body cannot be seen and removed with finger or forceps and the child is asphyxiating, the doctor should be prepared to stick a wide-bored needle through the cricothyroid membrane. More than one needle may be necessary.

Bronchi

Small children may inhale by choking on their food, or by playing games such as throwing peanuts (a particularly common offender) or coins in the air and catching them in the mouth. The child usually coughs, chokes, or gags at the time of inhalation. If there is not immediate significant airways obstruction the incident may be forgotten during a latent period of days or weeks, when only an occasional cough or slight wheeze is noted. Later the child may present with what is thought to be pneumonia, sometimes recurrent, or asthma, more marked in one lung than the other with obviously asymmetrical chest movement. Not all foreign bodies are visible on a standard chest X-ray, though the obstructed lobe will usually show up on an expiratory film or a lung scan. Treatment, and sometimes diagnosis, may require a bronchoscopy.

Stomach

Most objects will appear in the faeces without problem a few days after ingestion, but open safety-pins, hairpins, or needles (if they are still in the stomach as judged by an X-ray) may be better removed by prompt endoscopy, rather than allowing them the possible difficulty of negotiating the duodenum, although some surprising objects can do so. If stuck, perforation may occur, causing pain and vomiting, either at once or later. If the foreign body is considered innocent, the child's diet should remain normal, whilst waiting for the object to reappear. Laxatives are not given. Button batteries can be dangerous as they may contain potassium hydroxide (a strong alkali) and mercury, and referral may be wise in order to follow their progress through the gastro-intestinal tract by X-ray.

The eye

See chapter 15.

NOSE BLEEDS

The majority of nose bleeds can be stopped by sitting the child up and firmly pinching the nose for 10 or 15 minutes while he breathes through his mouth. If that does not work, packing the nose or cautery of a bleeding vessel may very occasionally be required. Recurrent nose bleeds are a common complaint and sometimes can be dealt with by cautery. Unnoticed bleeds are perhaps the commonest cause of haematemesis in later childhood and sometimes present as otherwise unexplained anaemia. Extremely rarely, nose bleeds may be the presenting sign of thrombocytopenia or other clotting disorders, or of hypertension, or renal failure, or of nasal telangiectasia as part of the syndrome of multiple telangiectasis when lesions may be seen elsewhere on the skin or mucous membranes.

Bibliography

Billmire, M. E. and Myers, P. A. (1985). Serious head injury in infants: accident or abuse? *Pediatrics,* **75**, 340–2.

Colver, A. F., Hutchinson, P. J., and Judson, E. C. (1982). Promoting children's home safety. *British Medical Journal of Clinical Research*, **285**, 1177–80.

Grayson, G. B. (1981). The identification of training objectives: what shall we tell the children? *Accident Analysis and Prevention*, **13**, 169–73.

Kemp, A. M., Mott, A. M., and Sibert, J. R. (1994). Accidents and child abuse in bathtub submersions. *Archives of Disease in Childhood*, **70**, 435–8.

Meadow, R. (1985). Management of Munchausen syndrome by proxy. *Archives of Disease in Childhood,* **60**, 385–93.

Mortality Statistics (1992). Review of the Registrar General on deaths by cause, sex and age in England and Wales, No. 19. HMSO, London.

Morton, R. J. and Phillips, B. M. (1992). *Accidents and emergencies in children*. Oxford University Press. (A particularly useful volume.)

Polnay, L. and Hull, D. (1993). *Community Paediatrics*. Churchill Livingstone, London.

Sibert, J. R. (1991). Accidents to children: the doctors role. Education or environmental change. *Archives of Disease in Childhood*, **66**, 890–93.

Vale, J. A., Meredith, T. J., and Proudfoot, A. T. (1986). Editorial. *British Medical Journal,* **293**, 1321.

Volans, G. N. and Byatt, C. M. (1986). Poisoning from domestic products. *Prescribers' Journal,* **26**, 87–97.

5 Psychosocial problems of childhood

The General Practitioner is a doctor who provides personal, primary and continuing medical care to individuals and families ... His diagnosis will be composed in physical, psychological and social terms. (Royal College of General Practitioners 1969)

Doctors always need to ask not only 'what is the matter with the patient?' but also 'why is this child being brought to me at this moment?' A rise in the frequency with which a parent brings the small child with upper respiratory tract infections is one indication of increased stress within the family. Not only do mothers in such circumstances have a lower threshold for consulting, but children living in stressed families are also more likely to develop minor infections. An out of hours call to see a minimally sick child who could well have been brought to the surgery during the day may be another indication of a stressed or disorganized family. Equally, the manner in which a child's physical problems are presented is an important indicator of family tensions. Perhaps one minor symptom after another is revealed to the GP, who is left with a feeling that, even if the consultation had gone on for another hour, the mother still would not have had the chance to express all her anxieties about the child. Conversely children are sometimes used as the key to open the door on a discussion of the mother's problems, leading to irritation in a GP who had planned for a short, snappy consultation. Sometimes the doctor only becomes aware of a fraught situation when he realizes that he has seen a young patient with minor symptoms six or eight times during the preceding year. In addition, frequent attending children are more likely to have emotional problems themselves.

There is another type of consultation, with young children, which should indicate that all is not well within the family: the 'chaotic consultation'—when the child or children start wrecking the surgery and the doctor is unable to get a clear idea of the problem from the mother. Has the child seemed ill or not? Is he vomiting or isn't he? Is he really off his food? A chaotic consultation may reflect a chaotic home life. If the doctor senses that there are emotional difficulties within the family, but does not know what they are or whether help is feasible, a discussion with the health visitor is useful, with a request for her to follow-up the family if she is not already doing so. However, health visitors will often be more aware of a family's situation than will the GP. Thus, when we discuss children with emotional difficulties it is with the knowledge that only a minority of psychosocial problems present to a doctor in a completely non-physical way.

Most families cope well with the problems and challenges of child rearing, but the doctor, especially in an inner city practice, daily facing the problems described in this chapter, can become disheartened and lose the enthusiasm to go on trying. Even if it is not possible to radically improve parenting, a lot can be achieved for these children by using the full resources of the welfare state and preventive child care services. Repeated minor and individually ineffective interventions, often to support the mother and make her feel cared for, rather than focusing directly on the child, may be cumulatively positive. Let us soldier on.

THE 'SNOWED-UNDER MUM'

Women from working-class backgrounds are more likely than middle-class women to respond to a life crisis by becoming clinically depressed (Brown 1978). Such women seem particularly vulnerable if they do not have supportive partners, if a parent died during their childhood, or if there are three or more young children in the family. At least one-quarter of women with small children suffer from symptoms which meet criteria for a diagnosis of depression. The GP may sense that this is happening to one of his families: the over-burdened mother who looks sad and appears likely to burst into tears or weeps in the surgery, or who shows lack of affect—perhaps effect would be a better word. There may be frequent consultations for relatively minor disorders, or an infant who fails to grow satisfactorily.

What can the GP do for these beyond giving them an opportunity to unburden? First, the receptionist is important in ensuring that the practice strategy for these families includes responsive and prompt access to the practice team. Secondly, GPs are often aware of the stress within families that may be the reason for frequent consultations. This knowledge may lead to an open discussion of, for example, lack of support from an alcoholic partner. Thirdly, if the family structure exists, he can sometimes help the mother get better support from her partner and other relatives, who may not realize how depressed she is. Fourthly, he can exploit the available professional network. Mother and toddler groups where mothers can drop in and share their experiences may be helpful. Doctors sometimes forget the stress of debt; the Citizen's Advice Bureau or Law Centre can advise on how to cope. Fifthly, it may be possible for teachers to reduce school pressures on a child if they know that the family is going through a particularly difficult period. Sixthly, if the problem is poverty or boredom at home, many mothers find it a relief to do part-time work, provided that satisfactory arrangements can be made for the care of the children. The whole family may benefit from the money and from the mother being able to get away from the home for a few hours at a time.

It is possible to overlook organic problems in the context of psychosocial pathology—not all cases of headache and vomiting, or urinary frequency are due to 'nerves'. Follow-up consultations for acute illnesses are advisable for sick children from these families. An over-burdened parent may not be a reliable observer or reporter of deterioration in her child's condition. Finally, the GP can avoid starting all but the most severely depressed mother on psychotropic drugs—as one patient aptly put it, 'brushing the dirt under the carpet'.

DOCTORS AND SOCIAL WORKERS

Like the media, doctors have an ambivalent attitude to social workers. On the one hand, they sometimes consider the social services pretty useless and resent their statutory position in child care, but on the other, they set impossible tasks and expect them to be carried out immediately.

The personalities of social workers and their jargon tend to clash with the attitudes of GPs, who are used to seeing large numbers of patients and making quick decisions on often inadequate information after a brief consultation. The views of one of the authors changed when he realized that he was in fact referring to social workers just those families whose psychosocial problems he personally found most difficult to help. Mutual trust is essential for a successful relationship. For example, the GP must be able to rely on the social worker not to divulge to the patient confidential information given by the doctor.

Co-operation between the social services and other agencies involved with abusing or very disorganized families is usually planned at a case conference, but it is difficult to put together a reasonable package of overall management if one of the most important figures, the GP, is absent. On the other hand, it is reasonable for him to ask for a case conference to be held at a time and place convenient for him and for it to be kept short. The GP may be the 'key worker':

Diane was aged seven and had been born with a congenital heart defect. The father took most responsibility for the care of the child because the mother was an agoraphobic alcoholic with aggressive tendencies. At the case conference called to discuss whether a Care Order should be applied for, the GP was the only person present whom the mother allowed into the flat and who had regular contact with the child and the father. It was agreed that he would be the 'key worker' to monitor the situation and to recall the case conference if the situation worsened unexpectedly.

ILL-TREATED CHILDREN

The Children Act 1989 and child abuse

The spirit of the act is that the wishes and feelings of children must be taken into account, allowing for their maturity and understanding, and it embodies a number of important principles (Table 5.1).

An Emergency Protection Order (EPO) issued by a magistrate lasts for eight days and can be extended once. It enables the local authority to remove a child

Table 5.1 The Children Act 1989

1. The welfare of the child is paramount in all court proceedings. Courts are required to deal with children's cases as quickly as possible.
2. Wherever possible children should be cared for within their own families.
3. Children should be kept informed about what happens to them. Older children have a legal right to be heard and to participate in the decision-making process or to initiate actions against parents or teachers.
4. Children should be protected by effective intervention if they are in danger.
5. Parental responsibility is always retained by both parents except when the child is adopted.
6. Families with children in physical, social or emotional need should be provided with professional help appropriate to their ethnic group, culture and religion to enable them to remain as a family unit.

from home when it is deemed that welfare, health or future development will otherwise suffer. An EPO can be challenged by the parents after 72 hours. **A Child Assessment Order** which lasts seven days compels parents to allow access to the child so that an assessment of his health and development can be undertaken. The order allows removal of the child from home but it does not give the local authority parental responsibility. The child (but not the parents on his behalf) can refuse to undergo medical examination even when examination has been ordered by the court. Thus when a child is brought to a doctor because of suspicion of abuse, permission to examine must always be obtained from the child when he is judged to have sufficient understanding. The Act also permits participation of parents, and of children of sufficient maturity in child protection case conferences (see below). Where there is proof that a child is suffering ill-treatment (physical, sexual or emotional abuse) or is beyond parental control, the local authority may apply for longer term powers with a **Care** or a **Supervision Order**.

Physical abuse

Families at risk

The following circumstances indicate that the child may be at risk of rejection, neglect, or physical or emotional abuse.

1. The mother repeatedly presents evidence that she is not coping. There are numerous consultations about minor or non-existent problems, or she fails to attend for routine care, and refuses to allow access to the health visitor or the GP—the 'snowed-under mum', only more so.
2. The mother has an unrealistic expectation of her child; rather than supply love to him, she expects that the child will love and care for her.

3. The mother confesses to intensely angry and aggressive feelings beyond those which are a normal feature of family life. The GP unfortunately must also be alert to the parent who has no intention of hitting her child but who threatens to do so as a means of levering more support out of the services.
4. The family living under conditions of overwhelming stress, for example, serious debt (often money owed to a 'loan shark'), appalling housing conditions, serious family illness or poor self-esteem, for example, following compulsory redundancy.
5. The mother was ambivalent about the pregnancy and, perhaps, requested and was refused a termination.
6. The parent received violent or inadequate care during his or her own childhood.
7. A previous child presented with unexplained bruises or the mother has been seen with a black eye or multiple bruises.
8. History of repeated unexplained infant deaths in the same family.
9. The mother is so depressed post-natally that she cannot recognize the baby's needs.
10. The parents belong to the group of mothers and fathers who are so alcoholic, drug addicted, psychopathic, or psychotic as to be completely unpredictable.
11. Another member of the family expresses concern that the parents are being violent or neglectful.

In general, babies who have suffered long separation from their mothers through preterm birth, neonatal disorder, or maternal illness, are at more risk. So are those who are slow to develop, have a chronic illness, are 'hyperactive', cry excessively or are perceived to have characteristics reminiscent of a disliked or violent partner.

Before the doctor decides to intervene he must evaluate whether the family's behaviour is outside an acceptable range, as there are children in rough households with adequate affection in which various members are hit from time to time as a 'disciplinary measure'. Often easing poverty is the central issue for them. However, even in these families any visible bruising ascribed to discipline should be taken seriously; very seriously if the child is a baby. There are other ways than violence of injuring a child which may be more preventable. Gross lack of supervision is an example, and may be evident in the way the child is allowed to roam unsupervised in the corridor while the mother consults.

A two-year-old, walking alone, drowned by falling into a canal. Previously he had fallen from a third floor flat and survived, and on another occasion he had been returned home to the police after being found wandering along the road. His brother had also been previously admitted for several months following severe scalds to both feet.

Diagnosis

Obviously most children seen in general practice with bruises and injuries have not been ill-treated, but the following features lead to suspicion: The story given is either implausible, perhaps blaming a young sibling or a pet, or very vague, or there has been an inappropriate delay in seeking medical help. The parents may have used a pretext for coming and have not pointed out an actual injury, half-expecting the doctor to note it; for example, 'He won't stop crying', when the child has an obviously fractured arm. Sometimes there is a story of brief unconsciousness, leading to an incorrect 'epileptic' train of thought, the parent seeming to suppress memory of a blow that could have knocked the child out. The account of injuries may be inconsistent with the child's motor development; for example, a large boggy swelling on the side of the skull in a 6-week-old infant being attributed to rolling off a bed.

The child should be fully examined from head to toe and the height, weight and head circumference plotted on a centile chart, since non-organic failure to thrive (see p. 88) may be a feature of an abused or neglected child. The demeanour of toddlers should be noted. They may seem unduly wary of adults, or apathetic. The size, shape, position and ages of bruises (red or violet initially, then blue-brown, and later greenish-yellow—it is not possible to time these changes as precisely as was once thought) should be noted. It should however be remembered that toddlers and preschool children often sustain bruises over lower legs, extensor surfaces of forearms and sometimes on the forehead as a result of normal minor falls and accidents. Fingerprint bruising on the face (four marks on the left cheek, one on the right), slap marks on the face and buttocks, grip marks on the upper arm where a child has been shaken, are all characteristic. So are crescent-shaped bruises due to human bites. Symmetrical perineal scalds may be seen in a toddler whose bottom is immersed in hot water as punishment for lack of bowel control. Deep circular burns with indurated edges, especially on the hands or feet, should raise the possibility of cigarette burns. The mouth should be inspected for evidence for a torn frenulum between the gum and the upper lip caused by a blow to the upper lip or when a bottle has been jabbed into the mouth. In more severe cases there may bony tenderness due to fractures or retinal haemorrhages from violent shaking.

Mongolian blue spots, familial fragile bones, and bleeding disorders have occasionally led to a false diagnosis. Because of public attention there is much anxiety lest the diagnosis may be missed, but over-suspicion can also do harm and on some occasions grave injustice.

The Munchausen syndrome by proxy (MSBP)

The GP may become uneasy about a sequence of unexplained episodes of illness in a child and begin to wonder if they are induced by a parent. Characteristically the mother (or occasionally another carer) may have an unfulfilled life or a history of psychiatric or persistent physical disorder. She may work in health care and appear appropriately concerned and even over-helpful. The father usually takes a passive role. There is often a history of a wide range of obscure signs or symptoms described but not seen: fever, fits, unconsciousness, bleeding, or rashes, resulting in multiple diagnostic and treatment procedures. Sometimes there are bizarre fabricated signs or investigations witnessed by others, for example, haematuria caused by the mother adding menstrual fluid to the child's urine. There is apparent 'cure' of the illness when the child is not in the parent's or carer's presence. Long-term follow-up of a selected series of such children suggested that, whether fostered or left with their parents, the long-term outcome was poor in at least half (Bools *et al.*, 1993). At its mild end MSBP merges with exaggerated concern or over-emphasis of trivial physical symptoms, such as the naughty child who is kept on a special diet because of 'severe allergy'.

Management

The GP should be familiar with the local child protection protocols (obtainable from the social services department), which should provide essential information, such as the names and phone numbers of social work teams and paediatricians with interest in child protection. The decision of how to proceed depends on the situation. Clear cut physical injuries or violent sexual abuse need both medical and social services referral promptly. This will inevitably lead to early police involvement. With more doubtful situations, possibly involving factitious disease, a discussion on the telephone with a paediatrician with a special interest may help to share the burden. The fact that the injured child has been brought to the doctor may mean that the parent wants help and is likely to acquiesce in the course of the action advised, even if it has to be presented in a somewhat oblique way, for example, 'Mary must go to hospital so that we can find out why she bruises so easily'. When the GP decides to admit such a child he must brief the hospital at a sufficiently senior level. Irritating problems may arise when the carefully orchestrated removal of a child from home to hospital is frustrated because an inexperienced casualty officer thinks the injury is unimportant and the child is sent home. It may help if a member of the practice team accompanies the parent and child to hospital.

It is more difficult to decide what to do with the commoner marginal case. An example is a five-year-old (not a five-month-old—always a serious matter) child with a black eye who is known to have come from a stressed family, but in whom violence has not been a previous issue. It is easier to avoid over-reacting if the GP and the health visitor can be honest with the parents about concern regarding future possible injury or neglect. Such honesty is easier if there has previously been a good relationship between parent and doctor. Good care for these families means being accessible and uncensorious in the face of often chaotic, demanding, and perhaps aggressive behaviour. Co-operation with other agencies, however uncomfortable, has to work well. If the injury is repeated, clearly it is necessary to involve social services.

Child abuse is a danger area for professional reputation. It is crucial for his own protection that the doctor keeps especially detailed notes. Communications with other agencies should be recorded, if verbal, and perhaps followed-up by letter. The GP has no more legal standing in a case of child abuse concerning one of his patients than any other citizen. The decision that a child should or should not remain at home rests with the courts, but if the child remains with the family the GP and health visitor may be involved in close monitoring of the situation.

A Child Protection Case Conference is convened by social services or NSPCC, ideally within eight working days of agreement to do so, to develop a management plan for the child and the family. The participation of parents and mature children permitted by statute can have an inhibiting effect on some professionals. A well prepared and efficiently chaired meeting can at least lead to improved co-operation between professionals and, by sharing responsibility, give them individually some protection from future criticism. However, conferences often last too long, occur at difficult times for the GP, and may lead to action being postponed 'until after the next case conference'. Several decisions must be reached at the case conference:

1. Is the child going to be registered as 'at risk?
2. Is the future management plan clear to everybody and are their individual roles agreed?
3. Who is to be the key worker responsible for monitoring the child's progress?
4. When is the situation to be re-assessed?

Disaster may occur in even the most closely supervised families.

The GP was called to see Luke on the boy's second birthday. He was lying face downwards dead in his cot. An autopsy revealed that he had been suffocated and the mother was later convicted. Luke had been admitted to hospital on several occasions with minor scalds and bruising and case conferences had been held. Subsequently the family had been visited by a health visitor and a social worker at frequent and regular intervals, and his mother had most weeks brought him faithfully to the baby clinic.

In view of experiences like this it is understandable that doctors who have seen a child neglected or ill-treated feel frustrated when the child is not compulsorily taken into care. Whereas there is evidence that children from very disorganized homes do better in terms of educational achievement and psychiatric adjustment in the medium term when taken into care, care proceedings have two great drawbacks. First, the mother will often quickly become pregnant again and be even harder to work with as a result of a previous care order. Secondly, it is clear that many teenagers who have been in care may still have great difficulty in integrating themselves into ordinary adulthood.

Terry was adopted into a middle-class family in early childhood. As a teenager he broke with his adoptive family and eventually settled with Annette. They had four children. One died of cot death, one was underweight and relatively neglected, one nearly died of gastroenteritis. Nevertheless, after intensive social work, they have gradually improved as parents; the surviving children are doing fairly well in a day nursery.

Child sexual abuse

Some sexual component is a normal part of all close human relationships and that between adult and child is no exception. The problem, however, is to define what is normal or abnormal, acceptable or unacceptable. Unfortunately there is little sound epidemiology in this area (Jones and Thomson 1991) and there are many dogmatic beliefs. There is a danger that current publicity surrounding the topic may make it more difficult for the GP or health visitor to make an objective assessment of the child with symptoms which may or may not be associated with sexual abuse.

In one study the prevalence of child sexual abuse in Great Britain was 93 per 1000 and of incestuous abuse 13 per 1000 (Baker and Duncan 1985). Girls appear to be more commonly involved than boys. Of 56 children referred to a clinic in London with this label, two-thirds were under ten and one-quarter under five (Furniss *et al*. 1984). In only one case was the sexual abuse by a stranger, and in 50 cases a relative—usually a father or step-father—was responsible. Hobbs and Wynne (1987) found that in 75 per cent of cases perpetrators were related by blood or family role and 25 per cent were teenagers.

Child sexual abuse may come to the attention of the GP or a member of the primary care team as a result of a disclosure from the child or member of the family, or through non-specific medical or behavioural presentations. It is not difficult to think of the possibility of sexual abuse when a child presents with genital problems, such as injury, blood-stained underwear, or a discharge which may be blood-stained. It is more likely to be forgotten when there has only been a change in behaviour, such as recent onset of school failure, an alteration in mood, or running away from home. A probable psychosomatic symptom, such as genital or rectal itching, or soreness, wetting, frequency, soiling, or recurrent abdominal pain may be the only manifestation of the problem. Sometimes the child is inappropriately sexually provocative or makes his or her dolls play in an overly sexual way.

If the child is brought to the GP with a definite allegation of recent child sexual abuse involving actual or attempted intercourse, the GP should not feel obliged to examine the genitalia, especially if the child is reluctant. It is usually better left.

In any case, for both forensic and diagnostic purposes, a detailed physical examination will have to be performed by an experienced doctor who will take the appropriate specimens; either a female police surgeon or a paediatrician (depending on local circumstances). Repeated examinations are undesirable. If the episode is recent, parents should put any items of underwear in a plastic bag and the child should not be washed until the specimens have been taken. If sexual abuse is a possible but unlikely cause of symptoms, then a brief examination of the genitalia may be appropriate. For example, vulvitis and discharge may be caused by a visible piece of toilet paper stuck at the vaginal orifice. Social services will need to be involved at an early stage if the diagnosis is a significant possibility. There is also abuse without attempted intercourse—the child being expected to witness, or participate in, masturbation or fellatio, for example.

More frequently, the doctor is faced with the decision of whether and how to raise the topic with a mother or child coming with an indirect presentation. There are various ways: 'Are you worried that anyone could have interfered with her?' or, more cautiously, 'In a small number of cases this sort of soreness is cased by sexual interference ...'. Many doctors will find it easier to discuss sexual matters with young children if the possibility of sexual abuse has already been brought into the open during the consultation. 'I know a girl who got sore because someone played with her private parts', 'Has anyone been playing with your bottom?' It is helpful to ask the mother what are the words they use for genitalia and bodily functions. If the child starts to describe the situation the doctor needs to make enough time to follow the situation through: 'Did he take his clothes off? What happened next? Did it hurt?' Again, detailed notes are essential. It is much better if the situation can be handled in the presence of a colleague, preferably female. Alternatively, with a young child, it may be more appropriate to discuss the suspicion with the health visitor who can make a more leisurely assessment. This is especially true if the doctor is male and the child female. A more direct, unembarrassed approach is needed with adolescents.

SOME COMMON PROBLEMS

Colic

Many babies have a regular fussing period, often in the evening, during which they are only kept reasonably content by constant nursing. If the infant has paroxysms of screaming, associated with loud intestinal gurglings and accompanied by drawing up the legs, he is diagnosed by the family as suffering from 'colic', a purely speculative aetiology for a rather clear-cut clinical syndrome which usually resolves by three to four months of age. Many causes have been suggested, including cows' milk allergy, either directly, or via cows' milk drunk by a breast-feeding mother. Excessive parental tenseness is considered by some to be important. Certainly the baby will sometimes settle gratifyingly when cuddled by the doctor who has been called out late at night because of incessant crying.

It is probably a problem which has many causes. If the pattern is not regular, or if it is of recent onset, or if the baby is unwell, other more serious diagnoses must be considered. These include meningitis, otitis media, urinary tract infections or injury. In rare instances, manipulating the mother's diet or changing the baby's milk may help. Colic can be a very tedious and demoralizing problem and, like constant sleeplessness, may very occasionally justify a short admission, especially if there is a possible risk of parental violence.

Sleeping problems

Is the child having enough sleep? The time to judge is not at night but in the day. If he is physically active, emotionally alert and able to meet the stresses of the day, he is getting enough sleep—whatever the parent's book may say. Video studies show that many young children wake during the night without seeking attention. In about one-fifth of families, waking becomes a bothersome problem. Parents may ask if it is due to disease; occasionally it is. The night cough of asthma, or painful otitis media may wake children. Very much more commonly there is no physical disorder. Regular broken nights week in, week out, can be immensely destructive to family life, especially if the parents have other pressures, such as unusual working hours. The issue should not be treated too lightly, hence the length of this section.

It is a useful general principle not to make waking up at night too pleasant for the child: an approach which can be helped by not bringing him too quickly into the living room or parents' bedroom when he wakes. One paediatrician recommends the parent to get up and make a cup of tea when the child starts to cry; it is less daunting to listen to crying when one is out of bed, and sleep may have returned by the time the tea is ready. Various other measures besides a sympathetic medical ear may help in the intractable case, although many waking toddlers will continue their pattern for several years. The most useful approach is to take the time to run in detail over the child's bed-time and night-time routines, as simple changes may on occasion lead to a major improvement. It is a great advantage if a sleepless child does not have to share his room with a sibling, otherwise the problem may escalate. The times to consider are the evening, the night, and the morning.

Difficulty in going to sleep

The number of hours a child needs to sleep depends on his age, his personality, and also, to some extent, on the amount of time he snoozes during the day. More placid infants tend to sleep more than lively, active ones, which may be some consolation to exhausted parents. A toddler may need to be roused from an afternoon nap so that he sleeps better in the evening. At any age, a child will not take kindly to being whisked away from the hub of the family and unceremoniously dumped into bed. The period of undressing and washing should be made a pleasant routine and even after he has been put into his cot or bed, parents may need to potter around nearby while he is drifting off to sleep. Sometimes the child will go through a repetitive routine—cuddling an object, rocking repeatedly, or thumb sucking. Many 6- to 12-month-old infants cry for a minute or two when put into bed but this usually stops quickly and the mother can leave the bedroom as planned. If she needs to return she should, if possible, try to comfort by voice alone. Children will usually go off to sleep while normal household noises continue; it makes a rod for the parents' own back if they introduce an artificial level of quietness.

The child who awakens during the night

It is not usually helpful to tell the mother to let the young child cry in the hope that, after four or five nights of prolonged screaming, the habit will be broken. It may not succeed, is rather cruel, and is not a workable solution if the family shares part of a house with other tenants. Unfortunately, many young children awaken at night for no obvious reason. They cry until a parent comes. In these cases, the rule should be to do the minimum that allows the child to go off to sleep again; if possible, a brief appearance in the child's bedroom, the minimum of handling, and a rapid exit once the child has stopped crying. Do not take him out of his room or the cot if it can be avoided. As part of the general strategy of attention to detail, the GP should search with the parents for any preventable cause of night waking. An infant may be uncomfortable because he is wet, dirty, cold, or hot. He may be disturbed because of some recent family upheaval or some change in normal routine. Some children get hungry or thirsty during the night and need to eat or drink at bedtime. Sometimes a bottle beside the cot will be a help. Some toddlers go through a period of awakening at night after a nightmare and deserve comforting, as do older children.

Night terrors are rare but quite alarming. By the time the parent comes into the bedroom the child is sitting up with open eyes, only half-awake but terrified, although the episode is forgotten by the morning. It may take a quarter-of-an-hour for him to settle down again and the parent may need to be reassured that the child has not had a fit. Night terrors, though sometimes precipitated by stress, are not usually associated with an emotional disorder. They occur more frequently in boys.

Sometimes a waking problem can be solved by not giving the child what he wants:

Peter was a two-year-old who insisted on his mother's presence twice a night between midnight and 5 a.m. His father was not acceptable, so for a few nights his dad went when he called. After a week of 'Mummy, mummy, only mummy', he stopped calling his parents at night.

Some children aged over three years can be induced to stop disturbing their parents with remarkably small bribes. In fact, judging from occasional successes in our own families, the minor bribe appears to be an under-employed tool in child rearing. The behaviour therapists would have us believe, and it seems correctly, that small, quick prizes are more effective than hopes of future bliss; pennies rather than bicycles.

Early-morning waking

If the early-waking child merely plays with his toys and sings happily, he should be left alone. Leaving a box of toys by the side of the cot that he can unpack and play with in the morning, and perhaps a drink and biscuit, can help. If he insists on coming to his parents' bedroom before they want him, one of them should promptly take him back to his own room; hopefully he will stay there.

In some cases very brief psychotherapeutic intervention for the parents of sleepless infants can be very helpful.

Defeat

Complete failure is not an uncommon problem in the management of the sleepless child. The promise of an occasional unbroken sleep may protect the family's sanity. Perhaps a relative can have the child for a night. Alternatively, the very intermittent use of a sedative, probably for not more than two or three nights in a row, may be considered, for example, trimeprazine tartrate (Vallergan) oral suspension 2 mg/kg, 30 minutes before bed-time, the dose to be increased to 4 mg/kg on subsequent occasions if the smaller dose is ineffective. It has been shown to work in a double blind trial when used in the, in our view, rather high dose of 6 mg/kg, but no significant toxicity was observed. There was no continued benefit after the drug was discontinued, but both treatment and control groups slept better by the end of the study (Simonoff and Stores 1987). When a family are at their wits end, sleeplessness may even justify a brief hospital admission.

Finally, rigid rules are wrong. Some families can cope only if the child sleeps in or beside the parents' bed for a year or two. In other families late evenings or early mornings shared with the child are accepted or even enjoyed. If the family are happy with an eccentric sleeping pattern there is no need for the doctor or health visitor to interfere.

The child who refuses to go to school

School refusal must be differentiated from truancy, which is the wilful avoidance of school, usually by disaffected teenagers who resent having to remain at school until they are 16 years old with no jobs to go to afterwards. The prognosis for future schooling of these children is bleak. Their parents may acquiesce, especially if there is the old-fashioned habit of keeping the child at home as a baby-sitter or drudge. There are large school-to-school variations in the rates of truancy. If illness is used as an alibi for truancy, management requires co-operation between the education welfare officer, the school, social services, and the GP.

True school refusal is:

1. Often claimed by parents to be really due to organic disease—a point of view colluded with, on occasion, by the GP, perhaps because of the intense way the child presents his symptoms.

2. A relative emergency; refusal once allowed to become a routine is rather difficult to overcome.

3. More often caused by stress within the home than at school.

The somatic disguise often means that the family doctor only becomes aware of the cause of the symptoms when he realizes how often the child has been absent from school. The key question is 'How many days off school has he had in the last term?'

Refusal often presents when the child starts school or soon afterwards, associated with anxiety about separation from the family, or later, when there is a move to secondary school, or at around 15 years. However, the problem may begin at any time with reluctance to attend school accompanied by symptoms of anxiety and panic when the time to go to school approaches. Somatic disguises include various aches and pains, feeling sick, lethargy, and low spirits, with perhaps diarrhoea and a variety of odd sensations. The symptoms may be most marked when the child has to go to school again after a week-end break, but sometimes a temporal association is not apparent. Diagnoses such as glandular fever, arthritis, ME, or 'severe' allergy are often considered. Quite often the problem is indeed triggered off by an intercurrent illness which has been allowed to dominate the management long after school refusal has become the real diagnosis.

While, in some children, the main anxiety is about what may happen at home when they are not there to look after their drunken or quarrelsome father, or their depressed or oppressed mother, in other children stresses at school are important, particularly when there are also underlying intrafamily problems. For this reason contact should be made with the school. Is bullying real as opposed to imaginary? Does the class teacher find this child difficult (the reciprocal of the child finding the teacher aggressive, and more easily asked of the head)? Is poor progress in class leading to despondency?

The cause at home of the child's symptoms may not be obvious:

Mary was a timid, thin girl of 13 who had already changed her secondary school once because of unhappiness. She still spent a considerable amount of time at home because of vague tummy and headaches. Three years later, her sister told the GP that the mother had a covert boy-friend and had been drinking heavily for several years.

The main goals of treatment are to get the child back to regular attendance at school and to identify and sort out any underlying problems. It will often be difficult for the GP to get parents to accept that their child's somatic symptoms are not due to physical disease, and sometimes a reassuring consultation with a well-briefed paediatrician may give the GP confidence to be firm about the child returning to school. Any plan of action is more likely to be successful if the doctor has the co-operation of both the head teacher, the parents and the school welfare officer.

If a young child's anxieties about leaving home are so severe that he refuses to go to school, it may be possible to make the situation more secure for him, both by discussing the underlying problems with him and with his parents, and by instituting practical measures that make the situation less stressful. A regular, reliable routine is important in reducing anxiety. Even a stoical child will be upset if he cannot rely on a parent's promise to be at the school gate in time to collect him at the end of the day. A child of eight or nine who has already started going to school and returning by himself can again be taken and fetched by a parent. It may be possible for him to come home or to telephone home at lunchtime. It helps if there is somebody at home during school hours so that the child can make contact if he feels anxious. He probably will not do this after he has checked once or twice that there is really someone there. Finally, early referral for psychiatric help will be necessary if the child does not quickly return to school.

Constipation

Parents are often worried if their baby passes small hard motions or goes for a few days without opening his bowels at all. Many healthy infants have periods of infrequent bowel action and if a breast-fed baby is changed to the bottle the stools become firmer and more formed. Some breast-fed babies may go several days without a motion. The mother of a 'constipated', well-nourished, healthy child who is gaining weight satisfactorily can be told to ignore the fact that the baby is only opening his bowels every two or three days. There are strong family belief systems about defecation, so it may be useful to ask the mother first what 'bowel troubles' she or other family members have, what damage she feels constipation is doing to the baby, and how she is managing the situation. A lot of interesting information may be obtained about her bowel anxieties and she, or the grandmother, may confess to attempting manual removal of faeces, a very rarely justified procedure. A glycerine suppository is more appropriate if the baby is in real pain during defecation, but this is unusual.

If the baby merely appears unduly uncomfortable at stool, increasing the amount of fluid drunk and making sure the feed has not been made up over-concentrated may be all that is needed. Traditionally, putting brown sugar in the feed is thought to help. In the weaning period prune juice can be helpful, as may increasing the amount of fibre.

An anal fissure may make a baby reluctant to pass a motion. Very rare causes of true constipation in the baby include hypercalcaemia, hypothyroidism, or Hirschsprung's disease. In the latter, chronic constipation may alternate with diarrhoea. Its hallmark is gross abdominal distension; the rectum is usually empty of faeces on examination but removing the finger may be followed by an explosive gush of faecal material and abdominal decompression. There may be a history of delayed neonatal passage of meconium or a positive family history.

Encopresis

The vast majority of children are 'clean' by the age of three years but 2.3 per cent of boys and 1.6 per cent of girls still soil themselves at eight years of age (Bellman 1986). Dirty pants are not always a sign of serious emotional upset. For example, temporary soiling may occur in younger children as part of the regressive behaviour seen when a sibling is born. Some children from a chaotic, socially deprived background, or without proper toilet facilities, may always have dirty underpants. In these children the soiling is a relatively minor part of the whole picture.

More significant is the typical encopretic child, perhaps brought because of teasing at school, who has overflow incontinence and liquid stools seeping round hard faeces in the rectum. The child refuses or fails to open his bowels and accumulated masses of faeces are palpable per abdomen. They are passed every few weeks as enormous tree trunks which may block the toilet. Soiling and the abdominal masses may then disappear for a week or so before the whole cycle is repeated. There may be a history of difficult confrontational toilet training or of pain on defecation before the process started. A sore, soiled, sticky anus may contribute to the child's continuing reluctance to go to the lavatory.

There are many management approaches; one is described in detail by Clayden (1992). Ours is based on the proposition that if the rectum is kept empty, the child will be clean. That in itself will act as positive reinforcement. There is no point on embarking on a treatment programme unless the child is willing to co-operate. As with enuresis, a system of rewards based on realistic achievement and of frequent contact early in the treatment process, together with attention to detail, are keys to success. The practice nurse or health visitor can become usefully involved. There are many different ways to keep the rectum empty. Usually even with gross faecal impaction oral laxatives (for example, bisacodyl 5 mg increasing to 10 mg nightly, if necessary, and later reducing to twice weekly) will gradually clear the masses. It will do this more effectively if they have first been softened with a few days of lactulose. A microlax enema may be helpful early on. A good bowel motion at least every 48 hours is needed to keep the child from soiling and is a useful target. Having got clean with the help of laxatives, the problem is to wean the child off them. This should not be attempted too soon. At this stage, plenty of fluids, a high-residue diet (bran in a form palatable to the child, such as cereal, biscuits, bread—perhaps chosen by him as having high fibre content by studying supermarket labels) prunes or raisins, plenty of time to go to the lavatory in the morning (perhaps with his Walkman), and making sure that access to toilets at school is available to the child and that he always carries lavatory paper, are all helpful. For some children, instruction on how to strain effectively helps as they may appear never to have really learnt how to push down on the perineum. The rewards should centre round the regular use of the toilet and the successful bowel motion, not on avoiding soiling; that will follow.

If therapeutic success is not achieved after a few months of frequent consultations for moral support in a child without obvious psychopathology, it may be worth considering referral to a child psychiatrist. Co-operation in management needs to be close as Nolan *et al.* (1991) reported that in a randomized trial of a laxative and behaviour modification programme (very similar to that we recommend) half the children were in remission at the end of one year compared to a third of those treated with behaviour modification alone.

Children who pass normal stools in abnormal places—classically the best settee—are an altogether different problem. In these, who are to be distinguished from ordinary soilers who hide dirty pants from their parents, the management requires early psychiatric help. The same applies to the ordinary encopretic in whom there is other evidence of disturbance, or in whom gross soiling is occurring without any real evidence of constipation.

Soiling is also a problem in a few children with organic disease. These include those with minor spina bifida, whose sphincter is abnormally patulous on inspection, some unfortunate children with ulcerative colitis, and, of course, the severely mentally retarded. Constipation associated with poor growth may rarely be a sign of hypothyroidism. More difficult is the very rare late presentation of Hirschsprung's disease. If the features of this disease mentioned above are present, particularly marked abdominal distension, referral to a paediatric surgeon for the definitive exclusion of very short-segment Hirschsprung's disease may be wise.

SOCIAL AND EMOTIONAL DEVELOPMENT

GPs are often consulted by parents concerned about some aspect of the behaviour of their young child. They may not be able to judge whether this is appropriate to the child's age or not unless they are aware of the normal social and emotional development of young children.

Even in the first few weeks of life, there is quite a complicated interaction between the baby and his mother, in which the infant takes an active role. He usually smiles first in response when he is about six weeks old, and long before that fixes his gaze briefly on her face when talked to. At about three months he is beginning to react to familiar faces by smiles, coos, excited movements and contented noises. A baby under the age of about six months shows little fear of strange people and places, and will respond in a similar, usually friendly, way both to his family and to people he does not know well.

By six months he will usually be more friendly and more at ease with a person he is close to. After this age, the infant will show that he is attached to a specific person—the one who gives him most loving and constant attention—usually, of course, his mother. This attachment will show itself in various ways. The infant responds to the mother in a relaxed, happy manner; he becomes anxious when she goes out of sight and he clings to her when he feels frightened. A toddler likes to be within sight or hearing of a familiar adult. In the long-term, if the favourite person is absent, most infants will get attached in a similar way to someone else.

After infancy, children need to develop relationships which persist even when the person concerned is absent. As the child matures, he behaves in a more secure manner, being less likely to cling to an adult and finding it easier to move away and explore strange surroundings. Nevertheless, in the second year he will still rush back quickly to his mother if he feels frightened or upset. Children raised in an institution are less likely to form secure 'bonds' and may show immature clinging and following behaviour beyond an age at which it is appropriate. Paradoxically, they may also appear pathologically friendly to strangers such as nurses or doctors. They may be very popular patients on children's wards.

Most three-year-old children can feed themselves and do most of their own dressing and undressing. They can take themselves to the toilet, provided somebody helps to wipe their bottom. They get satisfaction from having achieved control over their sphincters. A parent should allow them to help look after themselves, even though the processes take a long time. Negativism is a characteristic feature of the normal 18-month to 3-year-old child when they try to assert themselves and behave in a non-conforming manner, but they also want to please their parents and become anxious if they do not do so. At this age children live in an egocentric world and have little notion about sharing toys or adult attention. Conflicts between their wishes, which are often quite unrealistic, and those of their parents lead to tantrums—usually, but not always, in the child! Communication between the parent and child improves with the development of speech, helping the resolution of the innumerable conflicts. Tantrums lessen over the preschool years. As the two-year-old matures, he becomes aware of the differences between the sexes and more interested in sexual exploration. Masturbation is a common normal phenomenon in these preschool years.

The process of identification with the parents and their ideals and standards is thought to lead to the development of a conscience in the child, enabling him to decide what is right and what is wrong, what is considered good and what bad behaviour. Conscience is thus unlikely to be well developed in children from unstable, unloving homes, or institutions in which satisfactory parents with whom they can identify are absent. Similarly, children who are deprived of love in their early years may not be able to give or receive love later on in life. It is difficult for the clinician to assess the truth of this, but it certainly appears to make sense. For example, many parents who abuse their children appear to have either been in care or have been abused themselves in the past. The style of parenting, good or bad, loving or unloving, tends to recur again and again 'even unto the third and fourth generation'.

EMOTIONAL AND BEHAVIOURAL PROBLEMS

Emotional and behavioural disturbances in children are extreme or persistent examples of behavioural traits which are present in nearly all children at some stage of their development. The commonest are classified as disorders either of conduct or of emotions.

Conduct disorders

Most children occasionally take something belonging to their parents or another child, or occasionally truant for part of a day, but a child with a conduct disorder shows persistent antisocial or aggressive behaviour which does not respond to firm and confident handling. This behaviour takes various forms. Examples are the completely egocentric child who has no concept of the needs and feelings of others, the youngster who shows impulsive and reckless behaviour, and the young teenager who persistently truants without parental collusion and who may also lie, steal, damage public property, or abuse drugs. Delinquent behaviour in older children is likely to come to the attention of the GP because pressure from school, police, or other adults pushes the parents into action (Chapter 7). Sometimes such behaviour is normal for the family milieu in which the child is brought up.

Persistent aggressive behaviour, and conduct disorders plus hyperactivity and repeated truancy, especially from primary school, appear to have a particularly poor long-term prognosis. Conduct disorders are more frequent in boys than in girls.

Emotional disorders

An emotional disorder may be seen as a 'medical' problem because of physical symptoms of panic, nausea, diarrhoea, headache, or frequency of micturition. It is appropriate to feel tense in stressful situations, but abnormal tension is felt by some children who, like some adults, seem to have a high level of anxiety which becomes attached to any problem they come up against. Such children may have difficulty getting off to sleep and worry excessively about minor hurdles such as class tests. Anxious children may also be depressed, with inability to concentrate, a moany approach to life, and a lack of interest, often in association with severe school or family problems. Some are quite unable to get on with their peers.

A preschool child will often have irrational fears of the dark, or of certain animals, and this again can be described as abnormal if it is very persistent or interferes with the older child's ability to enjoy life. Alternatively, children who have persistent intrusive thoughts, often with prolonged and complicated rituals which must be gone through before they feel comfortable, are described as being obsessive or compulsive. Often the symptoms are not sufficiently bothersome to require intervention.

Harry, aged eight, always insisted that his parents straightened the bedside rug, put a half-full glass of water next to him, closed the curtains completely and folded back the bed cover before he felt comfortable enough to try, often with difficulty, to go to sleep.

A child may, under stress, lapse into behaviour that is more appropriate to an early developmental stage, such as obsessive clinging to a parent or bed-wetting. These may damage the child's self-esteem and make poor performance at school more likely.

Risk factors

Why do some children succumb to psychiatric disorders while others, in apparently similar circumstances, surmount their difficulties? The risk factors and those that apparently protect the child are neatly catalogued by John Pearce (1993) (Table 5.2).

Severe emotional disturbance is more likely to develop in children from homes where relationships are unsatisfactory for one reason or another, or where the mother is mentally ill. It should not be assumed that every difficult or unhappy child is a symptom of a family under stress. Sometimes the disturbance in the family, as well as in the child, is due to there being something physically wrong

Table 5.2 Development of psychiatric disorder

More likely	Less likely
Disrupted upbringing	Stable supportive background
Low IQ—as high as 40% risk with severe learning difficulties	High academic achievement
Specific developmental delay	
Communication difficulty	
Academic failure	
Low self-esteem	Positive self-image
Difficult temperament	Stable personality
Physical illness: 20% + risk with epilepsy; Slight increased risk with most other illnesses	

Adapted from Pearce (1993).

with him, or to his having a more specific psychiatric diagnosis. Short-sightedness, moderate deafness, and under-treated asthma can of themselves contribute to behaviour problems (Weindling *et al.* 1986). The child may be taking illicit drugs, sniffing glue, or drinking alcohol. Mild autism, with odd repetitive behaviour patterns and poor person-to-person contact, can be the true diagnosis. In general, the more odd the child in relation to the family's normal behaviour, the more indication for specialist referral. In terms of long-term prognosis, children with neurotic anxieties or phobias do better than those with conduct disorders coming from unstable or unloving backgrounds.

Child psychiatric referrals

The practice team of one of the authors includes a child psychotherapist who sees children with problems that have not got to a stage at which formal psychiatric referral would be considered. She attends the weekly child health clinic, spending part of her time standing by the weighing scales ready to chat to mothers and staff. Half the families she sees are referred by the health visitors. Many problems of parent–child interaction first surface at this time, which may be the most promising moment for intervention. This type of specialist help, kept within the practice, seems to be acceptable to many families who would not agree to an out-patient appointment.

It may be difficult to decide how seriously disturbed a child is, taking into account their stage of development and cultural background. As previously mentioned, many normal children have transient problems such as fears, nightmares, wetting, tics, or tummy aches, which should only be regarded as needing specialist treatment if they are severe and persistent, or are associated with other problems. Is the child functioning well or badly in the main areas of social life? Is he clingy or over-aloof? Over-shy or over-aggressive? Is he progressing at school? The disturbance may only be evident at times; he may be quiet and obedient at school and aggressive and disobedient at home, or vice versa. It is thus frequently important to seek information from school as well as from the parents and child before a decision whether to refer or not is made. There are some symptoms which are particularly worrying and demand urgent assessment. These include:

(1) persistent destructiveness;

(2) aggression leading to injury of others or themselves;

(3) age-inappropriate sexual behaviour;

(4) persistent withdrawal;

(5) bizarre psychotic behaviour;

(6) arson.

(Adapted from Pearce (1993))

Referral of children for psychiatric help is a difficult area for many reasons, and the initiative often seems to peter out before treatment is started or after one or two sessions. The parents may be antagonistic to the idea that their child, or indeed the whole family, might need psychiatric treatment. They may be too unstable to follow a regular regime of treatment. Some will be angry and impatient that no quicker solution to the child's problems has been offered.

Frequently, the GP has to feel his way slowly before suggesting that psychiatric help is needed. This may take months or even years. Ideally, he should wait until the suggested referral comes or almost comes from the parents. This usually happens either because the family is unable to cope with the child's disturbance or because society pressurizes the family, as when the teacher suggests a referral. Sometimes, however, it is the GP's responsibility to point out to parents that specialized treatment is indicated, even though they themselves have not realized this. On occasions, it can be valuable to refer the child prophylactically for therapy or counselling, for example, when the family is rocked by bereavement or breakdown of a marriage.

The ground for psychiatric referral must be carefully prepared. This means taking time to discuss with the family what a referral entails: that there will be a period of assessment, often over several interviews, often by members of a multidisciplinary team containing, in addition to doctors, educational and clinical psychologists, various forms of therapist and sometimes social workers, followed perhaps by regular treatment sessions which may go on for a year, or more. As much of the family as possible will be involved in the assessment and further information may be required from the school. Failure to prepare the ground properly may lead to a waste of everybody's time and energy; so will a service with a long waiting-list. The GP needs to bear all these factors in mind in negotiating with the family. An initial assessment in a child psychiatric outreach clinic in the practice may lead to a smoother more acceptable referral. The psychiatrist will also find the easy access to the primary care team an advantage.

There are several approaches to treatment. These include **psychodynamic therapy**, using talking and play techniques which aim to bring into the open conflicts, tensions, and anxieties that the child is not aware of, but which influence his behaviour. The hope is that by doing so, the emotional disorder becomes accessible to treatment. **Cognitive therapy** tries to encourage positive patterns of thought rather than ones which are dominated by the child's negative ruminations about a problem, and **behavioural therapy** aims at improving behaviour by concentrating on symptoms rather than their unconscious causes. It may be the behaviour of parents rather than the child that needs to be helped to change. Many therapists are prepared to be eclectic and select whatever treatment they consider appropriate. In any case, the personality and commitment of the therapist are often of greater importance than the particular type of treatment employed.

A family needs to be viewed as an entity rather than just the sum of its constituent parts. Members are interdependent—the behaviour of one affects the rest. GPs will instinctively agree with the increasingly accepted view that emotional disorders in young people are often the result of a dysfunctional family background. Treatment is more likely to be successful if the family as a whole is involved, with the aim of improving understanding, communication, and mutual caring. Sometimes a parent may have unrealistic expectations of how a child should behave, as with the depressed, apathetic mother who cannot tolerate the normal boisterousness of a three-year-old and describes him as 'hyperactive'. It may need to be explained to such parents that successful therapy for the child will often involve them in changed behaviour and that they, therefore, need to be involved in the enterprise directly. To accept a child for treatment as the sole patient is usually second best. However, family therapy may be difficult to sell to the parents unless carefully handled.

It is notoriously difficult to evaluate psychotherapy in randomized controlled trials. If therapy is fraught with uncertainty, what of prevention? There have been a number of programmes to train health visitors to work with young families to improve parenting skills and competence, in an attempt to reduce the amount of emotional disturbance. According to Cox (1993), the results are equivocal, partly because of bias in the selection of cases studied and a lack of control groups. Nevertheless, we have the impression that sometimes a well-timed word of praise or reassurance, or a comment putting another perspective on a problem, or supporting a half-formed idea for change in the mother's mind may lead to an altogether disproportionate long-term benefit—a very satisfying outcome from an eight-minute consultation.

Indications for in-patient treatment include a life-threatening disorder such as a severe depression, severe anorexia, florid psychotic illness, Munchausen by proxy, or investigation of a complicated set of symptoms, where the diagnosis is uncertain. For refuge during a family crisis, social rather than medical care is often more appropriate.

SEPARATION AND DEATH

Hospitalization of the young child

A week or two in hospital away from the family seems to do little long-term emotional damage to children from secure, loving backgrounds. It is the already disturbed child who is more at risk. On the other hand, there are many studies which document the severe short-term distress that any child may suffer on going into hospital, particularly if he is between the ages of six months and four years. This possible grief should be borne in mind when weighing up the decision whether to send the younger patient into hospital or not. Parents should also be warned that a child may show difficult behaviour when he comes home. At first he may seem to ignore or even reject them. After this he may be more difficult, demanding, and clinging. If they are forewarned they may be able to respond in a loving, rather than an angry way, and so help the child restore his equilibrium.

Paediatric wards are much happier places than they used to be. Most provide facilities for parents to stay the night. There are also books and videos describing life on a ward that can be shown to the child before a planned admission. A child can also be helped to cope with his stay in hospital if a parent can spend long periods of the day and, if possible, the night, with him, if he is allowed to bring in familiar toys, if other members of the family visit him regularly, and if the child is looked after by only a few of the numerous adults on the ward. Young children may regain their equilibrium more rapidly if they have already spent occasional nights away from home with friends and relatives.

Serious emotional difficulties are more likely to arise after recurrent admissions or, as mentioned above, in the child who is sent to hospital from an insecure background—just the sort of child who is likely to be sent into hospital for relatively trivial physical disease because of the disorder at home.

Divorce and separation

Marriage is becoming less popular and is being replaced by long-term relationships. About a third of all marriages are likely to end in divorce or separation, although re-marriage is commoner than it used to be, as is, unfortunately, a second divorce. Young couples in the early years of relationships are most likely to break up their relationship. As over half of broken relationships involve children, many under-fives are brought up by one inexperienced young parent, sometimes with the support of middle-aged grandparents. In other families there may be a series of living-in partners.

People often visit their family doctor with symptoms of stress or depression when their marriage (or long-standing relationship) begins to crumble. He is often in a good position to offer continuing support to a family going through this sort of crisis. If he realizes what is happening within the family, it may be helpful to concentrate not just on the adults but also to initiate a discussion of the effects of the disharmony on the children. Most children do not want their parents to separate even if there have been frequent preceding rows. They feel angry and upset, partly because they perceive their parents to be behaving in a selfish way, doing what *they* want to do rather than what the children would prefer. They may also feel responsible for their inability to avert the catastrophe, or even feel a sense of failure that they have not been successful mediators between the warring parents. If the relationship has irreconcilably broken down, parents need to discuss the situation openly with the children in a manner appropriate to the latters' understanding, and help them work through their inevitable feelings of insecurity and resentment.

Attempts are often made to use the doctor as supporting artillery by one or other of the couple, putting the GP with both parents on his list in an uncomfortable situation. Although impartiality is difficult to maintain in acrimonious break-ups, involved children are best helped if medical partisanship can be avoided and if, instead, the GP repeatedly emphasizes certain basic truths. First, in English law, children are not property or income. All parties, grandparents no less than parents, should be encouraged to follow the lead of the courts in aiming at what is best for the children, rather than what is fair to the partners. The court can direct a welfare officer, who is usually a probation officer, to try and resolve conflicts between the parents about the custody of the child. Marital 'fault', however serious, cannot be equated with parental unfitness and balanced off by placing the children with the other parent. Secondly, although custody is often granted to one parent or the other, rather than shared between both, regular and reliable access must be worked out at an early stage. Because of children's distress and bewilderment at this time, various problems with access may arise. The child may refuse to see an absent parent through resentment or through fear of offending the parent with whom he lives, or he may be difficult to handle after a visit. In these circumstances, regular letters or phone calls may help to bridge the gap, which should be as short as possible. The parent with custody should be strongly discouraged from building on a distorted situation of no access. It may help to remind them that, if the child does not come to accept recurrent contact with the absent parent early on, that parent may well be unrealistically overvalued later and the child may then reject the resident parent totally. Access should include regular weekly or more frequent visits, overnight stays, and holidays, ultimately including the parent's new girl- or boy-friend. However, the father (usually) may disappear from the scene, and occasionally, if one partner is aggressive or utterly unreliable, a complete break may have to be accepted. Sadly, it may need to be explained to the child that even if their parent's relationship should improve following the divorce, this does not mean that the couple will get together again. Marital therapy, in addition to helping a marriage *per se*, may also be of use if separation does nevertheless take place, as it often will. During therapy a climate of some mutual understanding and trust between the parents may develop—elements that are important for the children's continued positive emotional development.

Divorce profoundly affects a child's life. It may mean a new school and a smaller house when the proceeds of the marriage are divided. A lower income increases the likelihood of a mother working long hours. Adjustment to the parents' new partners, who may well have children of their own, may be difficult and slow. The long-term effects of divorce on children are uncertain, but may be less than in previous generations because our society is learning to adapt to this common occurrence. However, if there are symptoms of prolonged emotional disturbances in the children, such as delinquency, marked depression, deterioration of school performances, sexual promiscuity, or drug abuse, then referral for formal psychotherapy or counselling needs to be considered.

Death of a parent

It is difficult to separate the psychological impact on a child of the death of a parent from the associated practical consequences. The surviving parent will usually become withdrawn, depressed, and less able, for a time at least, to respond to his or her children's needs. The same may also apply following divorce or separation. The family may experience financial hardship or even break up, the children going to live with relatives or with friends. It is not surprising that there is an increase in later emotional disturbance, particularly severe depression, in people who have been bereaved in childhood. A sudden, unexpected death may have a more catastrophic effect than one that occurs at the end of a long-drawn-out illness. Poor parenting before or after the bereavement is probably an important contributory factor to later psychiatric morbidity (Bowlby 1980).

Children of five years of age or younger are probably able to understand that death is an irreversible process. They have, after all, seen dead flowers or animals, and have begun to witness second hand the death and destruction which are the hallmark of so much television. Many children at this age and older are able to mourn the loss of a parent in a way similar to that of the grieving adults. The younger the child the less able is he to sustain the mood of sadness for long periods. As children tend to live more in the present than grown-ups, there will appear to be periods of time when the child will seem to have forgotten his loss and be absorbed in the day's routine. However, at times he will be obviously depressed and sad, yearning for the lost parent. The grieving will be particularly intense when the child is feeling stressed for some reason or other, or when there is a new family crisis. Sometimes he will hope that the parent will become alive again and fantasize that this has happened as, indeed, do grieving adults. Sometimes he will feel guilty and, perhaps, responsible for the tragedy or angry with the dead parent for leaving, since the young child is unable to understand the lack of control that supposedly 'powerful' adults have over their fate. He may also be afraid that the remaining parent will die, becoming more clinging as a result and perhaps less able to express natural childhood aggression in case it damages the survivor. The child may also become afraid that he will suffer the same fate, becoming introspective and hypochondriacal as a result.

Jeremy, aged eight, had lost his mother four years previously. Whenever he felt even mildly unwell he used to go to his father saying 'Am I poorly, will I die?'

If it is known that the parent suffers from a fatal disease, it may be possible and beneficial to both the dying parent and the older child to prepare for the inevitable loss by discussion and preparing written material, videos, and tapes for later use.

The child's 'healthy' mourning will be helped if he is told promptly when his parent has died and his questions about where the body is are honestly answered in a manner tailored to his age and understanding. The dead person's fate—has she gone to Heaven?—should be discussed in a way which is in keeping with the family's beliefs; other courses are unlikely to be sustainable.

It is not harmful for the surviving parent to show grief in front of the child, even though this may be upsetting to other members of the family. How, otherwise, is the child going to understand that it is all right for him to show his emotions? After all, if the father has lost a wife and appears dry-eyed, trying to carry on as if the catastrophe had not happened, how can a child remain convinced that his parents were tied together by a bond of love and affection? In other words, the child should participate in the family's grieving, which in many cases will include attendance at the funeral and/or saying goodbye to the body. In the months afterwards, it should be made easy for the child to talk about his dead parent and to keep his memories. People are not perfect and children should be encouraged to retain a realistic memory of what the dead parent was like. Paradoxically, this may make it easier for him to build a new relationship with a step-father or a step-mother. But death is not a tidy business and the process of mourning will not go smoothly, however good the intentions of all involved.

Bibliography

Baker, A. W. and Duncan, S. P. (1985). Child sexual abuse—a study of prevalence in Great Britain. *Child Abuse and Neglect*, **9**, 457–64.

Bellman, M. (1986). Studies on encopresis. *Acta Paediatrica Scandinavica*, **170**(Suppl.), 1–154.

Black, D. and Cottrell, D. (ed.) (1993). *Seminars in child and adolescent psychiatry.* Royal College of Psychiatrists, London.

Bools, C. N., Neale, B. A., and Meadow, S. R. (1993). Follow-up of victims of fabricated illness (Munchausen's syndrome by proxy). *Archives of Disease in Childhood*, **69**, 625–30.

Bowlby, J. (1980). *Attachment and loss,* Vol. 3: Loss, sadness and depression. Hogarth Press, London.

Brown, G. W. (1978). Depression—a sociological view. In *Basic readings in medical sociology*, (ed. D. Tuckett and J. M. Kaufert). Tavistock Publications, London.

Caplan, C. (1986). Preventing psychological disorders in children of divorce: general practitioners' role. *British Medical Journal*, **292**, 1431–4.

Clayden, G. S. (1992). Management of chronic constipation. *Archives of Disease in Childhood*, **67**, 340–4.

Cox, A. D. (1993). Preventive aspects of child psychiatry. *Archives of Disease in Childhood*, **68**, 691–701.

Douglas, J. and Richman, N. (1984). *My child won't sleep*. Penguin Books, Harmondsworth.

Furniss, T., Bingley-Miller, L., and Bentovim, A. (1984). Therapeutic approach to sexual abuse. *Archives of Disease in Childhood*, **59**, 865–70.

Hobbs, C. J. and Wynne, J. M. (1987). Child sexual abuse—an increasing rate of diagnosis. *Lancet*, **2**(8563), 837–42.

Illingworth, R. S. (1983). *The normal child—some problems in the early years and their treatment*, (8th edn). Churchill, London.

Jones, D. P. H. and Thomson, P. J. (1991). Children's sexual experience—normal and abnormal. In *Paediatric specialty practice for the 1990s*, (ed. J. Eyre and R. Boyd). Royal College of Physicians of London.

Kempe, C. H. (1978). Sexual abuse, another hidden paediatric problem. *Paediatrics,* **62**, 382–9.

Nolan, T., Debelle, G., Oberklaid, F., and Coffey, C. (1991). Randomized trial of laxatives in treatment of childhood encopresis. *Lancet,* **338**, 523–7.

Pearce, J. (1993). Child health surveillance for psychiatric disorder: practical guidelines. *Archives of Disease in Childhood*, **69**, 394–8.

Royal College of General Practitioners. (1969). The educational needs of future general practitioners. *Journal of the Royal College of General Practitioners*, **18**, 358–60.

Simonoff, E. A. and Stores, G. (1987). Controlled trial of trimeprazine tartrate for night waking. *Archives of Disease in Childhood*, **62**, 253–7.

The Allit Inquiry. (1994). HMSO, London.

Weindling, A. M., Bamford, F. N., and Whittle, R. A. (1986). Health of juvenile delinquents. *British Medical Journal*, **292**, 447–9.

6 Growth and its problems

Growth is a very sensitive indicator of a child's well-being. There is rarely anything serious chronically amiss with a baby or a child who is growing well physically and mentally. Unfortunately, a healthy growth is not always found.

THE INFANT WHO FAILS TO THRIVE

Failure to thrive is a time-honoured phrase which merely means failure to gain weight at the expected rate. It is best diagnosed by plotting sequential weights, and, ideally, length and head circumference measurements (often overlooked) on a suitable centile chart. The weight of the child who is failing to thrive will fall across centile lines, or away from the second centile. In essence, the rate of growth is more important than a single weight measurement which lies below the second centile. Edwards *et al.* (1990) have suggested that the child's 'genetic weight centile' is achieved between four and eight weeks rather than at birth. This is a better predictor of his centile at 12 months than the birth centile, which is partially determined by maternal influences and the fetal well-being during pregnancy. Thus, infants who are small for dates due to placental insufficiency 'catch up', while those who are large for dates (e.g. infants born to poorly controlled diabetic mothers) may drop to a lower centile. Careful assessment is necessary of those babies whose weight drops further and further away from the second centile, as opposed to those who are 'constitutionally light' with steady growth below and parallel to it.

Whilst the majority of small babies, even if admitted to hospital for investigation, do not turn out to have an organic disease, they do require careful evaluation. In the United Kingdom the commonest reasons for a young baby's weight lying below the second centile are psychosocial difficulties (discussed below), genetic endowment, or congenital malformations, chromosomal disorders, or disturbed growth *in utero* associated with maternal disease.

Others have a treatable disease, and as babies who do not gain sufficient weight have rather little reserve, they need diagnosis without too long a delay. This is especially true if they have other symptoms in addition. Vomiting may mean pyloric stenosis, a hiatus hernia, urinary tract infection, or allergy—although not as often as it is diagnosed. Apathy may also mean urinary tract infection or a serious metabolic abnormality. Breathlessness suggests heart failure; persistently loose or greasy stools, malabsorption. Persistent diarrhoea, especially if associated with other infections, may rarely mean immunodeficiency or AIDS. Infants with cerebral palsy may fail to thrive because of difficulties with chewing and swallowing. Individually, rare disorders of infancy, such as renal failure, or cystic fibrosis, may present initially with poor weight gain as the most predominant symptom.

However, psychosocial causes of failure to thrive are more common than any of the above. In a study of 40 underweight children who were admitted to hospital, no adequate organic cause was found in well over half, but their mothers were often depressed (O'Callaghan and Hull 1978). In fact, 13 of the mothers had visited their GPs for depression after the puerperium. They were also of a lower socio-economic group than the controls. It is not surprising that depressed mothers often find it difficult to develop a warm, loving relationship towards the baby, or to be alert to his needs, with consequent effect upon his nurture. Increased support may forestall failure to thrive if it is realized that the mother is depressed, or was depressed after a previous confinement.

If a well baby is failing to gain weight properly, a satisfactory solution to this will often only be achieved if there is close co-operation with the health visitor. Having excluded abnormalities on physical examination and cultured a urine sample, efforts should be made towards supporting the mother by frequent contacts in order to improve her response to the child's needs. Sometimes the problem centres around feeding. Perhaps appetite is being blunted with a bottle of milk, rather than solids being given at the beginning of a meal. Often no further investigations are necessary unless progress continues to be unsatisfactory.

Feeding problems as a cause of failure to thrive

Obviously, many psychosocial difficulties may present as feeding problems, but sometimes the latter occur in an apparently well-adjusted family, often when the mother is very keen to breast-feed successfully. One of the, usually minor, disadvantages of breast-feeding is that it is difficult to be sure how much milk the baby is getting. Although most babies who are under-fed will be fretful and demand frequent feeds, a few appear to be contented though taking too little milk. Breast-feeding may take a couple of weeks to become properly established. Healthy, breast-fed babies in general often gain weight at a rate falling slightly below the centile line, for the charts were constructed in the heyday of artificial feeding with the early introduction of solids. One study suggested that two-month-old bottle-fed babies were larger and subsequently grew more quickly than breast-fed babies (Whitehead and Paul 1981). Nevertheless if the baby looks undernourished, as judged by wasted buttocks and loose folds of skin in the axilla and along the thighs, further evaluation is needed.

An occasionally useful approach is to test-weigh the baby for a day or two, though it is very easy to undermine the mother's confidence and often simple measures to encourage improvement of the breast-milk supply are preferable. Ideally, test-weighing should be done throughout one 24-hour period, as the baby may get lots of milk at one feed, especially the first in the morning, and only nibble on other occasions. It is important to ensure that the weighing scales used for this exercise are sensitive enough to detect the net increase in weight, which may range from 20 to 160 grams, before and after a breast-feed. This may necessitate one or two days' admission to the paediatric ward, and is seldom embarked upon. An average baby in the first month needs some 150 ml/kg per day (2½ oz/lb per day) but smaller babies often need rather more. After the first few weeks, if the baby is on the breast and taking too little, it is often said that it is impossible for the mother to build up her breast-milk supply and that supplementary feeding by bottle is necessary. However, removal of the supplementary feeds, frequent feeding, and use of the breast for pacification can allow the volume of milk to increase, even at a late stage, if the mother is keen and well supported. After all, some adoptive mothers can breast-feed.

Provided the formula milk is being prepared correctly and enough is being given, a bottle-fed baby who is growing poorly will usually either have something wrong with his health or his handling.

Organic disease as a cause of failure to thrive

Infants who continue to gain weight poorly or lose weight despite our efforts will usually need to be referred for paediatric assessment, unless they have an obvious intercurrent infection. A diagnosis of gastro-enteritis should be treated with suspicion; first, because prolonged diarrhoea and vomiting with poor weight gain will sometimes be the symptom of malabsorption or milk intolerance. Secondly, the GP himself may unwittingly contribute to continued failure to thrive by maintaining a false diagnosis of gastro-enteritis and recommending repeated courses of glucose–electrolyte mixtures (for example, Dioralyte), or persistent use of diluted feeds for a well infant whose frequent motions and occasional vomits are due to the problem of handling rather than to infection, or in whom there is a temporary post gastro-enteritic lactose or cows' milk protein intolerance (see page 212).

It may be comforting to realize that laboratory tests only rarely establish the diagnosis when a careful history and examination have failed to do so. Sills (1978) found that of the 2607 tests performed on 185 patients with poor weight gain only 10 established a diagnosis and only 26 supported one. Nevertheless, continued and increasing failure to thrive demands attention until the problem is either solved or spontaneous improvement occurs.

THE SHORT CHILD

Height is important in three situations: to check that height and weight are in proportion when dealing with an over- or underweight child—if they are wide apart further action may be needed; to monitor growth in situations where this is at risk, as in chronic disease or when the child is on steroids; and to pick out from the large number of healthy, short children the very few with pathological treatable short stature before it becomes irreversible.

How to assess height

At birth the average full-term baby is around 50 cm long. As shown in Fig. 6.1(a), there is a rapid growth for the first two years of life with an increase in length of around 25 cm in the first year and 10 cm in the second. Thereafter the average growth rate is 5 to 6 cm per year until around 11 years in girls and 12 in boys.

In girls, puberty starts with breast development, growth of pubic hair and with an increase in growth velocity which reaches its maximum one year later at around 12. Once menstruation starts, growth is slowing rapidly. Total growth over puberty is 6–10 cm. In boys, growth comes later in puberty and is at its peak around 14 when testes are two-thirds of adult volume, the penis is considerably enlarged and pubic hair is at stage 3–4 (see Fig. 6.2(a)). The mean age of onset of normal puberty has a wide range in both sexes (Fig. 6.2). The longer period of pre-pubertal growth in boys is responsible for the difference of 13 cm between the height of the average adult male and female. Significant growth stops between 16 and 18 years of age when the epiphysis of the growing bones fuse.

The individual's height is interpreted by plotting it on a centile chart, which allows the child's height to be compared with a population norm. In 1994, new growth charts (Figs 6.3–6.8) based on more recent cross-sectional measurement of children (published by Child Growth Foundation, 2 Mayfield Avenue, London W4 1PW) replaced those based on Tanner-Whitehouse standards of almost 30 years ago. The newer charts reflect the 'secular trend' in growth and maturation, that is, the tendency of children in this century to become taller and mature earlier, probably due to improvements in nutrition and environmental conditions. The new charts also provide nine instead of the traditional seven centile lines, with two-thirds of a standard deviation separating each pair of centile lines. The lowest centile line is the 0.4 line and the highest is the 99.6 line.

For height measurement to be useful in measuring growth over time it must be accurate. A wall-mounted stadiometer or, more cheaply, a Raven Minimeter height measuring tape, can be used (Raven Equipment, Ford Farm Industrial Complex, Braintree Road, Gt. Dunmow, Essex CM6 1HU). The Hall (1996) report recommends routine growth monitoring by measurement of a child's height at around two years or earlier in a co-operative child, and a further measurement between three and four years.

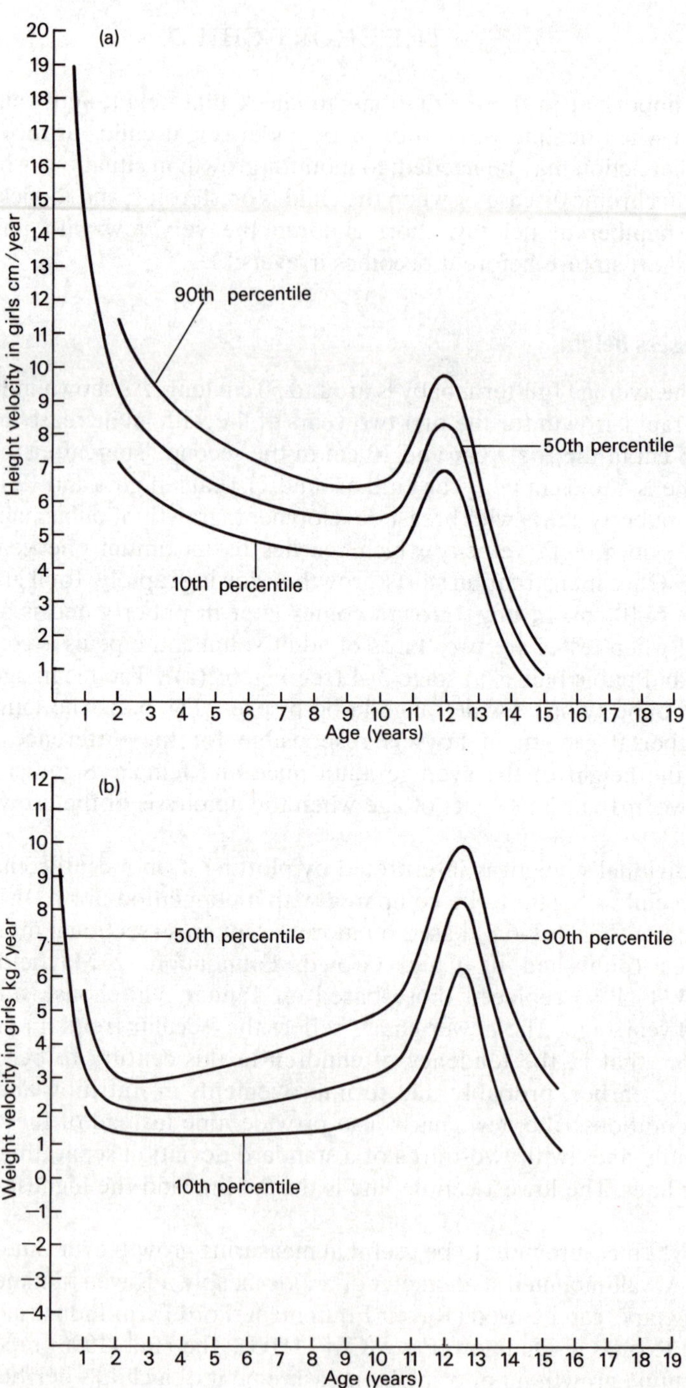

Figure 6.1. Height velocity (a) and weight velocity (b) in girls. From Tanner and Whitehouse (1976).

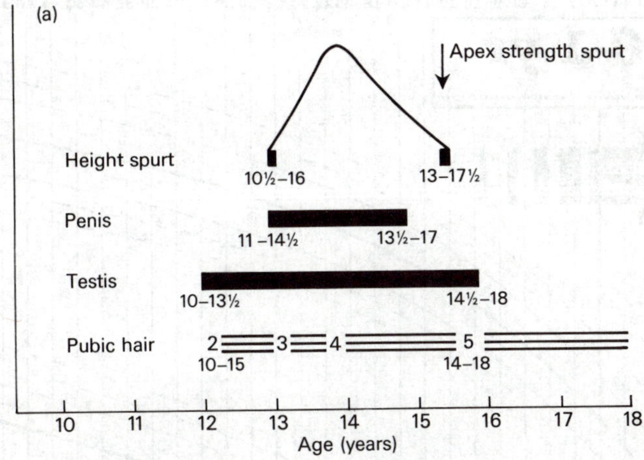

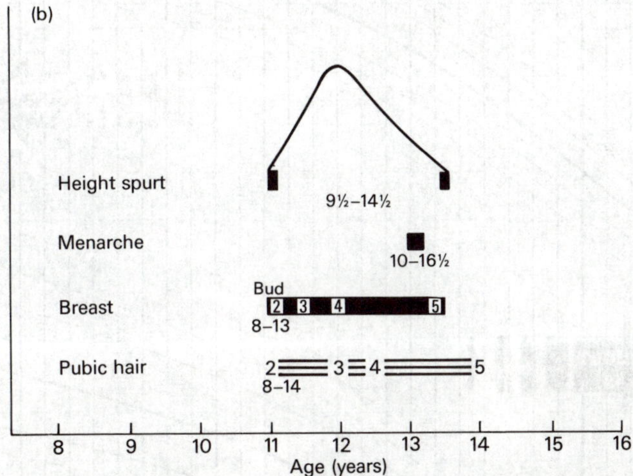

Figure 6.2. Sequence of events at adolescence in boys (a) and girls (b). An average boy or girl is represented: the range of ages within which each event charted may begin and end is given by the figures placed directly below its start and finish. From Tanner (1962).

The vast majority of these short children are healthy and it is rare to find undiagnosed disease in surveys of short children. Short parents are likely to have short children and that must be taken into account when assessing a child's growth. The parents' height needs to be measured (better) or estimated and plotted. For a boy, if the father's height is marked on to the chart at the 18-year level together with the mother's, after adding 13 cm to to her height to allow for the sex difference (13 cm is the mean difference between male and female adult height), their mean position denotes the mid-parental height. A range of 10 cm on either side of the mid-parental height represents the 9th to 91st

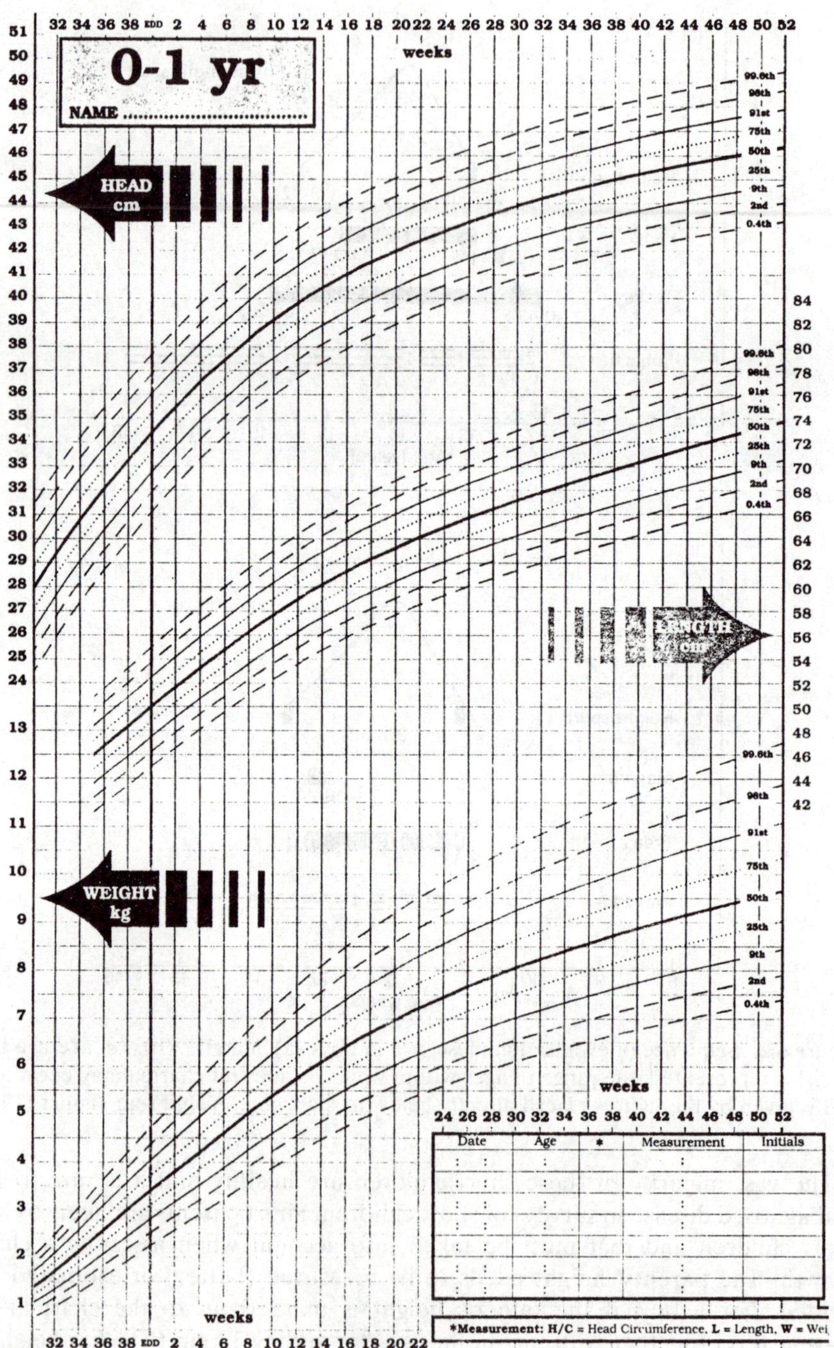

Figure 6.3. Girls growth chart (0–1 year). © Child Growth Foundation. Available from Harlow Printing, Maxwell Street, South Shields, NE33 4PU, UK.

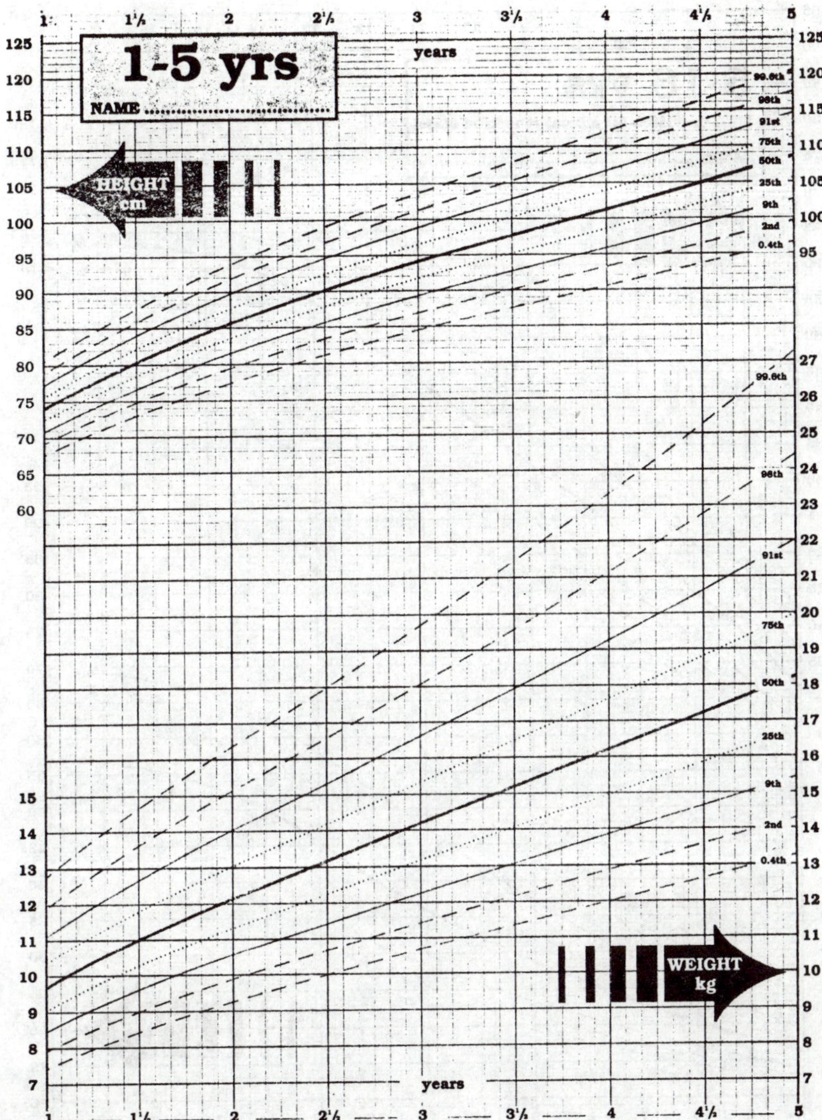

Figure 6.4. Girls growth chart (1–5 years). © Child Growth Foundation. Available from Harlow Printing, Maxwell Street, South Shields, NE33 4PU, UK.

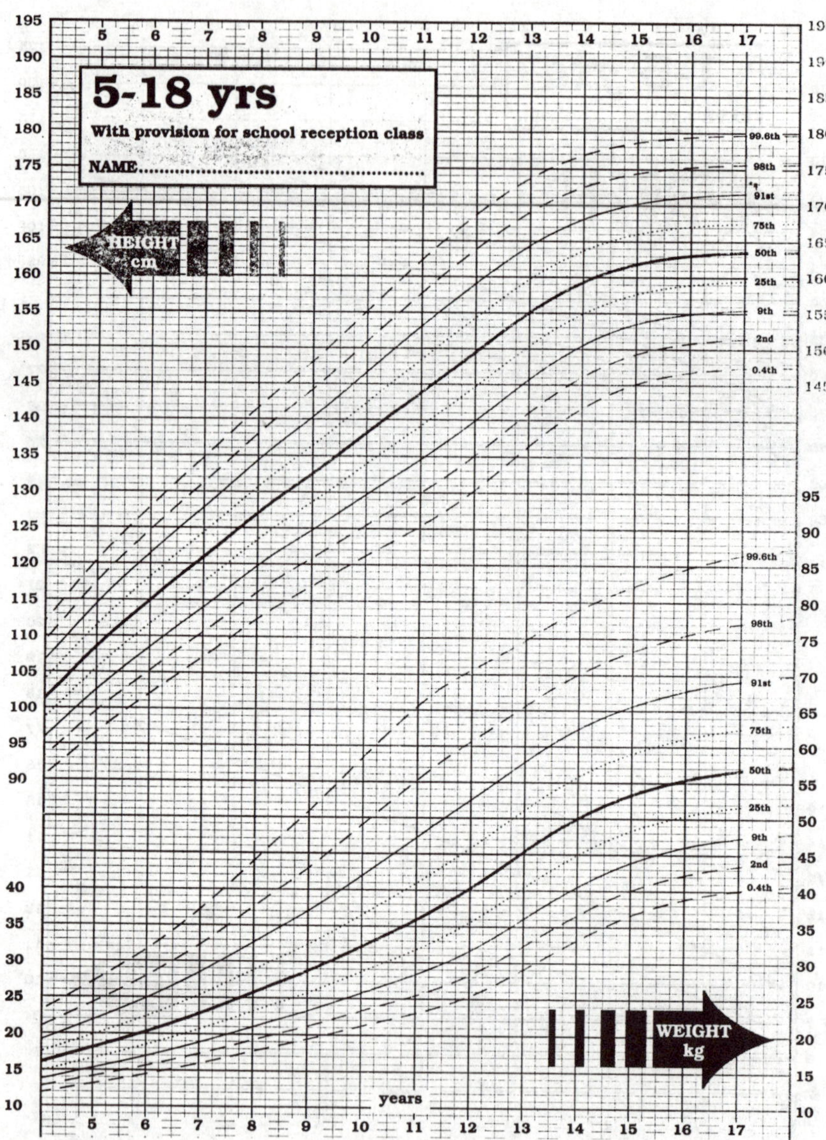

Figure 6.5. Girls growth chart (5–18 years). © Child Growth Foundation. Available from Harlow Printing, Maxwell Street, South Shields, NE33 4PU, UK.

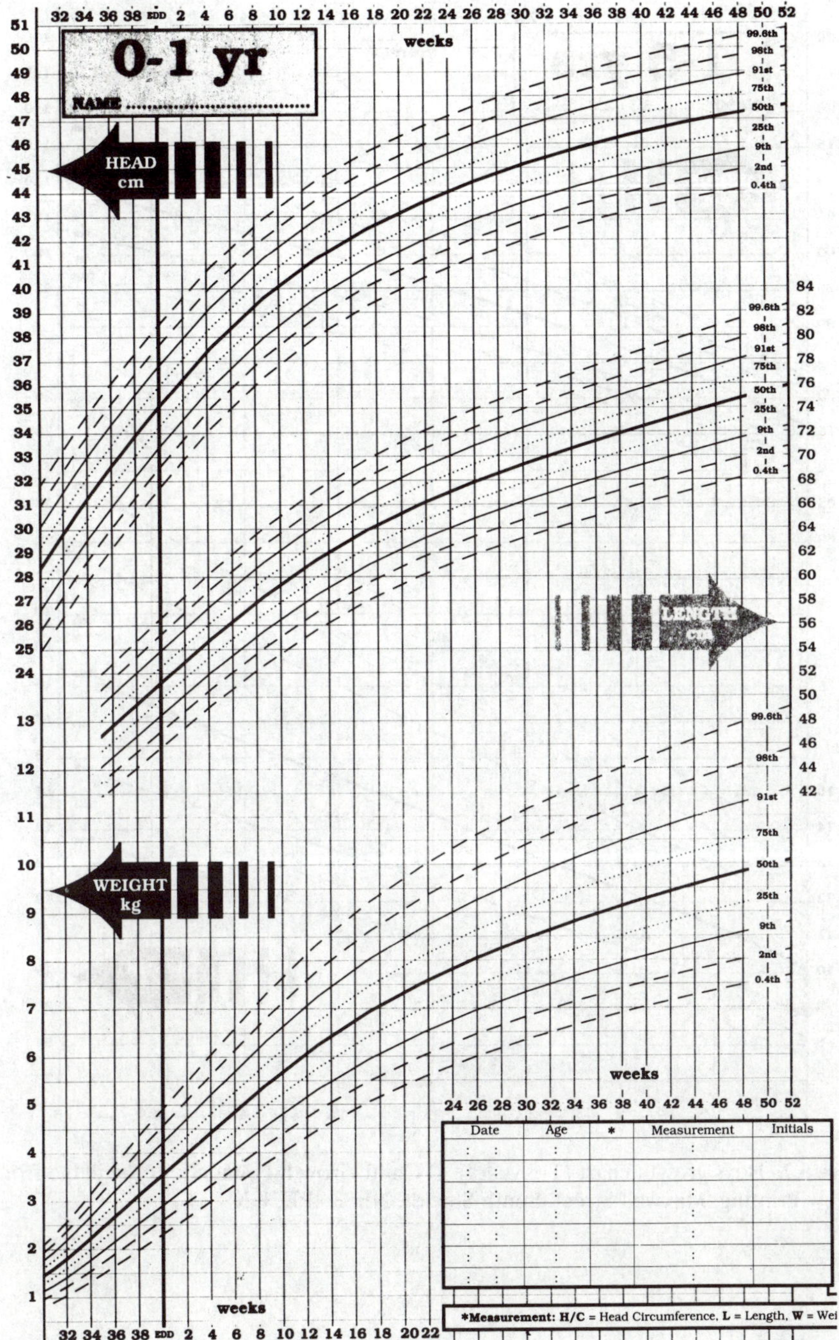

Figure 6.6. Boys growth chart (0–1 year). © Child Growth Foundation. Available from Harlow Printing, Maxwell Street, South Shields, NE33 4PU, UK.

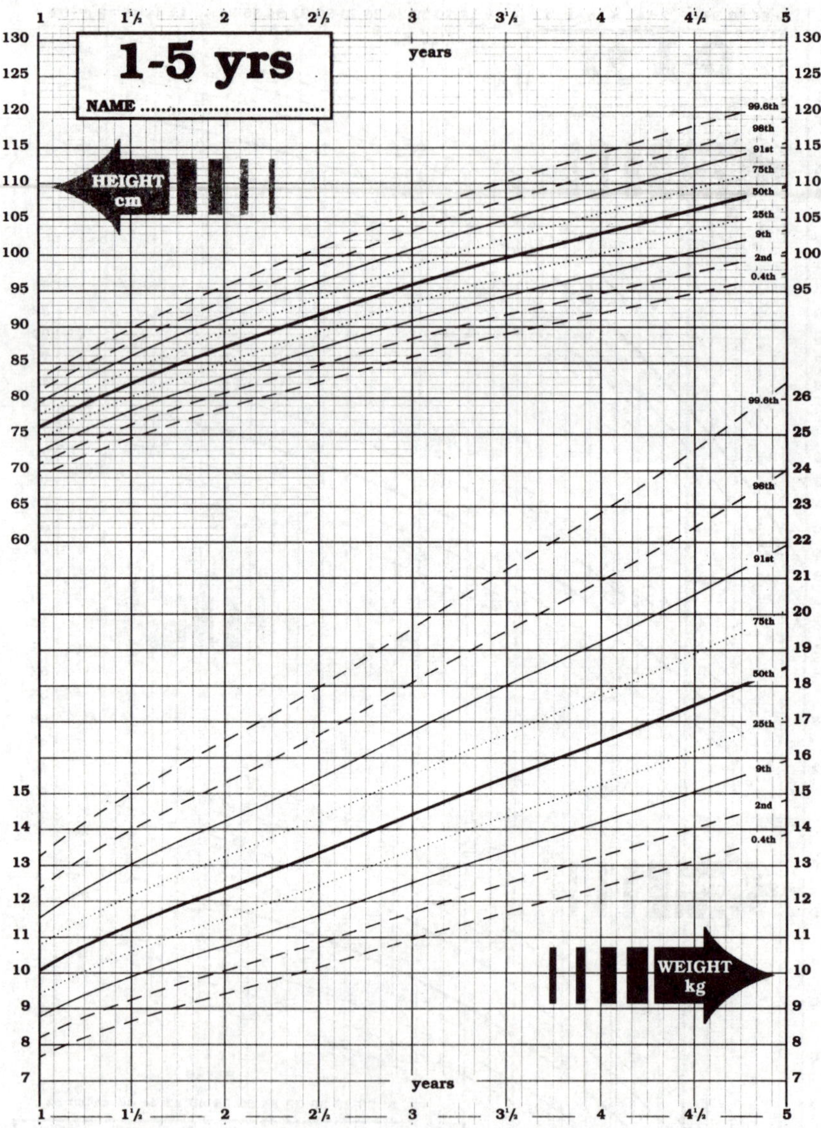

Figure 6.7. Boys growth chart (1–5 years). © Child Growth Foundation. Available from Harlow Printing, Maxwell Street, South Shields, NE33 4PU, UK.

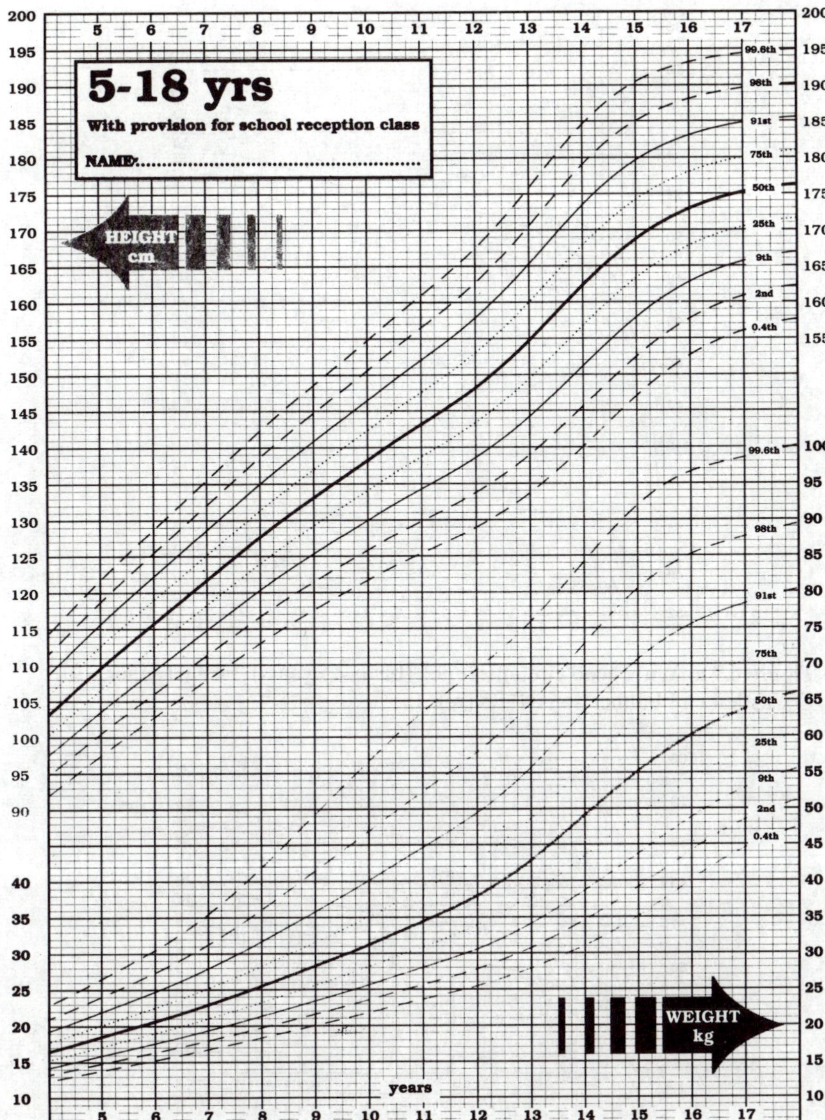

Figure 6.8. Boys growth chart (5–18 years). © Child Growth Foundation. Available from Harlow Printing, Maxwell Street, South Shields, NE33 4PU, UK.

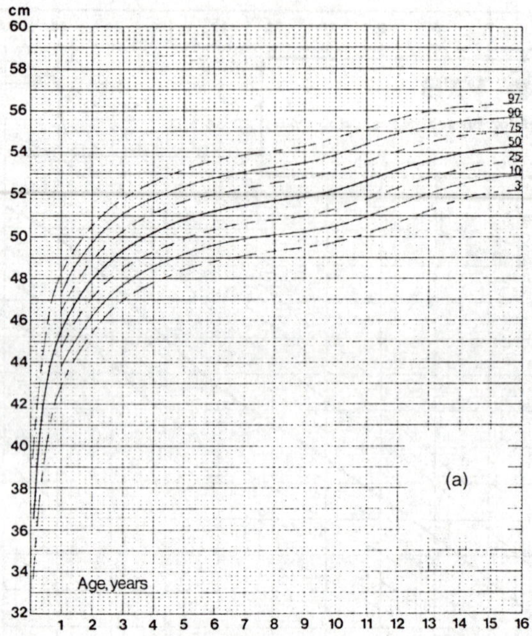

Figure 6.9 a. Girls head circumference (birth–16 years). From Tanner, 1978. © Castlemead Publications, 1985 (ref. 19).

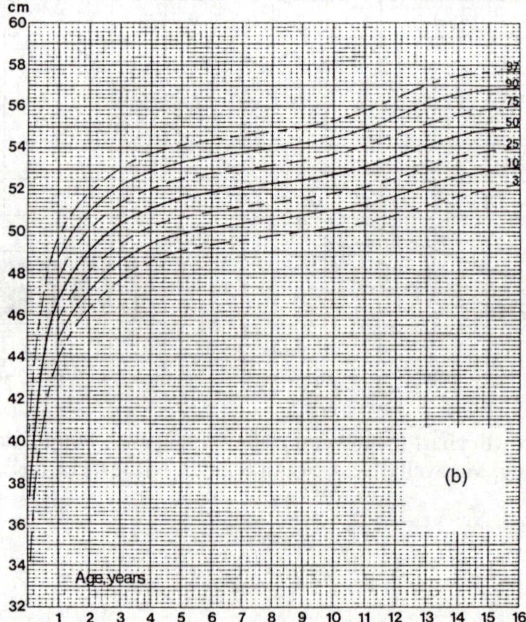

Figure 6.9 b. Boys head circumference (birth–16 years). From Tanner, 1978. © Castlemead Publications, 1985 (ref. 18).

Table 6.1 Causes of short stature and poor growth

1. Familial short stature
2. Constitutional delay in growth and puberty (CDGP)
3. Intrauterine growth retardation (IUGR)
4. Neglect/insufficient nutrition/emotional deprivation
5. Chromosomal abnormalities (e.g. Turner's syndrome)
6. Systemic illnesses (e.g. severe asthma, Crohn's disease, chronic renal failure, cystic fibrosis)
7. Endocrine disorders (e.g. growth hormone deficiency, hypothyroidism, Cushing's syndrome)
8. Cartilage and skeletal dysplasias (e.g. achondroplasia)
9. Steroids

percentile range for the son of those parents. For a girl the same can be plotted on a girl's chart, but subtracting 13 cm from the father's height. It should be remembered that parental short stature may itself have resulted from an inherited disorder or a similar early deprived environment. If in doubt it is important to re-check the height after six months and calculate the rate of growth (the height velocity, expressed in cm/year) (Fig. 6.1(a)). This represents the current dynamic of growth, whereas a single height measurement only gives an indication of previous growth.

Causes of short stature and poor growth

Causes 1 and 2 in Table 6.1 account for the majority of short children seen. Children with familial short stature often tend to be small for their age but have a normal growth velocity. Their bone age, an indication of skeletal maturity and remaining growth potential, is similar to their chronological age. They are likely to enter puberty and have a growth spurt at the normal age and obtain a final height appropriate to their parentage. There is no known treatment which will increase the final height of these children beyond this. CDGP is a common growth variant characterized by normal growth rate in infancy with gradual deceleration during childhood. These children are small for their age and their bone age is two to four years delayed. The onset of puberty is delayed: 14+ for boys and 13+ for girls. They have a normal growth spurt when it comes, and their final height is appropriate for their mid-parental centile.

Boys with CDGP are more likely to be overtly concerned and come to the GP about their short stature or delayed sexual development than girls. Some may become anxious, depressed and socially isolated, in spite of reassurance that they and their genitalia will grow to a normal size and that the latter will function satisfactorily. In a small proportion of these, intervention with low-dose anabolic steroid (Oxandrolone), or testosterone for three to six months, under the close supervision of a paediatric endocrinologist, can be considered to bring forward the timing of pubertal growth or sexual development without decreasing final height, whilst remembering the sound principle that normal variation should not be unnecessarily medicalized.

Insufficient food is the commonest cause of growth failure world-wide and this may also occur in Britain. Even in its absence, emotional deprivation of itself may cause growth failure through hypothalamic disturbance leading to impaired growth hormone secretion. Typically, these neglected children have a pale complexion, cold hands and feet, sparse hair and a sad expression. They often have a voracious appetite and in hospital they may eat food set aside for other children. They usually show spectacular 'catch up' growth when provided with an affectionate, caring, and nurturing environment.

Turner's syndrome (chromosomally XO or one of its variants, incidence 1 in 2500 births) should be considered in any girl presenting with unexplained short stature or absence of pubertal development. Other features include webbed neck, low nape of the neck/hairline, small lower jaw, broad chest with widely spaced nipples, a wide carrying angle of the elbows and coarctation of the aorta together with a history of puffy feet as a newborn. If the diagnosis is suspected, referral is indicated because growth hormone treatment may help with growth and oestrogen treatment can take them through puberty.

Children with almost any chronic disease, such as severe congenital heart disease, cystic fibrosis, diabetes mellitus, or chronic renal failure, often have retarded growth. Moderate or severe asthma, even in the absence of steroids, may slow the tempo of growth and delay puberty, but final stature is maintained (Balflour-Lynn 1986). Malabsorption, for example, from coeliac disease (page 213) slows growth, and in children with Crohn's disease growth failure may precede abdominal pain and diarrhoea.

Idiopathic growth hormone deficiency occurs in about 1 in 5000 births in the UK. The affected children are extremely small, 'podgy' and immature in appearance; the boys have a tiny penis. There is a progressive slowing of growth which usually becomes apparent after the age of two years. Treatment with subcutaneous growth hormone results in normal adult height, especially if treatment is started early, and some benefit accrues if started late. The costs of a course of treatment are, however, over £6000 per year and treatment needs to be continued until growth ceases—another drug not to be given for frivolous reasons! Referral should be made as early as possible if growth hormone is to be started while there is still time for an adequate response before puberty.

Cushing's syndrome, with hypertension, moon face, striae and trunk obesity is an even rarer cause. Short stature is an important feature of late onset hypothyroidism, which usually presents insidiously. However, careful enquiry may reveal symptoms of lethargy, constipation, and on examination, dry skin, bradycardia, cold peripheries, coarsening of facial features, and delayed relaxation of the ankle jerk may all be found. Thyroxine treatment results in catch-up growth.

Finally, the most important side-effect of chronic steroid administration in childhood is stunting of growth. Height should be carefully monitored and

Table 6.2 Reasonable indications for referral of a short child

1. When the height is below the 0.4 percentile (only 1 child in 250 will fall below this line).
2. When the height is well between the 0.4 and 2nd percentile, taking into account the size of the parents. Referral is more important if growth is slowing down as judged by repeated measurements.
3. When there is evidence of systemic disease, evidence of severe social or emotional problems, or of obvious skeletal malformation.

recorded on a growth chart in any child taking systemic steroids or high doses (>800 micrograms per day) of inhaled steroids.

PUBERTY

The normal age for onset of puberty is between 8 and 13 years for girls and between 10 and 15 years for boys. Figure 6.2 summarizes the physical changes of puberty. The numbers 2–5 for breast and pubic hair development refer to Tanner's 5-point scale (Tanner and Whitehouse 1976), 6 points in the case of male pubic hair. Like most such scales they are easy to remember; in effect 1 is no change from childhood, 2 a trace, 3 quite a large change, 4 almost adults, and 5 fully adult.

Pathological early puberty is rare and may be idiopathic or secondary to an endocrine or an intracranial pathology. Boys are more likely to have an underlying intracranial pathology, for example, a brain tumour, while in girls the investigations are usually normal. The GP should have a low threshold for referring a boy who begins puberty before the age of 10 years. The main problems with idiopathic early puberty are social in the short term, and, in the longer term, short stature because of early epiphyseal fusion after an abnormally early growth spurt. Extremely early puberty can be delayed with monthly subcutaneous injections of an analogue of gonadotrophin releasing hormone, which work by 'switching off' the release of gonadotrophins from the pituitary gland.

The most common pubertal problems presented to the GP are unequal breast buds, breast development in the male, and delayed puberty. A disc of mammary tissue in either sex may be so knobbly and mobile that the parents and indeed the GP may be worried about a tumour; it never is. Breast development in the male is common and harmless except for the rare presentation in this way of Klinefelter's syndrome with small, rather round testes, and unusually tall stature. The 47, XXY complement of chromosomes will be confirmed by culture. Individuals are usually azoospermic, and have in childhood a mildly increased incidence of language delay and clumsiness.

Late puberty is common. In well-nourished parts of the world delay is usually part of a family pattern. If children are showing definite signs of starting puberty by the age of 13 in the female and 15 in the male (see CDGP above), reassurance is all that is required. Beyond this age, or in families without a history of early puberty, reassurance should not be too whole-hearted. Pituitary disorders with short stature, and perhaps impaired visual fields and diabetes insipidus, or, in short girls, Turner's syndrome, or any chronic debilitating diseases mentioned on p. 101 may lead to delayed puberty. So may undiagnosed coeliac disease. It may be therapeutic, and sometimes diagnostic, to examine a teenager with real or imagined anxiety about his pubertal development. Boys tend to be worried about the size of their penis and girls about breast development. In girls, delay in menarche beyond the latter part of puberty in an otherwise well child can be a feature of emotional stress, anorexia nervosa (p. 112), or frequent vigorous exercise. Most girls of 16 who have not yet started their periods will be referred to exclude an anatomical problem, or a chromosomal, or endocrine disorder.

THE FAT CHILD

The naked child who looks fat to the GP is also likely to be obese by more sophisticated measurements. By the time he is 20 per cent above the average weight for his height and sex, he may be arbitrarily defined as being obese. Obesity is quite common in early infancy. Prevalence then decreases through childhood to increase again from the onset of puberty. Teenage girls are more likely to become fat than teenage boys. The belief that early obesity is a strong predictor of later adult fatness has come under increasing attack, but is sometimes true. Fat infants are more than twice as likely to become fat children as their slimmer peers, but 8 out of 10 will not be overweight by the time they start primary school (Poskitt and Cole 1977) and 40 per cent of overweight 7- to 11-year-olds become fat young adults (Stark *et al.* 1981). On the other hand most fat adults were not fat as children (Peckham *et al.* 1983). An obese child is likely to go through puberty a year or so earlier than his peers. His final height will only be average because of early cessation of growth.

Fat parents are likely to produce fat children, although it is difficult to separate the effects of inheritance from the effects of family eating habits. If the child sees his parents eating large quantities of fattening food, he will follow suit, particularly if he is accustomed to receiving sweets as a reward for good behaviour. For many overweight mothers a fat child is a healthy child and proof that he is well looked after. The fat child has taken in more calories than he needs and he may be aggrieved to find that many of his peers eat more than he does yet remain slim.

Some children eat too much because they are bored, or they are unhappy, or because in their families the giving of food is a major symbol of parental love. On the other hand, some become unhappy because they are overweight, being teased about their appearance at school and perhaps also at home. They become embarrassed when they have to change in front of other children and the fat adolescent may feel that he is unattractive to the other sex.

When the GP or health visitor notices that the infant is gaining too much weight, then is the time to strike and persuade the mother to give the child less to eat and less milk to drink—another reason for plotting the weight of infants on centile charts when they are brought to the child health clinic. However, too much professional obsession with obesity may have contributed to the present epidemic of borderline anorectic teenage girls; a sense of proportion is required, in both senses of the word. Advice on feeding given by the GP must correlate with that of the health visitor. An infant's thirst can be quenched with water rather than more milk, and he can be brought up without getting used to sugar being added to his feeds or drinks—which is good for the teeth also. It is usually unnecessary to introduce solid food before the infant is about four months old, when home-made purées of vegetables and fruit (which contain fewer calories than many tinned preparations) help to get the infant used to savoury rather than sweet foods. Breast-fed babies are less likely to be overweight than bottle-fed babies, perhaps because the former are not pushed to take a predetermined amount of milk.

Very few fat children require hospital referral. If the height of the fat child is above the 50th percentile, as it is usually in early childhood, and he is healthy and growing normally, then it is unlikely that his obesity is caused by a primary endocrine or metabolic disease. Short obese children, on the other hand, should be referred for further observation in order to exclude such rare conditions as hypothyroidism, or Cushing's syndrome due to a pituitary, or adrenal tumour, or to adrenal cortical hyperplasia. Prolonged inactivity, perhaps the result of a physical handicap, may predispose to obesity.

Attempting to achieve weight loss is a real misery for everyone and success cannot be maintained unless the patient and family are well motivated, and rarely even then. Worse, success implies a permanent change in eating habits.

The child may decide to lose weight to increase his allure at the time of puberty or when he finds he cannot cope with games. It is perhaps more satisfactory to aim for a constant weight while growth in height continues, rather than try to be too ambitious:

Elizabeth was aged 11, plump, and being teased at school because of this. Her father was also a stone overweight. Both went on a diet and lost weight satisfactorily. Unfortunately, Elizabeth regained most of this during the next year, but since she was well motivated because she was going through puberty, she was able to learn from this that she needed to keep a continuing eye on her diet and managed to develop an acceptable figure.

A discussion of the treatment of obesity tends to sound like the medical column of a women's magazine. Management is time-consuming and the ground has to be well prepared. If a community dietician is available she can take a considerable load off the doctor. She is also better at the job. There are two options, best taken up together: eating less and exercising more. The child may have to settle for walking to and from school and avoiding second helpings; anorectic drugs are contra-indicated. More usefully the family must be educated about food, rather than be given a rigid diet sheet containing mainly foods the child dislikes. It is useful for the mother or the child to record the food intake for a day before coming back for the next consultation. This provides a valuable basis for discussion, often making it obvious to the GP where the problem lies. The diet must start from where the child's present eating habits are, rather than from a theoretical conception of the ideal. But if he is found to be addicted to fatty foods it is important to explain to him why he should replace these in particular. A lot of families, and some doctors, do not realize that fats are twice as caloric on a weight basis as carbohydrates and proteins. A reduction of fat in the diet is as important as the sensible substitution of fruit, vegetables and low-calorie drinks for cakes, biscuits, and sugary cereals. The family's menu may have to change to support the youngsters' attempts to lose weight.

A formal low-calorie diet can be recommended only for children who are severely obese, want to lose weight, and are supported by their families. In the older child the aim should be the loss of about 0.5–1 kg per week and in the younger child half this. The weight loss will be most rapid in the first two weeks and the child must be warned, if he is not to become discouraged, that it will slow down thereafter. The intake will need to be reduced to 1000–1200 kcal daily. Weighing at the practice with encouragement to stick to the dietary regime may help to maintain momentum. Even if the child is motivated to lose weight it is difficult to stay slim. The latter requires a long-term commitment to revised eating habits, meals rather than nibbling, sensible foods, no second helpings. Well-educated families can find a comprehensive volume of calorie values for a wide range of foods, including brand names, very helpful. This can allow them to live flexibly with dietary treats within a fixed calorie intake.

Bibliography

Balflour-Lynn, I. (1986). Growth and childhood asthma. *Archives of Disease in Childhood*, **61**, 1046–55.

Edwards, A. G. K., Halse, P. C., Parkin, J. M., and Waterston, A. J. R. (1990). Recognising failure to thrive in early childhood. *Archives of Disease in Childhood*, **65**, 1263–5.

Hall, D. (ed.) (1996). *Health for all children*. Report of the Third Joint Working Party on Child Health Surveillance, (3rd edn). Oxford University Press.

O'Callaghan, M. J. and Hull, D. (1978). Failure to thrive as failure to rear? *Archives of Disease in Childhood*, **53**, 788–93.

Peckham, C. S., Start, O., Simonite, V., and Wolff, O. H. (1983). Prevalence of obesity in British children born in 1946 and 1958. *British Medical Journal*, **286**, 1237–42.

Poskitt, E. M. E. and Cole, T. J. (1977). Do fat babies stay fat? *British Medical Journal*, **i**, 7–9.

Sills, R. H. (1978). Failure to thrive—role of clinical and laboratory evaluation. *American Journal of Diseases of Children*, **132**, 967–9.

Stark, O., Atkins, E., Wolff, O. H., and Douglas, J. W. B. (1981). Longitudinal study of obesity in the National Survey of Health and Development. *British Medical Journal*, **ii**, 13–17.

Tanner, J. M. (1962). *Growth at adolescence*, (2nd edn). Blackwell, Oxford.

Tanner, J. M. and Whitehouse, R. H. (1976). Clinical longitudinal standards for height, weight, height velocity, weight velocity, and stages of puberty. *Archives of Disease in Childhood*, **51**, 170–9.

Whitehead, R. G. and Paul, A. A. (1981). Infant growth and human milk requirement. *Lancet*, **ii**, 161–3.

7 Some problems of adolescents

A group practice of 10 000 patients will contain on average 1500 between the ages of 10 and 20. In this chapter we discuss some of the features of consultations with adolescents, and some of their common problems not covered elsewhere in the book.

THE PRACTICE AND THE ADOLESCENT

Practice leaflets can usefully include a paragraph describing special services provided for adolescents plus reassurance that the under-16s can see their GP or other member of the team for a confidential consultation. This right has been firmly endorsed by the BMA, the GMSC, and the RCGP. Rare exceptions are if the young person is considered to be too immature to understand what is going on or to consent to treatment, or if the safety and welfare of a third person are at risk.

Some practices offer a 14- or 15-year-old a routine consultation to give them the opportunity to raise any topic they wish to discuss. Unfortunately those most 'at risk' are least likely to attend. Important health issues for adolescents include how to keep fit, information about inherited and other diseases, healthy diet and various themes surrounding pregnancy, birth control and concerns about sexual function.

The consultation is also an opportunity to inform the adolescents about local facilities for self-referral and, if appropriate, give information about the risks of smoking, excessive drinking, illicit drugs and unsafe sex. There is some evidence that the young person is more likely to be put off smoking by information on the immediate unpleasant consequences (smelly breath, stained fingernails) than by a warning of what might happen to them in 20 or 30 years. One objective of this consultation is to indicate that the young person is no longer to be treated as a dependent child, and has a right to see the GP of his choice. If the youngster is reluctant to consult his family's doctor, it may be useful to encourage him to see another doctor in a partnership who is not so clearly identified with the parents. Often this is a GP registrar who is perceived as belonging to a similar generation.

PATTERNS OF CONSULTATION

The arrival of a 12-year-old child alone, a 16-year-old with her boy-friend, or a 20-year-old with her mother are all interesting "physical signs". One advantage of the doctor fetching patients from the waiting room is that he can see who they have come with and how close they are. These observations can provide diagnostic or therapeutic openings. Is the 12-year-old waiting alone poorly supervised or being expected to be mature beyond his years? Even if a seemingly grown-up child of this age attends by himself he must still be considered to be in the care of his parents. This means that, unless the instructions given are relatively simple or unimportant, or the young person expresses a definite wish for the consultation to be confidential, the parents should usually be contacted, perhaps by a note given to the child. Contraception can be tactfully raised with the 16-year-old if it seems appropriate: 'Was that your boy-friend in the waiting room?' 'If at any time you would like to discuss any aspect of family planning with me please don't hesitate?' 'Of course, anything you say to me will be completely confidential.' Parental accompaniment of a 20-year-old may mean the topic of conversation is perceived to be embarrassing or potentially serious, or perhaps parent and child are over-entwined in a symbiotic relationship. The separation of parent and adolescent during a joint consultation may be achieved by sending the teenager through to the examination room to undress. Its value is not only to see the young person alone, he may even then be equally malcommunicative, but also to be able to tackle the parent. 'What do you think the problem is?'

Physical examination, especially if it involves exposure of the chest or examination of the genitalia, may be embarrassing to the adolescent, whose uneasiness may also make the doctor feel awkward, especially if he is of the opposite sex to the patient. Permission for examination should always be sought; female adolescents may prefer to be examined by a female doctor. A chaperone is advisable for any pelvic examination by a male doctor and, while it may be an ideal to examine the chest fully, the doctor should not usually argue with the patient who will only expose a minute amount of flesh or who is only happy for the back of the chest to be examined.

The GP will sometimes be asked for support by anxious parents of an adolescent perceived to be troublesome, because of intrafamily stress and parental exasperation generated by their inability to communicate with the teenager or influence his behaviour. Occasionally, questions about the parents' past may allow them to express their real anxieties. 'I didn't see my own parents for five years after our bust up when I left school ...'. A discussion of what adolescence is and of the physical and social changes that take place can be helpful. For example, the young person's attention gradually shifts from family to friends, who are initially usually of the same sex. There is often a great wish to be accepted by a group of peers (though this tends to break up spontaneously in later adolescence). The youngsters may remain loyal to one group through thick and thin, or they may change their allegiance as the months go by. Boys who mature late physically may not find life as easy as their early maturing friends—an additional problem if they are having other difficulties. They are more likely to be treated as children and to take a less assertive role within their peer group. The GP may need to explain that young people have to achieve separation from their parents, establish their own moral values, find a sexual identity, learn how to develop mature and loving relationships, and make plans for the future. They also have to re-establish the relationship with parents on a basis of equality rather than dependence—a difficult task for both parents and children, usually only incompletely achieved. Some families are too intertwined with each other, making it difficult for the adolescent to assert independence; others go to the other extreme so that the young person feels that he has no boundaries and nobody cares for him. There are important ethnic differences in parental expectations; for example, the older Asian teenager still has important responsibilities within the extended family (Chapter 9).

In so far as adolescents come to their GP at all when they are not acutely ill, it is often because of concern about their personal appearance, sometimes associated with sexual anxieties that they are too shy to refer to directly. As with any other patient, the real worry may only become apparent after initial symptoms have been presented and dealt with.

While there is often a refreshingly straightforward honesty about a teenager's medical requests, many adolescents find it difficult to be precise about their symptoms, and it is often difficult to elicit a chronologically accurate history. As a result the patient and doctor sometimes seem to be completely at cross-purposes, but this does not seem to stop the youngster returning for a subsequent consultation, as though nothing amiss had occurred. Occasionally, an obviously distressing symptom may be presented in an inappropriately offhand manner. A problem may also be presented in an intense and urgent manner at one consultation; a week later it will have subsided as an issue. Reassessment is often better than instant over-reaction by, for example, arranging an urgent referral.

The older doctor, especially, may need to remember that, however adolescents may express their individuality, it is important to treat them and their anxieties with seriousness and respect.

THE CHRONICALLY SICK ADOLESCENT

(see also Chapter 8 and sections on specific diseases)

There are at least three components to problems at this stage: normal adolescent turmoil constrained by the dependence of illness; the physical effects of puberty on disease control (e.g. oestrogens interact with insulin) and a tendency of doctors and parents to forget to give the teenagers enough information to manage their own therapy and to tailor it to their lifestyle.

It is important for the GP to encourage these teenagers to take as much control over the management of their disease as possible. This may not be easy, and parents may need repeated encouragement and support to overcome their natural tendency to be over-protective. The GP himself may forget how old the child is becoming because of the small size and delayed puberty of many chronically sick children. Self-reliance helps enhance self-confidence, decreases unnecessary dependence on the family, and makes it more likely that the youngster will take prescribed medicines. Non-compliance with treatment may be a recurrent theme. Perhaps there is a poor understanding about illness and how treatment will help (clear, preferably written, treatment plans are important). Side-effects of the drug or an unnecessarily complicated treatment schedule may be a problem. Most teenagers do not wish to be seen as different. This must be taken into account in planning a realistic treatment regime as well as frequency of follow-up. For example, inhaled steroids do not need to be taken in the middle of the day. Negotiation rather than instruction is the way forward. Sometimes, however, there is a bottom line which is not negotiable, such as the need for daily insulin injections for the adolescent diabetic. Other strategies can also help: coming to surgery with a friend rather than a parent; educational holidays, for example camps for adolescents with diabetes or asthma. Despite all this, some youngsters when old enough to decide for themselves may choose to reject, to a greater or lesser extent, the burden of life-supporting therapy.

CONDUCT DISORDERS

Conduct disorders often start in the middle years of childhood. The criteria for diagnosis are met by 4–10 per cent of adolescents. This wide range emphasizes the difficulty sometimes found in deciding whether the normal rebelliousness of a young person (perhaps with rather rigid and controlling parents) has become a conduct disorder. There are many forms: inappropriately aggressive and angry behaviour, various forms of delinquency such as stealing, excessive promiscuity and, as the increasing number of young people sleeping in city streets demonstrates, running away from home. Adolescents with conduct disorders are often alienated from their parents, especially if they have been subjected to physical or sexual aggression.

The GP is often at a loss to intervene helpfully in this social rather than medical arena, but it is worth bearing in mind that some badly behaved teenagers may be responding to the irritation of ill-health or minor handicap. Does he need glasses, asthma treatment, or even a hearing aid? Is he embarrassed by his enuresis or small stature?

EMOTIONAL DISORDERS

Young people, like adults, suffer from such well-recognized disorders as excessive anxiety, phobia or depression. Anxiety sometimes presents as panic attacks—difficulty in breathing, palpitation, tingling fingers, fears of impending doom, hyperventilation, perhaps prompted by an exam or other crisis. Often repeated reassurance that there is no physical disease is enough but, if the symptoms become fixed, psychological therapy rather than mood altering drugs is the route to go down. The prescription of a psychotropic drug to an adolescent should be a rare event. The occasional use of a β-blocker (not for an asthmatic) before performing at the school concert or a similar event may be an exception.

Adolescent depression appears to be on the increase. The onset is often insidious and the depression difficult to diagnose. However, several factors may alert the GP to the fact that the depressive symptoms are more than the expected mood-swings of a teenager. The depressed young person may lack self-esteem and self-confidence and believe himself or herself to be unloved and unlovable. He or she becomes increasingly withdrawn, with a failing academic performance, and complains of constant tiredness unrelated to physical activity, even though lack of sleep is often a feature. Headache, tummy ache, panic attacks, and other somatic symptoms are not uncommon, as is a morbid preoccupation with minor physical blemishes. There may be no obvious cause for the depression, but it is not unusual to find that there has been a preceding crisis—loss of a girl- or boy-friend, failure to achieve an important goal, separation of parents or death of a grandparent.

The GP should not feel afraid to ask a severely depressed teenager about thoughts of suicide. There are about 100 suicides annually in teenagers aged 15–19, a rising number, and some 10 in children under 15. Deaths of boys are three times more frequent than those of girls. This sex ratio is reversed for episodes of self-harm. All threats of suicide should be taken seriously. They may be more dangerous than the adolescent intends, perhaps because the life-threatening interaction between drugs and alcohol is not appreciated. Even if they appear to be an impulsive reaction to a family crisis, referral to psychiatric services is usually indicated. According to Barker (1983), the risk of suicide is greatest when there is poor communication with an isolated adolescent, or if there has been a long preceding period of depression, or a history of self-destructive behaviour—perhaps a previous suicide attempt in circumstances where it was unlikely that the person was going to be found.

General practitioner management of a possibly suicidal teenager is not very different from that of older patients—easy accessibility, seeking support from a colleague so that the burden is not borne alone, seeing the young person frequently, perhaps several times a week in the first instance. The objective is to show that the GP cares and that the young person is someone worth helping. If it is decided to prescribe an antidepressant this should be done in collaboration with a psychiatric colleague. It is often advisable to give the supply to the practice nurse, instructing the depressed young person to come every couple of days to collect a few tablets. Counselling is an essential accompaniment to medication.

When an emotionally disturbed youngster presents for help, it is often a more efficient use of a general practice consultation to concentrate on the 'here and now' rather than to rake over ancient history, although the latter will be a necessary prelude to any psychotherapy. As far as formal referral is concerned the issues are similar to those applying to younger children (p. 80), but advisory services with easy and informal access are fairly widely available and can be very useful for self-referral, perhaps following encouragement by the GP. Like other agencies, such as genito-urinary clinics which do not require a GP's letter before a patient is seen, fears of breaching confidentiality may lead to problems of communication between clinic and family doctor. Such problems are less likely if the doctor sends an introductory letter to the local 'walk-in' clinic he has encouraged a young person to attend. The teenager may be pointed in the direction of these advisory services directly, or indirectly through the parents. If the young person agrees, it is sometimes useful to see him and parents together.

PERSONALITY CHANGE—IS IT PSYCHOTIC?

Sometimes previously ordinary youngsters suddenly appear to behave bizarrely, stop working at school for no obvious reason, become isolated from family and friends, and may take an unexpected overdose. Consultations may leave the doctor bewildered: 'What on earth is he on about?' There are a number of possibilities to consider. Most commonly the change will reflect problems at home—parental tensions, alcoholism or abuse of illicit drugs such as excessive cannabis or LSD. The bigger the change from the previous personality, the greater the concern. Could it be schizophrenia?—'What are the voices telling you?' or organic disease, such as temporal lobe epilepsy with perhaps a history of earlier seizures, or even a frontal lobe tumour or unexplained hypoglycaemia?

EATING DISORDERS

Many teenage girls are preoccupied with their weight, and watch and worry about the amount they eat. It is often difficult to decide when extreme examples of this tendency should be identified as anorexia nervosa. Some depressed teenagers will eat less when they feel wretched, others will nibble or binge. In some, perhaps, anorexia is a more deep-seated emotional strategy to put off adulthood. Florid anorexia nervosa may present with weight loss, obsessive dieting, even though underweight, and, sometimes, with secret self-induced vomiting. The majority of severely affected patients are girls. The hallmarks of anorexia nervosa are a disturbed body image and the desire to achieve control over one's life by means of diet. Patients' fear that this control may be removed by the GP results in a degree of denial of the problem. Other features are amenorrhoea and, ultimately, the degree of emaciation—a very important objective element in assessing the severity of the situation. Risk factors for developing anorexia nervosa include a neurotic perfectionist personality, a lack of self-confidence and unhappy life events such as losses.

Most severe anorectics end up requiring in-patient psychiatric treatment, the mainstay of which is, at present, an enforced weight gain, but, for every one of these, there are dozens of thin girls whose preoccupation with slimming borders on the pathological. For this reason parents may be worried that their daughter is becoming anorexic, while the girl appears unconcerned. It may be difficult to gain and maintain the teenager's confidence and the doctor needs to tread a difficult path between taking on board all the parents' anxieties and colluding with the girl's denial. The result is often a compromise of incomplete assessment and partial surveillance.

Bulimia is usually considered to be less lethal than anorexia and is up to ten times more common. Again it is mainly girls who are affected. They try to regain control over their chaotic eating habits by episodes of bingeing followed by self-induced vomiting. In severe cases, the chaos may extend to other areas of their life—finance or sexual behaviour. Laxatives may be used to reduce weight and there may also be intermittent episodes of severe dieting. Again the problem is that the young person lacks self-esteem and is obsessed with their shape and size. Diagnoses may be difficult because of denial of a problem and body-weight may remain within the normal range. The classical signs of bulimia are parotid gland enlargement, followed by erosion of dental enamel from self-induced vomiting. The dilemma is again deciding when the situation is genuinely serious; many young women appear to vomit without justifying a serious diagnostic label.

Successful management ultimately depends on the active involvement of the patient and her family. If a significant eating disorder is suspected, assessment begins with a discussion about general health (are there any symptoms of diabetes, renal failure, malabsorption, inflammatory bowel disease or pituitary tumours?), energy, regularity of periods, and social and school life. During the initial physical examination any obvious loss of weight is noted as well as general development. Initial investigations should include urinalysis and any blood tests indicated by the history. As mood often improves and the obsession with weight diminishes as the young person gains weight, the GP can help by negotiating an eating pattern centring round regular, adequate meals taken with others to achieve this, rather than a stop-go policy. Regular consultation for sequential weighing and a chat will be necessary, but the GP may need to keep a record of when the next appointment is due so that he can contact the girl if she fails to appear. Serious anorectics may be very devious, drinking several pints before the consultation and putting weights in their pockets to keep the prying doctor at bay, so weighing in minimal clothes is advisable—if this is acceptable. If possible at least enough of the child should be seen to establish if there is unexpected emaciation, as shown by thin muscles and redundant skin folds. In less serious cases, it is probably better if weighing does not happen at every consultation. This enables the focus to be shifted from weight to a discussion of emotions. Deciding the right moment for referral may be difficult. An earlier discussion with a psychiatric colleague may be helpful, even if the young person refuses an out-patient appointment. Referral is indicated if weight loss is marked or continuing, the GP feels he is losing control of the situation, or there is evidence of severe emotional disturbance.

About five per cent will die from the effects of disease or, more often, suicide (Scarth 1993).

ABUSE OF DRUGS

As far as the family doctor is concerned, the drug-taking teenager is often an absent patient, unless young enough to be dragged along by upset or irate adults, or mature enough to have decided that the time has come to get off drugs, perhaps because he is uneasy about their physical effects. More often, parents come alone, having discovered that their son or daughter is sniffing glue or taking cannabis or something stronger. Sometimes, an inebriated child who has sniffed glue, drunk alcohol, or eaten psychedelic mushrooms is taken straight to casualty.

Counselling the parents on their own, includes describing the possible effects of the relevant substance and advising on how to avoid a confrontation that will lead to parent and child taking up entrenched positions. We offer to see, examine and discuss the issues with the young person in a non-judgemental way, the teenager having first been told by the parents that they have discussed his or her drug-taking with the doctor.

Teenagers consulting with vague physical symptoms may be taking cannabis or other drugs but be afraid to admit this, partly because the possession of these drugs is illegal.

Smoking and drinking

It is hardly surprising that so many young smoke or drink alcohol when they get such mixed messages from society. Though it is illegal to sell tobacco to youngsters under 16 and alcohol to those under 18, these laws are usually flouted. About a quarter smoke while 43 per cent of 15-year-olds in England and Wales drink in pubs. Girls are taking to tobacco more than boys, partly because smoking helps them achieve fashionable thinness.

Drunkenness is commonplace at parties for older teenagers and adds to parents' reluctance to be involuntary hosts to these events. Alcohol effects are well known and include central nervous system depression leading to uninhibited behaviour, including unsafe sex. Moderate doses will lessen anxiety and may cause talkativeness and exaggerated cheerfulness until the person drinking falls asleep. Deleterious effects of alcohol on driving include a prolongation of reaction time, which may be especially lethal when combined with the overconfidence of youth. Parents have to be prepared to fetch their son or daughter from a party or at least pay for a taxi home. However, in general, young people do seem to be more aware of the risks of drinking and driving than their parents were or even are. Direct death from alcohol poisoning is usually due to respiratory depression or inhalation of vomit. Danger signs of excess drinking include an increase in intrafamily stress; frequent absences from school; excessively rowdy behaviour in public; stealing; alcohol-related accidents or unexplained gastro-intestinal problems.

Solvent abuse

Ten per cent of all deaths of 15-year-olds are caused by solvent abuse—most often inhalation of butane gas lighter fuel (Esmail *et al.* 1993).

The GP was phoned. The 15-year-old patient had been taken dead to casualty from the local shopping arcade. She and her friends, while truanting, had settled down to inhale typewriter correction fluid thinner. She may have had a cardiac arrhythmia. Post-mortem showed hydrocarbons in her urine but no pathological changes.

Solvent abuse is usually by younger adolescents. Hydrocarbons in glues, petrol, and dry-cleaning fluids, model-making cement, typing correction fluids, propellant gas from aerosols, produce on inhalation similar effects to alcohol. The youngster first feels euphoric, then becomes dizzy with blurring of vision, feelings of unreality, disorientation and ataxia. Visual hallucinations may occur. Acute intoxication comes on very quickly and disappears soon after the sniffing stops. A mild 'hangover' may be experienced following the session. Most sniffers inhale the vapours from a tube or bottle, others from a polythene bag over the mouth or nose.

Acute intoxication without alcohol ingestion suggests solvent abuse. Parents may smell the chemical in the child's breath and there may be signs of glue on clothes, face or hands, or empty containers in his room. In those who use a bag, 'glue sniffer's rash' , similar to acne, may develop where the bag rubs the chin and the bridge of the nose.

Although the majority of glue sniffers remain healthy, there is a danger of death not only from suffocation but also from inhalation of vomit, from an accident or a cardiac arrhythmia. Solvents may cause acute kidney, liver, and brain damage, apparently related to individual susceptibility rather than to the amount of solvent which has been inhaled. It is reversible in most but not all. Involvement in various sorts of antisocial behaviour is common in solvent users.

Ecstasy (methylene dioxymethamphetamine—MDMA)

Ecstasy is consumed by a large number of predominantly young people at 'raves', parties and clubs. Increased vigour and awareness of emotions and friendliness may result. Unpleasant experiences include anxiety and panic and a 'hungover' feeling the next day. Physical effects include sympathetic stimulation and an increase in body temperature which can lead to fatal hyperpyrexia after energetic dancing in an overcrowded hot room. Maintaining fluid intake at parties is important. Like heroin and cocaine, ecstasy is a class A substance, which means that its use can carry heavy penalties.

Heroin and other opiates (junk, skag, or smack)

Heroin can be smoked and injected. Purity of street heroin varies, with the associated risk of accidental overdose from unusually pure supplies. Besides being analgesic and euphoriant, these drugs produce sedation and depress the respiratory centre, cough reflex, and heart rate. Pupils constrict, blood vessels dilate, and reduced bowel activity leads to constipation. Nausea and vomiting are common with the first dose, but tolerance and dependence quickly occur and many addicts can appear to function normally.

Opiate withdrawal can be very unpleasant indeed, but is not life-threatening. The patient develops aches and muscular spasms, sweating, yawning, rhinorrhoea, and a feeling of cold. He is very anxious and is unable to sleep. Diarrhoea and spontaneous orgasms may develop.

Cocaine and derivatives (coke, crack)

The highly addictive cocaine is 'snorted' like snuff. 'Crack', cocaine extracted from its hydrochloride salt, vaporizes when heated. It can therefore be smoked, affecting the brain in about half a minute. The drug-induced stimulation and euphoria may be followed by depression. Cocaine overdose may cause hypertension, fits, and cardiac arrhythmias followed by respiratory or cardiac failure.

Repeated use of cocaine may cause ulceration of the nasal septum, insomnia, loss of appetite, and tolerance to some of the drugs' effects. It is an expensive drug, so its use may well be associated with criminal behaviour to obtain money.

Cannabis (grass, weed, marijuana, hash, dope)

Cannabis smoking is now very widespread amongst teenagers and regarded by some people as a normal part of growing up. According to a recently published survey by the Institute of Drug Dependency, 45 per cent of young people have tried cannabis by the age of 16. In most parts of the world the drug is usually smoked as part of a hand-rolled cigarette, often combined with tobacco. Sometimes it is baked in cakes (hash brownies, etc.). The effects, which start a few minutes after the drug is inhaled, seem to depend on the user's expectations and preliminary mood. Especially when smoking in a group, there is a pleasurable feeling of relaxation, hilarity, talkativeness, and enjoyment of company. With larger doses there may be altered sensory perception. Some people describe apparent slowing of the passage of time.

First-time users may become ataxic and not enjoy the experience, and a few continue to experience unpleasant sensations with the drug. Cannabis causes tachycardia and red eyes. It is an anti-emetic of some therapeutic use during cancer chemotherapy. It can also prevent muscular spasms in multiple sclerosis.

Management

When there is no sign of social dysfunction, and pressure for change comes from the parent rather than the teenager, gentle discussion of the parents' alcohol or tobacco use may help to lower the temperature by putting the child's or teenager's occasionally sniffing of glue or use of cannabis into perspective. When drugs and alcohol present a more serious problem, various management strategies have been suggested to help young people 'kick the habit'. A necessary prerequisite of all of them is that the doctor is non-judgemental and that the teenager wants to change his behaviour or is at least ambivalent. It may be useful to start by asking for a description of a typical day or week so that the doctor can get some idea of how important the substance is. Is there true dependence—daily use or withdrawal symptoms, relieved by taking more of the drug? It may be worth exploring the positive and negative aspects of the drug for the young person concerned. It makes him feel good and helps him get on with his peers, but is expensive and the hangover after weekend drinking unpleasant. A description of potential mental and physical dangers may be helpful as long as these are not rammed down teenagers' throats. Perhaps that part of the consultation should be preceded by 'would you like me to tell you about some of the effects of these drugs on your health?' The dangers depend on how much of what drug is taken by which route:

1. Even moderate doses of a psychoactive drug will impair reaction time and make, for example, dealing with traffic or playing on a building site more dangerous.

2. Increasing tolerance leads to a shortened effect from a given dose, which may mean that more money is needed to buy more of the drug. It may be easier for the doctor and teenager to start by discussing finance rather than long-term toxicity.

3. Increasing doses of more powerful drugs, such as the opiates or perhaps even very heavy cannabis use, may lead to self-neglect and physical as well as emotional ill-health, even though many heroin addicts look perfectly healthy and be well turned out.

4. For those people who are immersed in the drug scene, the hazards of injection include infection ranging from local abscesses and phlebitis to septicaemia, hepatitis, or AIDS. The incidence of other sexually transmitted diseases is also high.

A physical examination provides reassurance for many young people anxious about their drug habit. Often nothing is found, but the opiate addict may have lost weight or show signs of complications of the addiction. There may be thrombosed veins with local cellulitis, and injection abscesses, signs of a chronic chest infection, hepato-splenomegaly, jaundice, or lymphadenopathy. An examination may also be important in confirming that a patient who says he is not injecting himself is telling the truth.

For opiates the standard management is replacement of the drug with a decreasing dose of methadone. It may be worthwhile prescribing a short course of this substance on one occasion, where the GP has a well-established relationship with the family, even if he is sceptical that the young person is committed to giving up the drug at this stage. When he is better motivated he may return to his GP for help. If abstinence is part of a contract between doctor and patient, screening urine for various psychotropic drugs including opiates, amphetamines and barbiturates and cannabis (which may be present for up to three weeks after use) can be part of an agreed monitoring plan. A urine check is also occasionally justified for clarifying the situation in a child or young adolescent with bizarre, unexplained symptoms.

Teenagers on heroin are usually referred to a drug-dependency clinic, unless the practice is in an area where there is good support for managing them in the practice—a new trend. Liaison between GP and clinic must be good so that the regime negotiated between the clinic and teenager is not undermined by the GP, for example, prescribing a benzodiazepine without agreement. One must be wary of being manipulated by this group of patients. Some drug-dependency units run outreach clinics in general practices. Shared care between the GP and the drug worker can be very beneficial. If there is no chance of the drug clinic being used, or if it seems inappropriate, the family or patient may find one of the local voluntary support agencies helpful. They range from simple 'walk-in' clinics to residential hostels. Information about local agencies given in the telephone directory may also be obtained from the Standing Conference on Drug Abuse (SCODA), 49 Copperfield Street, SE1 (tel. 0171 928 9500).

Schemes for providing intravenous drug users with sterile injecting equipment and free condoms will hopefully reduce their risk of hepatitis and HIV infection.

MENSTRUAL PROBLEMS

Irregular or infrequent periods during the menarche are not unusual. It may take a couple of years for ovulation to be fully established, although the girl may be fertile before this occurs. There may also be temporary menorrhagia before ovulation becomes regular, allegedly because of unopposed oestrogen secretion. Most girls with menorrhagia are reassured by an explanation combined, if necessary, with prescription of iron and dietary advice. Painful, colicky, lower abdominal dysmenorrhoea at the onset of a period is common in the early teens, sometimes associated with nausea, headache, or irritability. An analgesic should be tried first, the combined oestrogen–progesterone pill being reserved for those who also need contraceptive protection. Aspirin with codeine is sometimes helpful, as are non-steroidal drugs such as ibuprofen or mefenamic acid (Ponstan). These drugs work because of their anti-prostaglandin effect. Some girls will consult about a period problem when they really want to discuss contraception, and others may be concerned that they could be pregnant but be reluctant to voice this fear openly. This issue can sometimes be approached by the GP including a question about the menstrual cycle when asking about other bodily functions—'When was your last period; was it normal?' This can be followed by an invitation—'You know you can come here for contraception, don't you. It is completely confidential and you can see me or the practice nurse'.

TEENAGERS AND CONTRACEPTION

According to a survey from the University of Exeter, 40 per cent of teenagers in recent years have had sexual intercourse by the age of 16, with a third not having used contraception during their most recent intercourse. A third of the young people surveyed had, during their most recent sexual encounter, used the pill and a third used condoms. According to Guillebaud *et al.* (1993), the most common pattern of sexual activity amongst teenage girls is serial monogamy, including, perhaps, the occasional casual sexual encounter.

Some young people will go to the GP for contraceptive advice, but many will prefer to visit a youth advisory centre or a family planning clinic especially geared to the needs of young people, such as a Brook Advisory Centre—flexible times for consultation, sensitive non-hurried counselling, on the spot pregnancy testing, and, if indicated, rapid referral for abortion.

Methods of contraception

Many young people do not like condoms, complaining that pleasure is reduced and that they worry about the danger of it tearing. However, there is an increasing awareness of the risk of sexually transmitted disease, particularly HIV infection. Many couples will use condoms even if the girl is also on the pill. They may not be aware that condoms are available free at family planning clinics and some practices. They may be used at the beginning of a relationship and then discarded for the pill if the relationship continues. Many young people will opt for an HIV test before abandoning the condom.

The pill is the most popular form of contraceptive for young people. The advantages and disadvantages are shown in Table 7.1.

Diaphragms are less acceptable to teenage girls because they are more complicated to use. However, unlike condoms, they can be inserted several hours before possible intercourse. They give some protection against some bacterial sexually transmitted diseases. Intrauterine contraceptive devices (IUCDs) are not advised for young nulliparous women because of the increased risk of pelvic infection. However, the new progesterone-coated IUCD may protect against infection and thus may be a good alternative to the pill.

Many teenagers are unaware that the inappropriately named 'morning after' pill can be given up to 72 hours after unprotected intercourse. There is a 2–4 per cent failure rate per cycle (Guillebaud *et al.* 1993). An IUCD inserted up to five days after unprotected intercourse is a less satisfactory method, but still preferable to termination of pregnancy.

TEENAGE PREGNANCY

In 1991, there were 103 000 teenage pregnancies (about a third were terminated). Over 80 per cent of these births were to mothers who were not married though

Table 7.1 Advantages and disadvantages of oral contraception

Advantages	Disadvantages
Most effective contraceptive	Occasional nausea, headache and weight gain
Reversible	No protection from STD
May reduce heavy periods and pre-menstrual tension	Possible increase in the risk of vascular disease, particularly in women who smoke—a low risk in adolescence
40 per cent reduction in risk of developing epithelial ovarian carcinoma	Tiresome breakthrough bleeding
50 per cent reduction in endometrial carcinoma	Possible increase in risk of cervical dysplasia (but this may be more related to whether the teenager smokes or has several sexual partners)
Reduction in benign breast disease	
50 per cent reduction in the incidence of pelvic inflammatory disease (due to the progesterone effect on cervical mucus)	Incidence of breast carcinoma increase from 2 to 3 per thousand after more than 4 years of use of the pill (a first degree relative with a history of carcinoma of the breast is a relative contra-indication)
Reduces the incidence of uterine fibroids and endometriosis	Post-pill menstrual irregularity

Based on Guillebaud *et al.* (1993).

often living in a stable relationship (Social Trends 1994). Half of the pregnancies in under-16s and a third of those in 16- to 19-year-olds were aborted (Seamark 1994).

The GP's advice may be sought by a teenager, uncertain whether or not to continue with the pregnancy or just needing support. The doctor needs to make a careful assessment of the situation before presenting the pros and cons of any course of action. What is the father's attitude; is he likely to remain on the scene? Was the pregnancy the result of a casual affair, or of a couple of forgotten pills, or occurring in the context of a long-lasting relationship? A third of marriages that begin under these circumstances break down within a year. It may sometimes be necessary to raise the issue of whether drugs, alcohol, coercion, or even sexual abuse were related to the conception. If the girl decides to have a child, how will she cope with the inevitable restriction of her social life or with changes in her plans to continue at school or college? A baby may be visualized as a cuddly object able to fill an emotional gap in a young teenager's life. Will mother and child be able to count on a supportive family network or, indeed, has she become pregnant as an act of defiance or as a means of escaping from her parents? Will they be able to live with family or friends or will they have to move to a poky flat or 'bed and breakfast' accommodation provided by the council for the 'homeless'? Will she manage financially even with state support? The GP must respect the wishes of a teenager who is insistent that parents should not be told, perhaps because of the fear that she will be forced into a course of action which is against her wishes, be it an abortion or continuation of the pregnancy. She may, in fact, not realize that a termination can be arranged on the NHS

The GP should arrange to see a teenager a few weeks after a termination and actively follow-up those who fail to keep this appointment, to ensure that adequate contraception has been started. She may be bereaved even if she was sure that she did not want to continue with the pregnancy. It is important also to check that she is physically all right and to ask about the relationship with her boyfriend and possibly also her parents.

A single teenage mother frequently has problems in rearing her child or children and is more likely to become seriously depressed than her peers. If she lives in the inner city, stresses of that environment—decaying housing, unemployment, easy availability of drugs, and pervasive fear of violence—add to her difficulties. She may come from an unstable family background which gave her little experience of adequate parenting on which to model her behaviour. Some of these young mothers are welcomed with their babies into the grandparents' family and eventually mature into competent wives and mothers—for others, motherhood is a struggle throughout.

Mary had a 22-week termination of pregnancy when she was 16 years old. Two-and-a-half years later she became pregnant again and decided to keep the baby, partly because she thought she was going to stay with the father and partly because she had found the previous abortion such an unpleasant experience. She had been brought up in a family of four children. The father drank heavily and took little part in the children's upbringing and her mother 'slagged her off in front of other people'. After the birth of the baby, she went to live three miles away in a council house with her delinquent boyfriend. Unfortunately, the relationship quickly collapsed and she returned with her 3-month-old baby to a familiar neighbourhood, staying with young friends who provided warm, although rather intermittent, support. Mary visited her GP in tears requesting a housing letter.

These young people need intensive support from health visitors and often the social services. It is sometimes difficult to keep tabs on their movements, particularly if they are placed by the local authority in temporary accommodation. Their practice records should contain the names and telephone numbers of other professionals involved in their care. There may be a young mothers' group run by health visitors, and some community midwives have special antenatal sessions for teenagers who are pregnant.The GP needs to be on the look-out for signs that the mother is not coping and be aware that there may be frequent emergency calls. (See p. 62—'snowed under mums'.) Is the baby beginning to suffer physically or is the rumour that he is being left alone unattended for long periods true? If all the available services have already been mobilized, has the time come to discuss possible fostering? In any event, is the mother using reliable contraception?

SEXUALLY TRANSMITTED DISEASES (STD)

Early sexual intercourse and promiscuity are associated with an increased risk of adolescent STD; in addition the immature young person is, in any case, less likely to use a condom.

Classically, the adolescent girl with sexually transmitted vaginitis or cervicitis will present with a profuse, irritating, offensive, vaginal discharge. Dysuria may be present and vulval soreness with ulceration. Teenage girls tend to present late with pelvic inflammatory disease (PID). This in turn may lead to subsequent ectopic pregnancy or infertility. Not all vaginal discharges are pathological. The teenager may have focused on her normal vaginal secretions, a concern which can lead on to a discussion of issues arising from her sexuality.

In general practice, the commonest cause of an irritating vaginal discharge or vulvitis is vaginal candida, perhaps a particular problem for girls on the pill.

The infected boy is likely to have a urethral discharge, dysuria, sometimes balanitis or even penile ulceration. Sexually active adolescents appear to be particularly vulnerable to chlamydia, this obligate, intracellular bacterium being the cause of about 50 per cent of non-gonococcal urethritis. Doxycycline 100 mg twice a day for a week is the treatment of choice for chlamydia or non-gonococcal urethritis, with erythromycin as an alternative. Pubic lice, genital warts from the papilloma virus, genital herpes with multiple ulcers causing pain and a burning sensation, and scabies, are other sexually transmitted diseases.

If STD is a serious possibility, most GPs will refer the young person to a genito-urinary clinic, hopefully one with expertise in dealing with adolescents. This policy of referral may be a counsel of perfection for the older adolescent girl whose cervical swab grows only trichomonas. Those referred will get the full range of tests including vaginal and cervical swabs for trichomonas and bacterial vaginosis, *N.gonorrhoeae* and *Chlamydia trachomatis*. Genital ulcers will be cultured and examined for treponema and the herpes simplex virus. Rectal and oral swabs may be indicated and blood tests for syphilis, hepatitis B, and, in some cases, HIV. If a significant STD is confirmed, contact tracing is essential, as infected partners are often asymptomatic. Finally, if a boy is seen with genital herpes or warts, his girl-friend should be advised to have a cervical smear.

Bibliography

Barker, P. (1983). *Basic child psychiatry*, (4th edn). Blackwell, Oxford.

Black, D. and Cottrell, D. (ed.) (1993). *Seminars in child and adolescent psychiatry*. Royal College of Psychiatrists, London. (Gaskell—a comprehensive review of this specialty).

Confidentiality and people under 16. (1993). Guidance issued jointly by the BMA, GMSC, HBA, Brook Advisory Centres, SPA, and RCGP.

Cooklin, A. (1993). Psychological changes of adolescence. In *The practice of medicine in adolescence*, (ed. C. G. D. Brook). Edward Arnold, London.
Cowan, F. and Mindel, A. (1993). Sexually transmitted diseases. In *The practice of medicine in adolescence*, (ed. C. G. D. Brook). Edward Arnold, London.
Esmail, A., Meyer, L., Pottier, A. *et al.* (1993). Deaths from volatile substance abuse in those under 18 years: results from a national epidemiological study. *Archives of Disease in Childhood*, **69**, 356–60.
Farell, M. *et al.* (1993). In *The practice of medicine in adolescence*, (ed. C. G. D. Brook). Edward Arnold, London.
Guillebaud J., Shaw, J., and Gray, K. (1993). Contraception and sexual health. In *The practice of medicine in adolescence*, (ed. C. G. D. Brook). Edward Arnold, London.
Mortality statistics. (1992). Review of the Registrar General on deaths by cause, sex, and age in England and Wales. Series DH2. OPCS, HMSO, London.
Scarth, L. (1993). Clinical syndromes in adolescence. In *Seminars in Child and Adolescent Psychiatry*. (ed. D. Black and D. Cottrell). Royal College of Psychiatrists, London.
Seamark, C. J. (1994). Teenage sexuality and general practice. In *RCGP members' reference book, 1994*. The Royal College of General Practitioners, London.
Social Trends. (1994). No. 24. Central Statistical Office, HMSO, London.
Strang, J. and Edwards, G. (1989). Cocaine and crack. *British Medical Journal*, **299**, 337–8.
Viles, R. (1985). Gynaecology problems in adolescents. In *Progress in child health*, Vol. 2, (ed. J. MacFarlane). Churchill Livingstone, London.

8 Children with disabilities, and school health services

The World Health Organization has defined *impairment* as a pathological process affecting normal physiology or anatomy, *disability* as reduced ability to perform normal functions resulting from an impairment, and *handicap* as the consequence or disadvantage for an individual resulting from a disability or an impairment. Until the last decade mental handicap was defined by comparing a child's intellectual ability to that of his peers. Intelligence tests were a standardized means of measuring a child's mental age from which IQ could be calculated, by dividing the mental age by the real age and multiplying by 100. Thus the general development of a 10-year-old child with an IQ of 20 was equivalent to that of a child of 2 years. IQ scores formed the basis for planning for an individual's educational needs.

THE EDUCATION ACT 1981

The above approach has been abandoned following the 1981 Education Act, which was based on the report of the Warnock (1978) Committee. The recommended use of the term 'special educational needs', takes into account not only the child's particular disability but also his abilities and all other factors (for example, emotional, social and cultural) which may have a bearing on his progress. According to the Warnock Committee, up to 20 per cent of children have special educational needs at some stage during their school careers, the majority of whom can be educated within mainstream schools, with or without special extra provision; for example, a care assistant for a child with cerebral palsy. Others, for example children with visual impairment, may need to be placed in special units usually in or next to mainstream schools.

An important aim of this Act was to promote social and functional integration between pupils with and without disabilities. However, some disabled children may prefer to be in a special school to avoid comparison with non-disabled peers. A special school provides structured learning in small groups with a low pupil to teacher ratio. In some schools the child will also receive help from physiotherapists, occupational, and speech therapists.

The decision as to the best form of educational placement for the child is legally a matter for the local Educational Authority and not medical authorities, but a doctor will be asked to contribute to the decision-making process. About 2 per cent of children with severe or complex learning difficulties require a statutory assessment resulting in the issue of a 'statement of special educational needs'. This statement is based on reports and advice obtained from parents, teachers (including nursery school teachers), the GP and health visitor, the designated medical officer, educational psychologists, social services and other services if involved. The procedure encourages openness with the parents and the doctor may be wise to remember that any reports that he provides for this purpose may be shown to them. Following the 1993 Education Act health advice may be requested before the stage of assessment for a statement of special educational needs. Once this assessment process is formally started the final statement must be produced within 12 weeks.

If the GP is concerned about the education of one of his young patients, the most useful person to contact varies from place to place. In general, the senior clinical medical officer (SCMO) or community paediatrician with particular responsibility for special education is a useful starting point. Disputed decisions over educational arrangements may be taken to appeal and the statement must be reviewed every year.

THE CHILD WITH LEARNING DIFFICULTIES

Infants with moderate to severe intellectual handicap may present with a recognizable syndrome or malformation shortly after birth (for example, Down syndrome) or with global developmental delay which may become evident during child health surveillance. Often the parents are the first to suspect that all is not right, but individuals with mild or moderate learning difficulties may only be identified when they fail to keep up with academic work in school.

Commoner known causes of learning difficulties

Though many children with severe learning disability have Down or fragile-X syndromes no cause can be found for many of the remainder. Such children may show delay in all fields of development, but the picture can be very patchy. Delay is often greatest in the development of social responsiveness and communication but least in gross motor development. A Down syndrome baby may show normal motor development in early months of life. There is a wide range from those who have profound disability to those who pass leaving certificate examinations and are capable of employment.

The degree of interest and attention the baby pays to his surroundings is the most important point. Thus, a nine-month-old baby with developmental delay may sit on his mother's knee passively, paying only fleeting attention to any toy or brick he is presented with, making very little spontaneous attempt to pick the

Table 8.1 Commoner known causes of learning difficulties

Prenatal factors
Chromosomal/single gene defects (examples)
Down syndrome, fragile-X syndrome, mucopolysaccharidosis
Dysmorphic syndromes (e.g. William's syndrome)
Prenatal infections (examples)
Rubella, toxoplasmosis and cytomegalovirus
Other environmental factors (examples)
Drugs and alcohol, irradiation
Perinatal factors
Trauma
Hypoxia
Preterm birth and its complications
Postnatal factors
Trauma (e.g. head injuries, accidental or non-accidental)
Infections (e.g. meningitis and encephalitis)
Poisoning
Neglect, abuse and emotional deprivation

toy up himself. He may make a poor range of sounds and the examiner may be concerned that he is deaf because he fails to turn to auditory stimuli, or only turns very slowly, when in fact his hearing is normal. His mother may complain that he sleeps excessively, or remark that he is a very "good" baby, causing no bother because he does not cry as normal babies do to attract attention. All of these should alert concern. So should the persistence of a behaviour pattern beyond an appropriate age . Whereas a normal nine-month-old is usually able to chew, the learning impaired child may have great difficulties with lumpy foods and still be eating strained products. In the second half of the first year, infants put all objects into their mouths, but this mouthing usually stops during the second year. Its persistence is further evidence of function below the chronological level.

In contrast to the globally delayed child, an intelligent deaf child will show a lack of responsiveness to speech, but normal or increased visual alertness and ability to manipulate. A shy child in unfamiliar surroundings may not perform too well during developmental assessment: neither may one who is distracted by a toddler wandering around the room, or is chronically or acutely unwell. Drugs, such as antihistamines may dull the senses. In short, a firm opinion based on one examination may be inaccurate; further assessment is nearly always necessary, perhaps done in the home by the health visitor.

One of the most difficult problems to assess is how far inadequate home circumstances are contributing to developmental delay. Does the child have a remediable developmental delay secondary to being left all day in his pram and not played with, or, on the contrary, is he constitutionally delayed and possibly contributing to his own under-stimulation by not stimulating the mother?

As maternal depression or neglect is often an important contributory factor, psychosocial intervention, such as more support for the mother, a day nursery place or even temporary fostering or adoption, may be needed. It will have more chance of benefiting the child's development if arranged at two or three years of age rather than later when the child is not coping at school. Very occasionally, with an uncooperative family, care proceedings on the grounds that proper development is being avoidably prevented or neglected will be needed. The doctor, health visitor, and social worker may discuss the situation and decide that such intervention is likely to be inappropriate or counter-productive, undermining the mother's confidence without substantially helping the child.

Globally-delayed children are often very slow in gaining bowel and bladder control. A family history of learning difficulties and speech delay are much commoner in delayed children than in the general population. It is clear that genetic, physical, and environmental factors are closely interrelated in these children's problems.

Even though a precise biological cause cannot always be identified, there are several reasons for trying to make an accurate diagnosis. First, prevention is difficult without a knowledge of aetiology and some causes may recur in further pregnancies if preventive action is not taken. Secondly, a precise explanation of itself contributes to the parents' peace of mind, and, thirdly, treatment of some conditions, such as phenylketonuria, hypothyroidism, hydrocephalus, or lead poisoning, may prevent further deterioration even though reversal of established delay may not be possible.

Management of the child with learning difficulties

In most cases, specific treatment is not possible and management must be directed towards:

(a) Providing support for the family

The news that a child is intellectually impaired is devastating to parents and must be handled with tact and sensitivity. Though the initial information will usually come from the paediatrician, the GP may need to repeat it and gradually discuss the implications. There may be several difficult months or years of uncertainty before the exact diagnosis and extent of the child's problem become clear. The child will often have multiple problems, including sensory impairment, and good liaison between the GP, health visitor, social services, child development team and local consultant community paediatrician is essential in ensuring that the family is aware of all local help. Have they claimed all the benefits that they are entitled to? Do the family know the address of the relevant voluntary society? Are they aware that the local authority may pay towards the rental of a telephone? Respite care by a 'foster' family is sometimes possible during annual holidays or when there is additional stress in the family caused, for example, by illness or moving house.

(b) Appropriate education services

When possible these should be provided in local mainstream schools, especially in primary school with appropriate support. However, children with profound and multiple disabilities have needs which are most likely to be met in a special school.

(c) Providing treatment of associated problems

Many intellectually handicapped children will have other medical problems which may require treatment, such as congenital heart disease in children with Down syndrome. Others may have epilepsy, hearing or visual impairments, or orthopaedic disorders.

Paramedical staff, including physiotherapists, occupational therapists, and speech and language therapists, have an important role in assessment and management of these children. They may see the child at a local child development centre or provide peripatetic services (at home or at school).

DEVELOPMENTAL REGRESSION

Rarely, an infant not only fails to learn new skills but begins to lose those that he already has, while very rarely in an older child there may be an unexplained decline in school performance. Such developmental regression is seen in infants with space-occupying lesions, such as brain tumours or subdural haematomas; they may also develop a full fontanelle and an abnormally large head, together with neurological signs similar to cerebral palsy. It is also seen in children with severe biochemical disorders in which there is progressive damage to the brain.

One example is Tay–Sachs disease in which developmental regression proceeds to blindness, severe dementia, seizures, and death. In this condition, sphingolipids gradually accumulate excessively in the brain because they cannot be degraded; the necessary enzyme, hexosaminidase A, is missing from the cells. There are a number of such storage conditions and in most of them the diagnosis can be made from a blood sample by enzyme or molecular genetic techniques. Serious regression of development is also seen with the onset of infantile spasms (Salaam epilepsy), usually in the early months of life. These seizures can be easily missed at first, as they consist of episodes of repeated flexing of the trunk or nodding the head (p. 264). In the older child, frequent *petit mal* or other 'minor' convulsions may impair alertness and lead to regression. On the other hand, chronic anticonvulsant toxicity may produce the same end result. Subacute sclerosing panencephalitis is the commonest childhood degenerative disease in the UK, and preventable by full measles immunization of the child population (p. 152).

While mild degrees of developmental regression are seen in a child who has had a trivial illness or who is subject to a domestic upset, it is clear that more serious regression requires detailed investigation and may have a very serious implication for the child's future.

CHILD DEVELOPMENT TEAMS

Most health districts have a child development team to co-ordinate the care of children with special needs and contribute to the Educational Assessment procedure. Membership varies, but usually includes a senior clinical medical officer or community paediatrician, child psychiatrist, health visitor, psychologist, physiotherapist, speech therapist, and administrator. Other doctors, including GPs or medical or surgical specialists, and other professionals, especially teachers and social workers, are invited to case conferences when appropriate. Teams accept referral of children under 16 whose development is causing concern. After the child's needs have been assessed, a management plan is produced. Other functions include co-ordinating care with relevant statutory and voluntary bodies, and giving information and advice to other professionals and to parents. Members of the team sometimes act in an advisory capacity but at other times accept clinical responsibility for treating some of the children referred.

The range of disorders dealt with includes significant developmental delay, cerebral palsy, malformation syndromes, visual and hearing disability, or emotional problems associated with other disabilities. Family doctors and health visitors should bear the team in mind when a child is seen, who has a significant developmental disorder which will involve the skills of several different specialties.

HELP FOR CHILDREN WITH DISABILITIES

Organizations such as **Barnardo's**, **SCOPE**, and **MENCAP** provide support for parents and information about specific disabilities. Financial hardship may result both from reduced income (reduced overtime, deferred promotion or mother cannot go out to work) and increased expenditure (special diet and increased laundry costs). A social worker or a welfare rights officer, will be able to help the family with applications to claim financial benefits (which are their child's right) from the Department of Social Security and charitable bodies.

1. The **Disability Living Allowance** (DLA) from the DSS is payable to a child who needs help for more than three months with personal care, and/or getting around. There are two components to DLA:

(a) the **care** component if the child needs help because he is ill or disabled. There are three rates of care allowance depending on the degree of help needed and on whether night care is needed;

(b) the **mobility** component if the child is five or over and needs help with getting around. There are two rates of mobility allowance—one for those who are unable to walk and one for those able to walk but requiring supervision.

Parents whose child is receiving the care or the mobility component of the DLA can apply to be exempt from road vehicle tax and for the disabled (orange) car parking sticker.

2. Parents or guardians who spend at least 35 hours per week caring for a child receiving the DLA may be eligible for the **Invalid Care Allowance** (ICA). The ICA is taxable and is taken into account when claiming other benefits, such as Income Support. An adult accompanying the child with a Disabled Rail Card is entitled to travel half fare.
3. Needy families may qualify for **Income Support**, **Family Credit**, or loans from the **Social Fund**. The **Disabled Child Premium** is added to the Income Support if there is a child in the family receiving DLA.
4. Funds can be provided by the local authority to alter even a privately-owned house or flat to make it suitable for a handicapped child.
5. The Joseph Rowntree Trust administer the **Family Fund** on behalf of the Government to provide *ad hoc* financial aid for families with a severely handicapped child under the age of 16. Money is given for items such as washing machines, clothes and holiday expenses.
6. Social services may be able to put the families in touch with link families or family groups offering short-term respite care for the child when the family goes on holiday.

CEREBRAL PALSY

Much of what has been said above applies to cerebral palsy, defined as a group of disorders of movement and posture due to developmental defect or damage to the immature brain. Learning disability, seizures, and disorders of vision and hearing are often associated with cerebral palsy. However, children with cerebral palsy can be of normal intelligence. A good example was Christy Brown, the Dublin novelist whose book *Down all the days* (Brown 1970) gives a striking picture of the athetoid cerebral palsy from which he suffered (later made into the film *My left foot*).

Cerebral palsy is more likely after preterm birth or after poor growth *in utero*, perhaps associated with hypoxia during delivery or with neonatal hyperbilirubinaemia. Post-natal brain damage from meningitis, encephalitis, or head injury can also be responsible in 10 to 15 per cent of cases. Sometimes it develops despite an uncomplicated full-term birth and in at least two-thirds of these cases there is no obvious cause identified (Robinson 1991).

Children with cerebral palsy are relatively uncommon (2.5/1000) and the average GP will only look after one such child. It may be spastic, athetoid, mixed, or hypotonic in type. Spastic cerebral palsy is commonest and presents with delay in motor and often social development, or in milder cases, if one-sided, with failure to use an arm or dragging of a leg. There may be paucity of movement so that the affected baby lies relatively immobile. The hands are likely to be kept tightly closed beyond the age of three months and there may be evidence of increased extensor tone, so that when held face down he may arch his back with extension of the neck, giving the unwary doctor a false impression of good motor power. However on pulling to sitting from a face-up position there will be a gross head lag, as flexion is weaker than extension. There is increased muscle tone which can be shown at 4–6 months by holding the baby vertically. Normally the hips and knees are flexed, but in diplegic or quadriplegic spastic cerebral palsy they are extended and crossed—'scissored', because of adductor spasm—and this may lead to difficulties with changing of nappies in severe cases. Tendon reflexes are brisk, a difficult sign to evaluate, and primitive reflexes such as the Moro persist beyond the age of five months. If spasticity is hemiplegic the hand is more severely affected than the foot, and kept closed, or an object may be approached with the whole hand rather than with the index finger long after the other hand's approach has matured. In spastic diplegia, scissoring of the legs is particularly striking and secondary dislocation of the hip may occur.

Children who show signs of ataxic or athetoid cerebral palsy in latter years go through a period of generalized hypotonia in early infancy, the striking physical sign being the way the infant feels likely to slip through the hands when being held. Joints are also abnormally mobile. Hypotonia is usually followed by subsequent development of ataxia or athetosis. Hypotonia may be a feature of many other conditions such as Down syndrome, neuromuscular disorders, biochemical disturbances, such as hypercalcaemia, and vitamin D deficiency. If a child has definite hypotonia but normal or near-normal mental development, referral for accurate diagnosis is important for both treatment, when available, and for genetic counselling. There is a high risk of recurrence and a poor prognosis as with X-linked Duchenne muscular dystrophy. This presents as walking delay or falls, with difficulty in getting up again. Examination may show hypertrophied calves and increasing muscular weakness in boys. The serum creatine phosphokinase is very high. Spinal muscular atrophy, which is also progressive and ultimately fatal, presents most commonly in infancy with marked hypotonia, sometimes leading to repeated chest infection through difficulty in coughing.

If early motor development is abnormal, the GP should refer the child to a child development centre which can provide the comprehensive care that such children need. He should check every now and again that the child and his family have access to, and make use of, the relevant help. The management of cerebral palsy is directed towards maximizing function and preventing secondary disability and handicap. Physiotherapy provides very important support for the parents and will help the child make the most of his limited motor power and co-ordination and prevent contractures by promoting activity, good posture and appropriate chairs etc. Physiotherapists have confidence in handling severely disabled small children in ways that encourage the parents to do the same. They will also advise on the appropriate mobility equipment and appliances, such as buggies and walking aids. Orthopaedic procedures are occasionally helpful for the correction of fixed contractures and for joint dislocations if this will improve function or reduce discomfort. Speech therapy is important for children with difficulty in verbal communication. Visual problems including squints, hemianopias, and reduced visual acuity, and helped by glasses, occur commonly. About a third will have fits.

Even in child development centres the staff come and go, and the GP, together with the health visitor, may need to be major figures of constant sympathetic support.

SPEECH AND LANGUAGE DELAY

Speech and language are complex neurological activities, so it is not surprising that children with cerebral palsy or developmental delay are usually slow to talk. Delayed language is also seen as a normal variant, as well as in deaf children, and very rarely as a symptom of autism or, as an isolated handicap, developmental aphasia. Some normal two-year-olds will only use a dozen or so words, others deploy more than two hundred.

By his first birthday the average baby babbles continually and understands simple commands associated with gestures. He imitates an adult's vocalization, and knows and turns to his name. He may say one or two words with meaning. Six months later he uses a number of single words and understands many more but may still jabber, using a wide range of inflections and sounds. The majority of words are nouns and are used rather loosely to cover other objects in the same category: 'daddy' for 'man', 'pussy' for 'dog'! By the second birthday he understands most of what is said to him. Two or three words are joined together and there is more grammar: not 'Daddy', but 'Daddy home now'. The child refers to himself by name, and constantly, and sometimes tryingly, asks what everything is. Lisps, misarticulations, and frank stammering are a normal variation at this age, but should gradually lessen over the next year or two. Early speech may be difficult for anyone except the doting parents to understand. Normal children tend to repeat what is said to them until they are about two-and-a-half-years-old.

By three years all but 3–4 per cent utter appropriate three-word phrases. Usually the child has a large, mostly intelligible, vocabulary, but many words are still mispronounced. Questions are often of the 'where?' and 'who?' variety, while by four there are many beginning with 'why?' Signs of a possible problem in speech or language development include failure to turn to sounds made nearby at six months, saying only half-a-dozen single words at 21 months, speaking in two-word phases at two years, speech unintelligible to family members at two-and-a-half, and having no small sentences by the age of three.

Acquiring language requires someone to listen to, adequate hearing, thought, and motor activity. If things are delayed the doctor must ask himself: Do the parents fail to talk to the child or speak different languages? Is the child deaf? Is there a learning difficulty? or (and rarely) is there a problem in making the co-ordinated movements necessary for speech? Most commonly one is dealing with an isolated delay in speech development in a developmentally normal hearing child. Speech delay is commoner in boys and socially disorganized families and may be one of the first steps along the road to subsequent educational failure.

It is easy to overlook partial deafness, perhaps from glue ear, as a cause of speech delay. The child may respond normally to moderate or loud signs, and the speech problem will be unexplained unless the child's difficulty in distinguishing between quietly spoken sounds is appreciated. Testing of hearing is discussed on p. 30. The normal, intelligent, severely deaf child will be alert and active, watch faces intently and understand gestures, though he shows no response to sound and does not understand what is being said to him.

On rare occasions delayed speech may be a presenting feature of mild cerebral palsy. Exceptionally rarely, the non-communicating child may be autistic. The most striking feature of autism is inability to recognize other human beings, including the parents, as persons rather than as objects. These children are not cuddly and may spend many hours in solitary, stereotyped play, often failing to make eye-to-eye contact. They also may perform curious repetitive rituals or mannerisms. Most end up very disabled, but occasionally children have islands of talent that can be tapped with patient special education. Very occasionally, children can have isolated aphasia in the presence of normal hearing, intelligence, motor function, and psychological behaviour. Such a child can be taught some degree of speech through years of intensive speech therapy. In its severe form it is a major handicap.

The doctor should clearly exclude deafness early. This done, evaluation by the health visitor at home may well clarify the problem as speech delay. How much do the parents play and talk with the child? Is the mother depressed? Does she go out to work leaving the child with a child-minder who has to look after several other children, so that he receives little verbal stimulation? Children who come from families where the parents do not speak English are unlikely to speak the language until they start nursery or school. Somewhat delayed acquisition of speech may be a small price to pay for the ultimate ability to speak two languages. However, if such a child has one of the other problems mentioned above, the difficulty will be compounded. The two to two-and-a-half-year-old child who is definitely behind with speech development may be worth referring to a speech and language therapist, who can both advise the mother on how to enrich the auditory input to the child, and also make a more precise measurement of the child's verbal development—a useful baseline when interpreting progress over the following year or two.

THE SCHOOL HEALTH SERVICES

School nurses, supported by parents, teachers and the school doctor, play a key role in delivering school health services. They are registered general nurses and many are also registered sick children's nurses. An increasing number have also completed a post-graduate specialist school nursing course. The nurse will be involved in health education, in counselling, and in providing help with social problems, as well as screening for disorders of vision, hearing, posture, and growth. Each school usually has an attached school doctor who will see children selected for a school entry medical, children referred because of concerns about their health, and children being assessed under the Education Act. These doctors are supported by a community paediatrician.

The important elements of a school health programme include:

(a) **Child health surveillance in school**
Routine screening for growth, vision, and hearing problems by school nurses still continues in most areas, but routine medical examination at school entrance is being replaced by a selective system. Children are selected for examination if problems are identified at a health interview conducted by the school nurse, or if the teacher, parent(s) or GP are concerned about the child's health. It is important for the GP to pass on information on problems identified through child health surveillance to the community child health services, where it can be stored on the district child health computer system.

(b) **Immunization**
Some GPs give the preschool boosters, but not usually BCG.

(c) **Health promotion**
This includes counselling about healthy eating, exercise, smoking, alcohol, and drug misuse, sexual health (including family planning advice and HIV/AIDS) and accident prevention. This is best carried out by teachers, with school nurses providing information and resources.

The school nurse and doctor can help in organizing the school day of children with asthma, epilepsy, or diabetes and enabling teachers to cope with their anxieties about these youngsters' fitness to join in different activities. Nurses and doctors attached to secondary schools need to be well-versed in the problems of adolescence: anxieties about their body and/or sex, smoking, drugs, and anorexia. School doctors do not see children routinely but will be consulted by teachers, parents or school nurses when problems occur in school.

The world of educational medicine is separated by too wide a gulf from primary care with ignorance of each other's role.The school nurse or doctor (whose name can usually be obtained from the Community Trust) is helpful when a GP is faced with a problem in which the school figures overtly, school refusal, or poor educational progress, or when difficulties at home may be affecting progress at school. Occasionally it is quicker for the GP to speak to the head teacher or the year head direct, having first discussed this with the parents and perhaps with the child if he is of secondary school age.

School doctors sometimes initiate immunizations, physiotherapy, speech therapy, or attendances at special enuretic or obesity clinics, as well as referrals to hospital departments, ideally with the GP's knowledge and approval. They also collaborate with the educational psychologists, education welfare officers, career service, and the Further Education Funding Council (concerning school leavers with special needs).

POOR PROGRESS AT SCHOOL

General practitioners are not very often consulted about children who are making slow progress at school. This is a pity because a general medical view quite often has something to offer, and sometimes the general practitioner's own knowledge of the family situation makes it obvious where the problem lies. We are really talking about children whose progress is not up to family expectations. There are also children from deprived homes who are underachieving. A number of questions arise:

1. Is the child suffering because of family disorder or illness; is he tired through lack of sleep because of nocturnal asthma, or because noise and overcrowding are also affecting his ability to concentrate on homework?
2. Is this school refusal? Is he staying at home inappropriately, minor illness being used as an excuse?
3. Is he very unhappy at school because of friction with other children, or with a particular teacher, or because he cannot follow the lessons?
4. Is there a problem with vision or hearing?
5. Is he unwell or on any medication which is affecting his ability to concentrate? Could he be having *petit mal* or absence seizures? Is he hypothyroid?
6. Has he had a previously unnoticed minor degree of cerebral palsy? Is there excessive clumsiness or poor co-ordination? Has low intelligence been overlooked?
7. Could he have a specific learning disorder with disproportionate difficulty in handling letter recognition or mathematical symbols? Looking at the child's writing and arithmetic in the context of their age and intellectual ability may give a clue.

After an initial consultation, liaison with the head teacher, the school doctor, or the educational welfare officer may be needed. If the parents or the GP feel that a child's educational performance is not matching up to his ability, the head teacher will usually be willing to arrange for the child to be seen by one of the Education Authority's educational psychologists. They play a major role in the assessment of children with learning difficulties and in advising about their special educational needs. An opinion from an independent educational or clinical psychologist, can occasionally be helpful in providing advice on appropriate schooling or career choices to parents who are willing to pay for it. Sometimes, however, if it appears to be a more general emotional or behavioural problem, a referral to a child psychiatrist, if possible after liaison with the school, is better.

Bibliography

Brown, C. (1970). *Down all the days*. Secker & Warburg, London. (Cerebral palsy from the inside.)

Polnay, L. and Hull, D. (1993). *Community paediatrics.* Churchill Livingstone, London. (A good resource for the areas covered by this chapter.)

Robinson, R. (1991). Cerebral palsy. In *Paediatric speciality practice for the 1990s*. (ed. J. Eyre and R. Boyd). Royal College of Physicians of London.

Warnock, M. (1978). *Special educational needs.* Reports of the Committee of Enquiry into the Education of Handicapped Children and Young People. HMSO, London.

9 Ethnic groups

Britain has become a multi-racial, multi-cultural and multi-lingual society. Naturally this has implications for the planning and delivery of health care.

Irish migration to Britain on a large scale began in the eighteenth and nineteenth centuries followed by Jews from eastern Europe and then, amongst others, Poles, Italians, Germans and Ukrainians, Greek and Turkish Cypriots. The most recent large migration was that of people from the Indian subcontinent and the West Indies. This began after the Second World War as a response to the demand for labour in Britain. Migrants in smaller numbers include the Maltese, Chinese, Vietnamese, and Iranians. In addition, the majority of more recent arrivals from Africa are political refugees from Somalia, Ethiopia and Zaïre (French speaking). In 1992, there were an estimated 25 000 asylum seekers in Britain, a third from Europe, mainly the former Yugoslavia (Social Trends 1994).

In this chapter we discuss the larger more recently arrived groups, on the assumption that the cultural practices of populations who have been settled in Britain for a longer period are more widely known. These groups now include British-born children and grandchildren.

The 1991 census for the first time included a question on ethnic group. Just over three million people described themselves as belonging to an ethnic minority, forming about 6 per cent of the UK population, and 10 per cent of births. The largest group (1.4 million) originate from the Indian subcontinent. The average age of recently settled ethnic groups is usually less than that of the rest of the population (Table 9.1). Almost half the people of Bangladeshi origin in Britain are under 15.

It is characteristic of most migrants that, when they choose to settle, they do so in groups. There is a desire to be part of a familiar and supportive network of fellow migrants and their families and a wish to be separated from an unfamiliar and perhaps hostile host population. Almost a third of potentially economically active Pakistani, Bangladeshi, and Black individuals were out of work in 1993, compared to 10 per cent of Whites (Social Trends 1994). Many live in overcrowded circumstances with relatives who are established residents. Refugees may have to stay in homeless family units or 'bed and breakfast' accommodation. The difficulty migrants have had in adjusting to life in this country has been compounded by racial harassment—perhaps part of a general increase in violence in present-day Western society.

Table 9.1 Self identification of UK population by ethnic group (1991)

Group	% under 15 in group	Total number
Black Caribbean	21.9	500 000
African	29.3	212 000
Black others	50.6	178 000
Indian	29.5	840 000
Pakistani	42.6	477 000
Bangladeshi	47.2	163 000
Chinese	23.3	157 000
Other Asians	24.4	198 000
White	19.3	52 million (including 800 000 from other EC countries)

Source: Office of Population Censuses and Surveys; General Register Office (Scotland).

The vast majority of first generation migrants hope to come, work for a time, save money, and return home, but the final return generally recedes. Some families are divided for years—when re-united there may be marital difficulties and emotional disturbance in the children. Difficulties at school may arise from language problems or if the child finds it difficult to respond to parental pressure for academic success. Conflict at home may arise if the cultural milieu at school is different from that of the family. Their educational level is usually poor initially and there is often a language barrier. Once they have brought the rest of their family to join them, they lose their 'niche' at 'home', just as have families from Britain who now live in Australia, Canada, or South Africa. Children born in Britain grow up to identify themselves as both British and Pakistani, or British and Caribbean, as well as Africans. Characteristically, the first migrants were men, subsequently joined by their wives or fiancées. Migration is often a chain process in which those already established abroad assist the passage of others and help them to get settled, so that peoples from particular places have become established in distinct areas of Britain.

The first generation generally attempt to instil in their children the language, way of life, and moral standards of 'home'. The children may work long hours in family businesses after school, with the girls also working in the home. They may attend ethnic and religious schooling in addition to keeping up with their British school work—a potentially stressful overload. Religious centres and ethnic grocers flourish. The need for a separate ethnic identity may be less pronounced in the second generation. Children assimilate the norms of the host society in addition to those of 'home', and they often become the link between the environment and their parents. Inter-generational conflicts are likely to arise between adolescents and their parents, sometimes over courtship and marriage. Many young are content to accept their parents' guidance or to achieve a compromise; nevertheless, the ability of parents (particularly from British Asian societies where many marriages are arranged in varying degrees) to obtain suitable partners for their children may be curtailed.

MEDICAL ENCOUNTERS

Because of the first generation mother's 'encapsulation', she has few real encounters with the indigenous population. When one does take place, it has particular significance for her. The quality of the contact with a receptionist will set the tone for the consultation and many practices make considerable effort to ensure non-English speaking patients feel welcome and understood by, for example, appointing practice staff from the major local ethnic groups. Training sessions for receptionists should include instructions on how to handle individuals who have difficulty in communicating in English and on the naming systems of ethnic groups in the practice area. For example, Chinese, Hindu, Sikh, and Muslim naming systems are different from those employed in northern Europe. It is often simplest to ask an individual what he would like to be called. This is then recorded on the front of the notes, and if necessary a phonetic transcription written next to it. Additionally, Muslim women do not take the husband's name after marriage, it may be necessary to write 'wife of (husband's name)' in the medical records. The naming systems of people of Afro-Caribbean or Mediterranean origin are similar to that employed by the British and members of other groups have also made efforts to conform. The practice leaflet and literature for patients will usefully be written in relevant languages for the minority who can read their native language while being unable to speak English (Tuffnell *et al.* 1994). However audio or even video tapes may be a better method of providing health information. Literature may be obtained from the health education department of the local Community Trust. These organizations may also provide skilled interpreters. In some districts there are also advocacy services provided by members of ethnic groups to represent the interests of people from their communities who come into contact with the medical profession.

There are a few other specific points relevant to a consultation with non-English speaking patients.

1. Due to the imbalance of power between many health professionals and ethnic minority patients, there is an onus on the professional to facilitate good verbal communication by (Mares *et al.* 1985):

   (a) Correct pronunciation of the patient's name.

   (b) Allowing more time for the consultation.

   (c) Speaking slowly and clearly in simple but correct English.

   (d) Writing full case notes to avoid having to repeat questions at future consultations.

(e) Asking the patient to repeat back items of information given by the doctor; these can usefully be written down for the patient to take home.

(f) Trying to ensure that the patient sees the same health professional at each consultation.

If linguistic difficulties make communication impossible, it is better, except in an emergency, to make another appointment when an interpreter is available. Ideally, these should be *trained* to convey and relay information accurately. Usually another member of the family is used as an interpreter, but parents may be reluctant to talk about sensitive issues in front of their English speaking children.

These points may be perfectionist in the context of a busy surgery but malcommunication is not only a waste of everybody's time, but can be positively harmful.

2. A teenage Asian girl may not wish to be examined by a man and may prefer to return when a female doctor is available.
3. Most of the first generation migrants come from societies where infant mortality was high during their own childhood, and they may be disproportionately anxious about their children's illness.
4. Some tend to formulate anxieties or problems in unusual or inappropriate ways: 'he is weak, for a thin boy'; 'the doctor will give you an injection if you don't eat better'. A similar threat is also used by some native British parents.
5. There are some specific details of the use of language that may lead to misunderstanding. For instance, many languages (including Latin) have only one expression for both forms of the superlative; that is, 'very much' and 'too much'. Many Indian and Cypriot migrants innocently use the one form or both. Thus, 'too much pain doctor' which may be perceived by the doctor as an irritating form of coercion, is often simply intended as a description of 'a lot of pain'. No doubt, there are many other examples.
6. The disparity between health care in the country of origin and that in Britain can cause difficulties in adjusting to the British system of care, which includes not only cure of acute illness but also ongoing management of chronic disease.

Children brought up in Britain obviously have different health beliefs, perceptions, expectations, and behaviour patterns from their parents, whose upbringing was elsewhere. Finally, the practice should be aware of services for local ethnic groups—both community support groups and specific counselling organizations.

Health problems on arrival in the UK

Some children who come and join their parents or come on their own, especially if refugees, may be small, poorly nourished, with iron deficiency. They need to be screened for tuberculosis (chest X-ray and tuberculin test), for various intestinal parasites (see p. 213) and for immunization status. A full blood count may be indicated. A disproportionate number of Africans and Chinese carry hepatitis B. Orphans from Romania and children from sub-Saharan Africa may be HIV positive.

Acute illnesses include malaria (p. 165), typhoid, and diphtheria. Some refugee children have seen relatives killed in front of them and suffer the nightmares and terrors of post-traumatic stress.

Holidays in the country of origin of the family are increasingly common. Immunization and other prophylactic advice may be needed and a travel history is often relevant.

Mohammed, aged 10, had headaches and rigours on return from Bangladesh. He had been staying with his grandmother in a village and drinking well water. His blood film showed that 10 per cent of his red cells had *Plasmodium vivax* parasites. Apparently he had not been advised by the travel agent to take antimalarial prophylaxis. The family had not consulted the practice nurse for pre-travel immunization.

BRITISH ASIANS

By common usage the term is restricted to families originating from the Indian subcontinent. There are, of course, many other British Asians of Chinese and other descent (Table 9.2).

The population of the Indian subcontinent is immensely diverse in terms of genetics, language, religion, and cultural practice. In Britain they are often loosely and incorrectly lumped together as Asian immigrants. Most migrants are of rural origin and originally emigrated so as to assist their extended families at home. There are also some professionally trained people, for example doctors, who originally came to study and finally settled; about 20 per cent of general practitioners are of Asian origin.

Diversity was increased by the arrival of East African Asians; generally educated business people with western-type schooling. They had middle class skills and standards and were commercially successful in East Africa, but had to leave either for political reasons or because of discrimination in employment.

The Asian tradition of relying on the extended family for support may be difficult to sustain and for many migrants no longer exists, so when problems arise, both men and women may feel isolated, without the array of sisters, brothers, aunts, and uncles that normally would support them. This cultural dislocation can cause depression, which tends to be expressed in physical symptoms.

Many Asian marriages are still arranged, but the pattern is variable and evolving. For example, boys marrying whom they wish is often tolerated, but a girl may be expected to make a traditional marriage with a husband selected by her parents. If the clash of expectations leads to early marital breakdown, an isolated, depressed, unsupported mother in temporary accommodation may result. She and her children may become cut off from the rest of the family because she has not conformed to their expectations.

Table 9.2 General characteristics of British Asians

	East Africa	India	Pakistan	Bangladesh
Religion	Hinduism, Islam, Sikhism	Hinduism, Sikhism and some Islam	Islam	Islam
Language	English, Gujarati, Punjabi	Hindi, Punjabi, Bengali, Gujarati, others	Punjabi, Pushto, Urdu, others	Bengali, some Urdu
Diet	Some vegetarian	Some vegetarian (may be strict) Hindus no beef	Strict dietary laws for meat only Ritual slaughter 'Halal' No pork or alcohol Fasting during Ramadan	
Particular diseases	Thalassaemia G6PD	Thalassaemia G6PD Rickets (Strict vegetarian diet; little exposure of skin to sun)	Thalassaemia G6PD Rickets	Thalassaemia G6PD Rickets
		Iron deficiency (late weaning on to low iron foods) TB (neonatal BCG recommended) Malaria and intestinal parasites and pathogens		

Modified from Black (1989).

Consanguineous marriage, especially in some Muslim groups, is common. Fifty per cent of marriages in the British Pakistani community are between first cousins and the figure appears to be rising (Darr and Modell 1988). It often has beneficial social consequences by, for example, enhancing the position of women within the family. In a consanguineous marriage, both partners have a common ancestor. This increases the chance of the birth of an infant with a recessive disorder because children inherit some identical gene sequences from both parents. Consanguineous marriage does not significantly affect the likelihood of handing on a dominant or X-linked condition. Though the diseases that will most commonly emerge are the haemoglobin disorders, consanguineous marriage favours the appearance of rare recessively inherited diseases. A detailed family tree is advisable for these couples before they embark on a pregnancy. If there is evidence of possible genetic disease, referral to a clinical geneticist is important. If the condition proves to be inherited, it may be possible to offer prenatal carrier testing and prenatal diagnosis. The total risk of stillbirth, neonatal or childhood death, or congenital malformation, is about 2.5 per cent in the general population. According to Harper (1988), when a couple are first cousins without evidence of a genetic disorder in the family, this risk is increased by an additional three per cent.

Other issues are summarized in Table 9.2.

BRITISH AFRICAN-CARIBBEANS

This group has been settled in the UK long enough to produce an adult second and third generation. In the West Indies, family organization tends to be matriarchal, originally developing as a result of breakdown in family life during slavery and subsequently maintained because of continuing poverty of the community. Child rearing was often independent of the father (or fathers), the family backbone consisting of the mother, who generally worked, and the grandmother who looked after the children. There was from the start, almost equal immigration of both sexes from the Caribbean.

In Britain, the family structure is becoming closer to the indigenous pattern. However, as the grandmother may not be available in this country, some children are looked after by child-minders while the mother works.

Many, though not all, born in the UK consider themselves British, though they are very aware of their roots in the Caribbean and especially Africa, their original homeland. Relatively cheap intercontinental air travel means fairly regular visits to families abroad. Religion and church-going are an important part of life and many members belong to specific Caribbean Christian churches or to the Church of England. The Rastafarians, mainly young African-Caribbeans, are named after Ras Tafari, former Emperor of Ethiopia. Many Rastafarians are vegetarian, others may eat meat, except pork which is considered unclean. Some men, women and children do not cut or comb their hair and it forms naturally into dreadlocks, which are sometimes covered by a woollen hat known as a tam. Marijuana is smoked by many members of this group.

Sickle cell disease and its variants and glucose G6PD deficiency are important problems in patients of African-Caribbean origin, though not as commonly seen as in those from Africa, probably because of earlier mixed ancestry in the Caribbean. Umbilical herniae, sometimes quite large, are often seen in infants. Keloid formation in scars is common.

AFRICANS

Their reason for being here and their social and family lives are quite different from those of British African-Caribbeans. Until 10 years ago, the majority came to Britain as temporary students, often to gain higher qualifications because of the paucity of advanced education in West Africa. In the end, most of them achieved their objective, returning home qualified for a professional career. They did not have grants and had to earn their living, so it could take years to achieve the required degree or diploma. Many brought their wives, who also wished for further education, and naturally many of these couples had children while they were here. In accordance with West African customs, some relinquished their children for temporary fostering. This did not imply any parental rejection or neglect. There is now a diminished return of students to Africa because of economic and political problems in their native countries.

Female circumcision of pre-pubertal girls is prominent in some North African cultures. The extent may vary from clitoral removal to sub-total vulvectomy with attendant scarring, incontinence, and haematocolpos. Female circumcision is illegal in the UK, but a girl who has been circumcised elsewhere may have urological problems inexplicable until the genitalia are examined.

BRITISH CYPRIOTS

Cypriots are a major ethnic group in London with smaller communities in other big cities. They represent a cultural 'half-way' house between the east and west. Between 1957 and 1967, 10 per cent of the Cypriot population emigrated to England. Although there are still important language and cultural differences, this group is now very integrated into British society. This is because not only has the present generation grown up in England, but also there had been rapid and parallel social and economic change in Cyprus. Most British Cypriots visit Cyprus on holiday and many now take jobs or retire there. They are in a sense trans-European commuters.

Cypriot social life is still based on the extended family which includes all relatives by marriage and may be so large as to merge into the whole community. Parents expect to influence to some extent the marriage choice of their children. Marriage outside the community is not frowned upon and about 20 per cent are with English partners.

Their expectations of medical services are high, and in particular they expect to be screened for haemoglobin disorders; 17 per cent of Cypriots carry β-thalassaemia trait.

Bibliography

Black, J. (1989). Child health in a multi-cultural society. *British Medical Journal.*

Darr, A. and Modell, B. (1988). The frequency of consanguineous marriage among British Pakistanis. *Journal of Medical Genetics,* **25**, 186–90.

Harper, P. S. (1988). *Practical genetic counselling*, (2nd edn). Wright, Bristol.

McAvoy, B. R. and Donaldson, L. J. (ed.) (1990). *Health care for Asians*. Oxford General Practice Series, No. 18. Oxford University Press.

Mares, P., Henley, A., and Baxter, C. (1985). *Health care in multi-racial Britain*. Health Education Council/National Extension College, Cambridge.

Nesbitt, A. and Lynch, M. A. (1992). African children in Britain. *Archives of Disease in Childhood,* **67**, 1402–5.

Social Trends. (1994). No. 24. Central Statistical Office. HMSO, London.

Tuffnell, D. J., Nuttall, K., Raistrick, J., and Jackson, T. J. (1994). Use of translated written material to communicate with non-English speaking patients. *British Medical Journal,* **309**, 992–3.

10 Infectious diseases

THE SICK CHILD AT HOME

If the ill child wants to stay in bed, fine. Otherwise there is no reason why he should not sit in a chair, or lie on the sofa watching TV. Some parents of young children find it helpful to put aside a box of toys that are only brought out if their child is unwell. Teenagers may enjoy quietly listening to their personal stereo. Sick children feel ill at ease and behave in a more dependent, immature way—they may feel more comfortable sleeping in the parents' room for a night or two, or vice versa. Previously clean and dry toddlers may revert to wearing nappies.

Fever in infants

It is sometimes difficult to decide whether an infant is just a bit miserable or genuinely unwell. A carefully measured temperature provides objective evidence; it is also a useful method of monitoring progress during an illness. A rectal temperature should be taken if an accurate reading is important. Morley *et al.* (1992) studied 937 healthy infants under six months and found that the upper limit of rectal temperature in a healthy baby was 37.9 °C. Reassuringly they concluded that the risk of rectal perforation whilst taking the temperature was less than one in two million, though a plastic, digital thermometer used correctly (baby supine, bulb lubricated with KY jelly, and gently inserted in the rectum for one minute) is faster and safer than the traditional mercury and glass one.

Fluids are much more important than food for the feverish child. Parents need to be reassured that their child will not come to any harm if he does not eat for a few days; 'not eating is the body's natural response to an infection'. Feverish children are likely to be miserable, hot, and uncomfortable and there is no evidence that reducing their temperature slows recovery. Paracetamol (not more than four times a day—dose from BNF) will usually ease aches and pains and is a more effective method of lowering the temperature than tepid sponging, fanning, or the removal of clothes. It is a toxic drug and half empty bottles should not be left lying around. If the child appears to be better, the antipyretics should be stopped to assess whether he has really recovered from the febrile illness or not. In any case a relatively cheerful child with a mildly raised temperature does not

Table 10.1 Period of infectivity of some infectious diseases

Disease	Period of infectivity
Hepatitis A	3 weeks, from 2 weeks before the jaundice appears
Measles	At least 7 days after the first symptoms
Mumps	Several days before the onset of symptoms until the swellings have subsided; usually 7–10 days
Pertussis	First 4 weeks of the illness
Rubella	Onset of symptoms to the 4th day of the rash
Varicella	1 day before the rash until the crusts have dried (usually 7–10 days). The scabs are not infectious

Adapted from Krugman *et al.* (1992).

need paracetamol. Most of the common childhood infections are contagious and as the period of greatest infectivity is usually before the diagnosis is made, non-immune members of the family will often catch the infection in spite of attempts to prevent it. Simple hygienic precautions are reasonable: a separate towel and flannel for the child with gastro-enteritis; a warning to vulnerable playmates to stay away whilst the child is acutely unwell. Brothers and sisters do not always easily accept diversion of parental attention to their sick sibling and, if they are old enough, they can be involved in care of the invalid.

The family will find it helpful to be given clear instructions on indications for contacting the doctor again. The indications depend on the type of illness: the child with a respiratory infection who becomes more breathless and wheezy, develops persistent earache or remains toxic for more than another couple of days; a one-year-old with watery diarrhoea who has not improved by the next morning; the child with otitis media who is not getting better 48 hours after the original consultation; the baby who presents with pyrexia of unknown origin (PUO) whose fever does not settle within a day or two needs to be re-examined, and a urine cultured.

The GP is often involved in negotiating return to school or nursery. Most children who have had a respiratory infection but who have been afebrile for a couple of days can return, irrespective of the presence of a cough, or the need to continue a course of antibiotics. The stools of an infant with bacterial gastro-enteritis will need to be free of pathogens before he goes back to the nursery. Older children who have had a more prolonged illness may cope better with only half-time schooling for the first week. If a child has to remain off school for several weeks (more common with a fracture than an infectious illness) he is entitled to free home tuition.

The period of infectivity of some of the commoner infectious diseases is shown in Table 10.1 Excretion of small numbers of organisms may extend over a longer period.

Table 10.2 Causes of prolonged, unexplained fever in children

Signs	Possible disease
Chest infection	Viral or bacterial pneumonia including tuberculosis, mycoplasma and psittacosis (from parrots and some other birds), influenza
Skin rashes	Viral infections Juvenile rheumatoid arthritis Kawasaki's disease, Lyme disease
Lymphadenopathy hepatosplenomegaly or splenomegaly alone	Viral infections Infectious mononucleosis Toxoplasmosis Cytomegalovirus HIV infection Brucellosis Leukaemia, lymphoma Juvenile rheumatoid arthritis Malaria
Loin pain and tenderness	Pyelonephritis
Lower abdominal tenderness	Crohn's disease Pelvic abscess (missed appendicitis)
Acute tenderness and swelling of limb or joint	Osteomyelitis Septic arthritis
Subacute arthritis	Juvenile rheumatoid arthritis Leukaemia, neuroblastoma
Jaundice	Hepatitis Leptospirosis
Tachycardia and systolic murmur	Bacterial endocarditis
Well child, no fever recorded by GP	Munchausen by proxy

UNEXPLAINED FEVER

Most children with a prolonged fever have an unusually persistent viral infection, a patch of pulmonary consolidation, or an undiagnosed urinary infection. The range of other possibilities is wide (Table 10.2) and we suggest the following approach to the problem of a child who has had fever for a week or more, with no obvious localizing symptoms or signs pointing to a diagnosis.

The history should be taken again in detail, with particular reference to the start of the febrile illness and to the following points:

1. Are there any minor symptoms to which not enough attention has been paid; for example, cough (pneumonia, tuberculosis), diarrhoea (abdominal pathology), or dark urine (hepatitis)?

2. Has the child been fully immunized?

3. Has there been any contact with anybody with a possible infectious disease or with pets?

4. Have they been abroad (or had contact with a person who has recently returned from overseas)? Had they taken malarial prophylaxis and had relevant immunizations?

5. Has the patient been taking any drugs recently that may be either causing an allergic response or modifying the usual symptomatology of a disease?

6. Is there any past illness that may have relapsed?

It is necessary to examine the whole body surface; perhaps a rash has been missed or the conjunctivae may show an early icteric tinge. If a group of lymph glands are enlarged the area they drain should be examined carefully, as well as a search made for any other lymphadenopathy or splenomegaly. Otitis media may be relatively asymptomatic in a younger child. Occasionally, children with pneumonia have only a slight cough with a patch of crepitations or diminished air entry in one lung field.

The tachycardia of fever may be associated with a soft systolic murmur. Rarely rheumatic fever may cause it, though this more usually presents with an acute arthritis. A rectal examination should be considered if there are abdominal symptoms and should cause little upset if done with gentleness. It may disclose a spurt of watery diarrhoea, or the local tenderness of a pelvic abscess.

If the spleen is considerably enlarged, tropical infection, leukaemia, lymphoma or juvenile arthritis are possible. The limbs and joints should be examined thoroughly for tenderness and swelling. As always, it is crucial to assess the child's general health. Most serious causes of fever are associated with weight loss, anaemia, and wasting of subcutaneous tissues.

No examination for PUO is complete without a urine culture, and at the same time the urine should be checked for bile. It is also reasonable for the GP to initiate the following investigations in any child with a PUO and good veins:

1. Chest X-ray.

2. Thick and thin blood films if there has been any travel to an area where malaria is even a remote possibility.

3. Bacterial culture of throat swab and of faeces if there has been diarrhoea or tropical travel.

4. Full blood count, erythrocyte sedimentation rate (ESR) and Monospot, bilirubin and transaminase estimation (may be very high in hepatitis), an extended Widal (for typhoid and brucellosis), antibody test for cytomegalovirus (CMV) and toxoplasmosis, and indeed a blood culture if suitable media are available. All of these can be done by many laboratories on 10–15 ml of blood.
5. Tuberculin test.

Further investigation depends on the results of the first set, the progress of the patient, and on how skilful the GP is in taking blood from the child. If the laboratory can store a specimen of the serum early in the illness, this may be useful as a base-line from which subsequent antibody tests can be assessed.

Even if a diagnosis is not established through these tests, most children with a persistent fever will have no serious organic disease. However, the occasional ill child with a prolonged fever, especially if anaemia or a high ESR are also found, may eventually turn out to have a malignancy, Crohn's disease, juvenile rheumatoid arthritis (joint involvement may come later), or other important pathology. It can be useful to ask a mother to record the child's temperature morning and night for a limited period, in order to provide an objective record. Frequent consultation about a low-grade fever in a well child may reflect familial rather than microbiological pathology or alternatively factitious illness.

VIRAL INFECTIONS

Some viruses of clinical importance in childhood in the UK are listed in Table 10.3. Basically a virus is a piece of nucleic acid containing genetic information that, in the extracellular or virus particle phase, is surrounded by a protective coat of protein. The protein and nucleic acid constitute the nucleocapsid, which in some cases is in turn surrounded by a lipid envelope. There are considerable variations in the chemical and physical properties of the nucleic acid genomes. In some viruses the genome is DNA while in others it is RNA.

Certain viruses, such as measles, mumps, chickenpox, and herpes simplex usually, but not always, produce a rather standard clinical picture, though the severity of the disease will be very variable. Other syndromes can be caused by one of several different viruses. Examples include aseptic meningitis, pharyngitis, conjunctivitis, myalgia, hepatitis, and febrile skin rashes. 'Glandular fever', although usually caused by the Epstein–Barr virus, is occasionally seen with other viruses. Many virus infections produce a 'non-specific febrile illness' with or without respiratory tract involvement. Viruses are also responsible for most attacks of gastro-enteritis.

The only two infections commonly seen in paediatric general practice in which a bacterial cause appears to predominate are urinary tract infection and otitis media.

Table 10.3 Classification of some viruses seen in UK practice with their common clinical manifestations. Several viruses have numerous subtypes (for example, Coxsackie, adeno, ECHO, and rhino viruses)

Classification		Manifestation	
RNA	Myxovirus	Mumps	Parotitis
		Measles	Rash; cough and fever
		RSV[1]	Bronchiolitis; otitis media
		Para influenza 1,3	Croup
		Influenza A,B	Fever, respiratory symptoms
	Picornavirus	Enterovirus	Skin, mouth, gut, CNS, heart and liver involvement
		Polio	
		Coxsackie	
		ECHO	
		Hepatitis A	
		Rhinovirus	Colds
	Rubella		Rubella
	Reovirus	Rotavirus	Gastro-enteritis; mild respiratory symptoms
	Retrovirus	HIV	AIDS
	Flavivirus	Hepatitis C	Acute and chronic hepatitis
DNA	Pox	Molluscum contagiosum	Pearly papules
	Hepadnavirus	Hepatitis B	Acute and chronic hepatitis, asymptomatic virus carrier
	Herpes	Herpes simplex	Stomatitis and cold sores
		Varicella–zoster	Chickenpox/shingles
		Cytomegalovirus (CMV)	
		Epstein–Barr	Mononucleosis
		Herpes virus 6	*Roseola Infantum*
	Adenovirus		Respiratory; diarrhoea; rarely cystitis
	Papilloma		Warts
	Parvovirus	B19 virus[2]	*Erythema infectiosum*; aplasia in haemolytic anaemia, e.g. sickle cell; arthritis

[1] RSV = respiratory syncytial virus.
[2] There are other human parvoviruses.

The incubation period of measles, mumps, German measles, and chickenpox is approximately two to three weeks. Following the introduction of the MMR vaccine the first three are becoming rare diseases. There is something to be said for allowing young children to mix with friends who are infected with chickenpox, as children are usually less severely affected than adolescents or adults.

MEASLES

This highly infectious illness is transmitted by airborne droplets. The incubation period is approximately 10–12 days. It is seldom subclinical. Previously it was a common disease, with annual notifications between 1940 and 1968 varying between 160 000 and 800 000. By 1993 over 90 per cent of children between the ages of one and two had been vaccinated, and only 10 000 cases of measles were notified in 1991—one affected patient for every three GPs. However, because of fears of an epidemic of measles amongst school-aged children not given the MMR vaccine, there was a measles/rubella immunization campaign in 1994.

The child develops an increasing fever, and symptoms of tracheitis or early bronchitis (often leading to an unnecessary prescription of antibiotics) before the rash appears. Koplik's spots on the inside of the cheek are often present during the prodromal phase or early rash phase, but unfortunately they are sometimes not at all obvious. The diagnosis is made by the GP who arrives to find a usually unimmunized, unwell, coughing, feverish child with sore eyes and a blotchy face. The typical maculo-papular rash starts on the head on about the fourth day of the illness and rapidly spreads down the trunk. At first the spots are discrete, then they coalesce. On the whole the more severe the rash, the iller the patient. After two or three days it fades in the same order as it appeared, leaving brownish stains which may look purpuric—in fact thrombocytopenia can occur. As the rash fades, the symptoms subside and the patient improves. Once the rash has developed, the diagnosis is usually easy, although mild measles may be erroneously diagnosed as rubella. Measles occurring in vaccinated children is usually less severe than in the unprotected, and the rash may be atypical.

Drug eruptions are sometimes morbilliform but do not usually evolve from above downwards. In scarlet fever the macular rash is much finer (see Table 10.4, p. 162). A rubella rash is pink and non-confluent. With diminishing experience of the disease, certainty of clinical diagnosis is decreasing. Diagnosis can be confirmed by antibody detection in blood and even saliva.

Common complications of measles are purulent conjunctivitis and acute otitis media—more than the mildly red ear-drum which is part of the disease. Croup can also occur. A rarer complication is bronchopneumonia, which should be suspected if the child is getting worse rather than improving, and is becoming tachypnoeic with a worsening cough two or three days after the rash has fully developed. Gastro-intestinal symptoms such as vomiting and diarrhoea are sometimes seen.

Post-infectious encephalomyelitis is very uncommon, usually, but not always, beginning some two to seven days after the rash appears. It varies in severity from a mild drowsiness to profound coma, with death or residual disability. Extremely rarely, subacute sclerosing panencephalitis (SSPE) develops 5–10 years after an attack of measles, with progressive dementia, neurological deterioration, and death. Measles in pregnant women can be a problem but is very rare. There may be a small risk of measles-induced fetal malformations (Hanshaw *et al.* 1985).

There is no specific treatment. The child should be given plenty of fluids. Paracetamol may make him more comfortable.

Jim, a six-year-old boy with Down syndrome, developed measles. His unmarried mother was hardly able to cope with him when well. By the time he was seen the rash was extensive, he was extremely miserable and both eyes were stuck closed with severe purulent conjunctivitis. His mouth was sore and he had impetigo around the lips. He was refusing to drink and showing signs of early dehydration. His chest was clear on examination. The child recovered after about a week with intense community support.

Otitis media should be treated as described on p. 192. Broad spectrum antibiotics should be given for measles pneumonia, since a variety of pathogens may cause this complication, including penicillin-resistant staphylococci. Post-contact prophylaxis is discussed on p. 39.

MUMPS

Mumps can be a difficult disease to diagnose, partly because, in one-third of cases, infection is subclinical, and mild cases also occur. The parotid swelling is often better seen than felt. The incubation period is usually 16–18 days. In a child the prodromal stage of malaise may only last a day or two, or may not be noticeable at all. He then usually complains of pain around the ear with, perhaps, discomfort on chewing, and, by the next day, has developed parotitis. One or both of the parotid glands may be involved and tender; sometimes the submandibular glands are also swollen. When they are the only glands involved it is difficult to be certain that mumps is the diagnosis. The size of an enlarged parotid is very variable. The swelling is below and in front of the ear; inability to place a finger in the groove between the mastoid process and the jaw is a useful sign. In early and mild cases the doctor will have to rely on the parent to assess whether their child's face is more swollen than usual, especially if the child is a chubby toddler with more than a fair share of lymphadenopathy around the angle of the jaw. The opening of the parotid duct may be unduly prominent and reddened—not a very useful diagnostic sign. After the first two to five days the temperature subsides and the patient usually feels better, although the swelling may take longer to go down. Children are not usually unwell for more than about a week.

The problem is to decide whether the vaguely unwell child with a slight tender fullness below the ear has mumps or not. Indeed, it is often not possible to be sure of the diagnosis without a contact history, or until a friend or sibling develops more obvious disease two or three weeks later. There are other common causes of swelling around the jaw. An alveolar abscess presents as a brawny, tender swelling, under, and lateral to, the mandible, between the angle of the jaw and the chin. There may sometimes, but not invariably, be obvious caries. Lymph node enlargement (with or without abscess formation) either of the tonsillar gland below and behind the angle of the jaw, or of the submandibular node half-way forward along the mandible is another possibility.

Mild CNS disease is commoner in mumps than in chickenpox or measles and is rarely serious. It may develop before the parotitis, with it, after it, or instead of it. The patient will usually have headache, vomiting, photophobia, and perhaps slight drowsiness, together with high fever and a stiff neck. He will usually be sent to hospital for a diagnostic lumbar puncture to exclude other causes of meningitis, unless the brave GP is confident that mumps is the source of the problem. The vast majority get completely better without any long-term after-effects.

Orchitis is rare before puberty. After puberty about 25 per cent of infected males develop it, and it can be very unpleasant. As with parotitis, clinical orchitis ranges from a mild ache in the testis to the full-blown picture The badly affected young man gradually becomes toxic with considerable malaise and a high fever. The testis may be very swollen, painful, and excruciatingly tender, with the scrotum becoming red and oedematous. Orchitis remains at its peak for two to four days and then gradually subsides, unless the other side becomes involved, when the cycle may be repeated. According to Krugman *et al.* (1992), even when both sides are involved (which occurs in about 10 per cent of those affected) and bilateral testicular atrophy supervenes, there is no firm evidence that sterility occurs.

Some children with mumps complain of upper abdominal pain and vomiting which lasts a couple of days; frank pancreatitis with severe epigastric pain, tenderness, and fever is very uncommon, as is nerve deafness. Manson *et al.* (1960) found that in 501 pregnant mothers infected with mumps there was no increase in fetal abnormalities.

Most children are satisfactorily managed with adequate fluids and mild analgesia. For mumps orchitis strong analgesia may be needed to enable the poor patient to get at least a few hours sleep.

CHICKENPOX

Varicella virus causes both chickenpox and shingles. The primary infection is chickenpox, and shingles develops if re-activation of the virus occurs. The incubation period is usually 14–16 days. In adults and in some children there may be a prodromal stage of one or two days with general malaise, fever, headache, and sore throat before the appearance of the irritating and pleiomorphic rash. Classically, each spot goes through the phases of macule, papule, vesicle, pustule, and scabbing. Usually by the time the doctor sees the patient, most of the rash is in the vesicular stage, which is fortunate, as it is difficult to be certain of the diagnosis unless blistering of the rash has started. Involvement of the trunk and abdomen is usually predominant but the scalp, limbs, and mucous membranes are also affected. Spots often occur in the scalp and new lesions continue to appear for up to a week. The disease varies in intensity, from a well child with half a dozen spots to one who is very unwell with a rash that is almost confluent. Permanent scarring from chickenpox is more likely if there has been secondary infection.

Diagnosis is usually easy, except in mild cases when the patient may have to be seen again a day or so later to look for vesicles, but some other rashes may be mistaken for chickenpox. Coxsackie infections (p. 164) can cause a vesicular febrile illness. Insect bites may cause vesicles, but not constitutional symptoms, and are, in any case, more likely to be papular than vesicular, though there may be a tiny vesicle in the middle of the papule. They occur more often on the limbs than the trunk, are less likely to cause a widespread rash, and unlike chickenpox, lesions are not seen on the mucous membranes.

The commonest complication of chickenpox is secondary skin infection, usually the result of scratching. The pathogens are usually staphylococci or *Streptococcus pyogenes*. A very rare complication is varicella pneumonia which is more common in adults. Many affected patients recover quickly, although X-ray changes (nodular opacities) may persist for several weeks or longer. Post-infective encephalitis is the most common of the rare CNS complication (less than 1:1000 cases). The outlook for patients with cerebellar signs of ataxia, tremor, and nystagmus is better than for those with convulsions and coma. Reye's syndrome presenting with persistent vomiting and increasing drowsiness, within a few days of the chickenpox, is extremely rare (1 in 11 000 cases) thanks to the avoidance of aspirin.

There is a slight association of chickenpox with serious congenital malformations summed up by Hanshaw *et al.* (1985) as 'a very remote risk, one that most families would most likely be prepared to take'. However, if a perinatal mother develops varicella the risk to the baby is strikingly dependent on the precise timing of infection (Krugman *et al.* 1992). With maternal infection between five days before and two days after delivery the baby may develop fulminating chickenpox in the neonatal period because it is unprotected by any specific antibody from the mother. Of such antenatally infected babies who develop the disease (5–10 days after birth) one-quarter die if untreated. By contrast, those babies who develop the disease earlier will have had a chance to receive maternal antibody before birth and have a low mortality. Those babies who catch the disease from their mother and develop it later in the puerperium are also at lower risk. In the event of perinatal maternal infection or exposure of a non-immune mother to chickenpox, expert advice should clearly be immediately sought particularly as other sources (*Immunisation against infectious diseases* 1992) give somewhat longer time periods of high risk. Prophylaxis with varicella–zoster immune globulin (VZIG) and treatment with acyclovir may be needed. Fortunately, 95 per cent of women have had chickenpox before pregnancy.

In ordinary circumstances management of chickenpox is simple. An attempt should be made to isolate the child from his peers, only if their parents feel it is an inconvenient time for them to contract the disease. He should have his nails cut short, and use his own towel and flannel. Calamine lotion is traditionally used to ease the irritation; an antiseptic cream such as cetrimide may help mildly infected lesions. If there is more severe secondary infection, flucloxacillin will be needed.

In children with HIV infection, or who are on steroids, or on chemotherapy for malignant disease, or who have leukaemia or a lymphoma, varicella may be very serious with haemorrhagic lesions, prolonged infection, dissemination, and even death. It is also dangerous in children with thrombocytopenia. If such a child develops chickenpox or is even in contact with it, the hospital clinician involved must be urgently consulted by the GP. VZIG should be given within two days of exposure. Acyclovir started within 24 hours of the onset of the rash is the drug of choice for varicella in the immunocompromised and indeed for anybody with severe or life-threatening infection. According to Krugman *et al*. (1992), second attacks can occur but are usually mild unless the child is immunocompromised.

SHINGLES

Shingles are due to reactivation of the varicella–zoster virus lying dormant in the sensory ganglia of the spinal cord or brain. It usually affects adults though it is by no means rare in children. The vast majority of cases appear to occur in otherwise healthy individuals, though immunocompromised individuals are particularly at risk of severe disease. According to Isaacs (1992) non-immune people may develop chickenpox from shingles; the reverse is uncommon.

In children the disease is usually mild. There may be a prodromal phase of a day or two of malaise and discomfort in the affected dermatome though this is less likely than in adults. Crops of macules and papules develop, not crossing the midline. The rash may become vesicular and crust and be associated with enlargement of the regional lymph nodes. There may be too few lesions for the GP to be certain whether he is dealing with herpes zoster or herpes simplex. In the former the skin around the rash may be hypersensitive. The child may take a week or two to recover. Acyclovir would only be needed in children with a severe infection or underlying disease, or if the ophthalmic division of the trigeminal nerve is affected, in which case the child will need to be referred.

RUBELLA

Primary rubella infection in childhood is a trivial disease. Many ECHO and Coxsackie virus infections can produce a similar picture and a definite clinical diagnosis should not be given casually to parents and patients. Such a diagnosis will very often be wrong, leading to inappropriate confidence in immunity during a future pregnancy.

Smithells *et al.* (1990) reported that the average annual number of cases of congenital rubella fell from 69 in 1970–74 to 23 in 1985–87 and there was a tenfold decrease in the number of rubella-associated terminations of pregnancy. Forty-one per cent of affected children had multiple defects and thirty-nine per cent a single one, usually deafness. Only half the mothers had a history of a rubella-like illness. Seven mothers of affected children had previously been immunized, but it was not possible to say whether there had been reinfection or failure of immunization.

Cataracts, malformations of the heart, and deafness are the best known complications of fetal rubella. Hearing loss, which may occur alone, ranges from severe disability making normal schooling impossible, to a mild loss detectable only by audiometry. CNS symptoms such as abnormal irritability, with or without occasional fits, and mental retardation may also occur. In addition, there may be hepatosplenomegaly, neonatal thrombocytopenia, and a long list of rarer complications. Post-natal infection in infancy is rare because of transplacentally acquired antibodies. Congenitally infected infants may excrete the virus for many months and are a continuing hazard to non-immune pregnant women.

The disease has an incubation period of 14–21 days. It is not highly infectious and prolonged contact, such as occurs in the home, is usually required for transmission. A quarter of cases or more are subclinical. The prodromal phase, which may not occur in children, is characterized by symptoms of a mild upper respiratory tract infection, with perhaps a feeling of gritty eyes and a slightly sore throat. The fine macular rash, paler pink than measles, starts on the face and rapidly descends down the trunk before fading after a day or two. It may end up as a diffuse redness. It may be absent altogether. There is usually cervical lymphadenopathy beginning a day or so before the rash appears. This particularly affects the posterior cervical and suboccipital glands, but this is not as useful a physical sign as is sometimes believed, as it also occurs in other viral infections and scalp infections.

Complications of rubella are unusual in children, but arthralgia and acute arthritis, the commonest complications for adults, may be seen in adolescents and it is worth warning parents about this. Joint symptoms usually occur within a week of the rash appearing and subside within two weeks, although they may last longer. Thrombocytopenia may be seen during convalescence but is rare and has a good prognosis; encephalitis is very rare.

The GP is often faced with a patient in early pregnancy who either has a rash or more commonly has been in contact with someone who may have rubella. Maternal rubella infection in the first 8–10 weeks of pregnancy damages the fetus in up to ninety per cent of cases, this risk falling to about 10–20 per cent by sixteen weeks (*Immunisation against infectious diseases* 1992). Even if antenatal testing in a previous pregnancy suggested that they are immune, pregnant women should be re-tested; nearly all will turn out to be immune. When rubella is suspected in a pregnant woman two serum samples should be taken, the first within two to three days of the onset of the rash, or following the contact, and the second eight to nine days later, to see whether antibody has developed. Recent infection is indicated by IgM rubella antibody which persists for only about four weeks. Normal human immunoglobulin is of doubtful value, and should be reserved for exposed pregnant women who would not wish to consider a termination; 750 mg is given as soon after exposure as possible.

HERPES SIMPLEX AND OTHER VIRAL MOUTH LESIONS

A florid sore mouth in an ill child is almost always primary herpetic gingivostomatitis. Some milder mouth lesions may be part of characteristic syndromes caused by certain Coxsackie viruses. One of these is herpangina, in which vesicles restricted to the fauces and soft palate rapidly ulcerate and heal over a few days. Another is hand, foot, and mouth disease, in which vesicular lesions in the mouth, which ulcerate, are associated with macules, papules, and vesicles on the hands and feet. Very occasionally it is part of the Stevens–Johnson syndrome associated with a vesicular, erythematous, papular rash in a toxic child.

Herpes simplex

Herpes simplex viruses are amongst the most common infectious agents affecting children. They are able to persist throughout the host's life, which gives the virus great evolutionary survival value—nice for the virus but a bore for the patient with recurrent cold sores. There are two serotypes: HSV-1 is commoner in childhood and usually affects sites above the waist; HSV-2 more usually affects the genital area. The virus can be quickly cultured from a swab sent in a suitable transport medium.

The incubation period of a primary infection is about a week and though most are asymptomatic, gingivostomatitis is the commonest clinical manifestation. This may be mild and resolve in a few days, but a child can sometimes be toxic for up to two weeks with a high temperature and acute misery because of his very sore mouth. He is reluctant to drink as well as to eat and there is a possibility, particularly in the younger child, of dehydration. The severely affected child's breath smells and he is constantly drooling, spreading the virus to nearby skin, which can develop satellite lesions. Numerous small, shallow ulcers can be seen on the gums and elsewhere in the mouth. The gums are particularly inflamed and often bleed. Cervical lymphadenopathy is common. Practically always, someone is concerned lest leukaemia be the diagnosis. It almost never is. Recurrent cold sores are, of course, a common sequel.

If the child is kept at home a health visitor or district nurse can be very helpful in instructing the mother on the maintenance of oral hygiene, and in keeping up the morale of the family during this very unpleasant illness. The child may find it easier to drink through a straw. Ice-cream or very cold drinks may be acceptable when everything else is refused. Many children are treated at home, but hospital admission may be advisable for some younger patients if the family's social situation precludes adequate domiciliary care, or if the child is not getting enough to drink.

Another form of primary herpetic infection requiring prompt referral is herpetic keratoconjunctivitis with a red, inflamed eye, sometimes with satellite vesicular lesions, and dendritic ulceration of the cornea, which is stained green by fluorescein. Permanent scarring can occur.

An unwell child with a red, ulcerated perineum and enlarged inguinal glands may have herpetic vulvovaginitis. If this occurs in the infant it is likely to be confused with an infected nappy rash. If the diagnosis is confirmed then sexual abuse needs to be considered, especially if, following a request for virus typing, the laboratory confirms that the virus is HSV-2. Primary genital herpes, followed by recurrent HSV-2 infection may occur in sexually active adolescents. If suspected it is important to test for other sexually transmitted diseases.

If a woman has active genital herpes when delivery is due, most obstetricians recommend a Caesarean section to reduce the risk of infection of the baby, as neonatal herpes can be a severe, disseminated, sometimes fatal illness. A paternal penile herpetic lesion developing in the last month of pregnancy is an indication for culturing the mother's vaginal and cervical secretions. Severe disseminated neonatal infection may occur if the baby catches HSV-1 from a mother with a primary infection or, if the mother is not immune, from a nurse with a cold sore. Children who have severe eczema may also get dangerous attacks of primary herpes (p. 221).

Acyclovir is an effective antiviral agent which inhibits the synthesis of herpes simplex or varicella–zoster DNA. Few side-effects have been reported but we do not use it for mild or localized lesions. Oral preparations are effective for the treatment of moderate or severe primary herpetic infection of the skin or mucous membranes, though sometimes intravenous therapy is preferable. Its use for bothersome recurrent lesions is not yet fully established. Acyclovir ointment may abort a recurrence when applied in the prodromal (tingling) phase.

INFECTIOUS MONONUCLEOSIS

Most infections in childhood and adolescence are probably mild or subclinical and these produce immunity. Three-quarters of young adults have antibodies to the causative Epstein–Barr virus (EBV), one of the herpes group of viruses which has also been implicated in Burkitt's lymphoma. In general practice, glandular fever is seen most commonly in the 15–24 age group, followed by children between the ages of 5 and 14. It is rarely diagnosed under the age of five. The incubation period is probably between four and six weeks. The disease does not appear to be very infectious, although the saliva may contain virus for several months after an attack. Some 25 per cent of household contacts become infected or develop antibodies.

Children with overt infection are usually feverish with lymphadenopathy, particularly in the cervical region, and splenomegaly. The throat is often very sore. The illness usually goes on for two to four weeks. In the adolescent the clinical picture ranges from a patient with malaise, a low-grade fever, and little lymphadenopathy to the more worrying angiose type, when the throat is acutely inflamed with patches of white exudate. These may coalesce to form a thick plaque, and in the most severe cases the throat and fauces become enormously swollen so that patients find it difficult and painful to swallow, and talk as if there is a large object in their mouth. Occasionally breathing is impaired; almost the picture of diphtheria. Various types of rash can occur—erythematous, maculopapular, morbilliform or even urticarial. Infectious mononucleosis may also present as a pyrexia of unknown origin (PUO) or may mimic infectious hepatitis. In a small number of patients there will be signs of a neurological disturbance, such as viral meningitis or polyneuritis. Rupture of the spleen, a surgical emergency, with shock and shoulder-tip pain can occur but is very rare, as are other complications such as pneumonitis, orchitis or thrombocytopenic purpura.

The most important test is the Paul–Bunnell test for heterophil antibodies against sheep red blood cells, or the less laborious, but usually satisfactory Monospot test, based on agglutinins against horse red cells. The antibody titre usually reaches diagnostically significant levels by the second week of the illness and gradually disappears over the next three to six months. Sheep cell agglutinins occur in other conditions such as hepatitis, serum sickness, leukaemia, and Hodgkin's disease. If the first test is negative it may be worth repeating in a week or so, together with a request for EBV antibodies if the patient shows no sign of recovery. Occasionally the Monospot may be falsely negative. A blood count in infectious mononucleosis will show an absolute increase in the number of lymphocytes, many of which are abnormal. A smaller number of atypical lymphocytes may also be found in the blood of healthy people or in patients with a variety of infections, including hepatitis from other viruses, and rubella.

The vast majority of patients make a complete recovery without treatment. Children very rarely complain of the prolonged debility that occurs in some older patients. This has, in any case, been shown to be less likely if the doctor emphasizes the likelihood of full recovery within a few weeks of the time of diagnosis. If respiratory obstruction is threatened in the severe angiose form, steroids may be helpful in reducing both the duration of the fever and the size of the tonsils (Bender 1967). Prednisolone 40 mg is given on the first day and tailed off over a week. Oral penicillin (not amoxycillin which may cause a rash and is less specific than penicillin for tonsillitis) will almost certainly have been given to the patient who presented with tonsillitis, before the diagnosis of mononucleosis had been confirmed.

Parents of sick children should be warned that although the illness is usually mild it may be somewhat drawn out, keeping their child off school for two to four weeks. However, he should be encouraged to return when the temperature and sore throat have subsided and he has been feeling better for a day or two, even though at this stage he will probably still have some enlarged lymph glands and a palpable spleen.

Cytomegalovirus (CMV), another of the herpes group of viruses, is a cause of Paul–Bunnell negative glandular fever. It can cause the same symptoms and signs, namely lymphadenopathy, hepatosplenomegaly and a fever. Atypical lymphocytes usually occur as do abnormal liver function tests. Like glandular fever it can occasionally cause prolonged malaise and clinical hepatitis. The virus can be fairly easily cultured from the urine, or a rising antibody titre against CMV can be demonstrated. CMV infection can also be acquired from transplanted organs and blood transfusions. Most post-natal infections are asymptomatic; overt infections are particularly likely in immunosuppressed children. About 1 per cent of non-immune pregnant women become infected during pregnancy, but the fetus is damaged in only approximately 10 per cent of these. CMV is nevertheless the commonest viral cause of mental retardation (Best and Banalvala 1990) and is also a cause of congenital deafness. CMV damage to babies usually follows a primary infection during pregnancy. It may occasionally occur after a reactivated maternal infection. The infected child may excrete the virus for a long time; hygienic measures may reduce the risk of spreading the infection to carers.

Toxoplasmosis is another infection which may mimic glandular fever but with especially prominent lymphadenopathy. It is a protozoan intracellular parasite found in many animals, but sexual reproduction and spore production occur only in the intestine of the cat. Most infections are subclinical. Once acquired, the organisms encapsulate in various tissues and usually remain latent except in the immunosuppressed. It is a curious coincidence that either cytomegalovirus or toxoplasma infection in pregnancy may damage the unborn fetus, even though the organisms are completely different, one being a virus, the other an intracellular protozoan parasite.

It is important to think of toxoplasmosis if a woman develops a temperature during pregnancy, particularly if it is accompanied by a “glandular fever” type illness. The risk of toxoplasmosis may be reduced if pregnant women who have pet cats, cook both their own meat and that given to their cats thoroughly, and wear gloves when cleaning out the cat litter.

The picture of congenital toxoplasmosis also varies, ranging from fetal or neonatal death to a mildly affected child with normal intelligence but poor sight because of retinal damage. Treatment with spiromycin kills the organism but this drug does not cross the placenta and therefore cannot eradicate fetal infection once it has occurred.

ROSEOLA INFANTUM (EXANTHEMA SUBITUM)

This not very infectious illness, caused by the human herpes virus type 6, is seen in infants and toddlers. There are three or four days of high fever in a relatively well child, often without symptoms of an URTI. As the fever subsides, a macular or maculo-papular rash develops. This usually first affects the trunk, then sometimes spreads to the face and limbs. It fades after a day or so. Often the child has some lymphadenopathy. *Roseola* may be one of the commoner reasons for leaping to the false conclusion that every child who gets a rash after penicillin is allergic to the drug. He may have had *roseola infantum*, though it is difficult to be certain. Febrile convulsions may occur in association with *roseola*.

ERYTHEMA INFECTIOSUM (FIFTH DISEASE; SLAPPED FACE DISEASE)

This illness (caused by parvovirus B19) may be subclinical but can cause a fever from which the patient quickly recovers, followed a week or so later by a rash. Cheeks become bright red and flushed and this is followed by a lacy maculo-papular rash on the trunk and limbs. The rash may fluctuate in intensity over some weeks before it finally disappears. Painful swollen joints may follow, particularly in adults. By the time the rash appears the child is no longer infectious.

Parvovirus infections can have serious implications for children with a shortened red cell survival (thalassaemia or sickle cell anaemia), causing an aplastic crisis with a dramatic fall in haemoglobin. Parvovirus in pregnant women may affect the fetus, causing a miscarriage or stillbirth with hydrops fetalis secondary to intrauterine anaemia in 9 per cent of cases (PHLS Working Party 1990). Congenital anaemia can occur.

SKIN RASHES

Very many febrile viral illnesses are associated with skin rashes and it is often possible to guess which group of viruses is responsible. Even urticaria may have a viral aetiology. On the whole, relatively well children who develop a short-lived, roughly symmetrical, macular or maculo-papular rash are likely to be suffering from a virus infection. Some of the commoner causes of non-vesicular rashes are shown in Table 10.4.

Other causes of non-viral febrile rashes include septicaemia, Henoch–Schönlein purpura, juvenile rheumatoid arthritis, drugs, and various tropical diseases.

VIRAL HEPATITIS

Jaundice in children after infancy is usually viral, although haemolysis, biliary obstruction, or drug toxicity are also possible. Most cases follow hepatitis A infection, a few hepatitis B, and others Epstein–Barr, cytomegalo-, or other viruses.

Table 10.4 Erythematous rashes in childhood

Maculo-papular and erythematous rashes[1]	Likely cause
Reddish brown maculo-papules; may become confluent; spreads from face downwards; fades leaving brownish stain; sick child. Preceded by Koplik's spots and conjunctival and respiratory symptoms	Measles
Pink discrete macules; spreads rapidly from face to rest of body; non-irritating; usually gone in three days; child not very ill; no staining	Rubella Coxsackie ECHO
Discrete pinkish red macular rash; starts from trunk and spreads to rest of body; lasts for couple of days; as rash develops sick child improves	*Roseola infantum*
Bright red flushed cheeks; followed by maculo-papular rash on limbs and trunk; lace like appearance; relatively well child. Joint problems in adults	*Erythema infectiosum* Parvovirus
Fine papular or punctate erythema; may be most marked on neck and in axillae and groin; flushed face with circumoral pallor; desquamation after about a week; tonsillitis and raw red tongue	Scarlet fever
Red, raised, indurated area with palpable margin; toxic child	Streptococcal erysipelas

[1] Drug eruptions may mimic any of the diseases mentioned. (Modified from Krugman *et al.* 1992.)

Hepatitis A

This is usually a mild disease and is common in childhood, with an incubation period of 15–40 days. Most have anicteric disease—'gastric flu'. A urine test for bile may explain this illness. Some proceed from malaise, nausea, anorexia, and upper abdominal discomfort to frank jaundice with pale stools and dark urine. The small 27-nm diameter viruses may sometimes be found on electron microscopy of the faeces. Estimation of anti-hepatitis A antibodies in serum is more widely available. IgM can be detected when the patient becomes unwell, and disappears after about eight weeks.

Patients are infectious for two to three weeks before and one week after the onset of jaundice. Hepatitis A does not lead to a carrier state or cause chronic liver disease, and case fatality rates are less than 0.1 per cent in children, although the disease can be more severe in adults.

Before and during the icteric phase the concentration of conjugated bilirubin rises sharply in the plasma and bilirubin will appear in the urine. Urine testing for bile is simple and useful. The plasma alanine transaminase activity is enormously elevated even if jaundice never develops. The serum alkaline phosphatase activity is not very helpful in childhood hepatitis because its normal range in children is wide. If blood is taken, it is worthwhile trying to establish the causative agent by requesting hepatitis B antigen, and hepatitis A antibody, and perhaps also a Monospot test and a CMV antibody titre. In jaundiced children with an enlarged tender liver and occasionally a palpable spleen the illness usually lasts, at most, a fortnight. Children recover more quickly than adults.

The child may eat what he wants. Enforced bed rest is unnecessary. Remembering that hepatitis A is usually spread by the faecal–oral route, it seems sensible to advise the family to wash their hands after going to the lavatory and before preparing food. Normal human immunoglobulin gives a high degree of protection against hepatitis A when given prophylactically—the earlier in the incubation period the better. It should be offered to any household contact of the index case who has not already had the disease (0.02–0.04 ml/kg; 0.06–0.12 ml/kg gives longer protection for up to about six months). It is not yet known whether hepatitis A vaccine is effective in reducing the risk or severity of infection in close contacts. Maternal hepatitis A infection in early pregnancy does not seem to be associated with an increased incidence of congenital abnormalities, although it may be followed by miscarriage or premature birth. An attack of hepatitis A gives immunity only against hepatitis A.

Hepatitis B (serum hepatitis)

Although infection with hepatitis B virus (HBV) usually follows a blood transfusion or the injection of other blood products, in adolescents, tattooing or sexual intercourse may be responsible. Immunization is advisable for medical and nursing students. The incubation period is two to six months.

For those who wish to interpret the laboratory tests, it is worth knowing something about the submicroscopic morphology of the virus. It consists of an inner core with the core antigen HBcAg and an outer coat with the surface antigen HbsAg; this latter appears in blood early in the course of the disease. The e antigen HBeAg seems to be the best marker for infectivity and its persistent presence is associated with chronic disease and a potentially infectious patient. Hepatitis B tends to be more severe and prolonged than hepatitis A, although it is often clinically indistinguishable and in many instances asymptomatic. It may be associated with urticaria or arthritis. Its onset is likely to be less acute than hepatitis A. Up to 10 per cent of patients go on to a chronic carrier state. This may be associated with liver damage, ranging from minor cell changes to chronic active hepatitis, cirrhosis and hepatoma. Increasingly mothers-to-be are routinely tested for hepatitis B. If the woman is a chronic carrier or develops hepatitis B during pregnancy, especially in the later stages, there is a significant risk of hepatitis developing in the baby in the first six months of life. While this is sometimes asymptomatic, it can cause permanent liver damage, liver cancer, or death in later life. Hepatitis B infection in the mother does not appear to lead to congenital malformation. A combination of HBV specific immunoglobulin plus hepatitis B vaccine has been shown to be effective if given on the day of birth. The initial dose of the vaccine is likely to be given in hospital, with the GP responsible for ensuring that the infant receives follow-up doses six weeks and six months later.

Without this prophylaxis there is a 90 per cent chance of the infant becoming a chronic carrier.

Many non-A, non-B episodes of hepatitis are due to hepatitis C, which produces a similar picture to hepatitis B. Other viruses which may affect the liver include the Epstein–Barr virus, cytomegalovirus and herpes simplex. Other commonly acquired viral infections may also transiently affect the liver.

ENTEROVIRAL INFECTIONS

This group of RNA viruses, which include poliomyelitis, usually live in the gastrointestinal tract and produce a great variety of symptoms and signs. The commonest clinical picture in children is a non-specific febrile illness lasting on average three to four days after an incubation period of one to five days. The child is likely to have painful muscles and perhaps mild respiratory and gut symptoms. Enteroviral pharyngitis, tonsillitis, conjunctivitis, vomiting, and diarrhoea are also common. Viral meningitis is discussed below. Herpangina, hand-foot-and-mouth disease, and epidemic myalgia are Coxsackie infections. Rashes similar to rubella are seen with these and with ECHO viruses. So are petechial rashes which should, in an unwell child, raise the possibility of meningococcal septicaemia. Neonatal enteroviral infection is often a mild disease, but sometimes it is disseminated, with vomiting, breathlessness, and collapse from cardiac and hepatic failure leading to death.

Epidemic myalgia (Bornholm disease)

This is usually caused by Coxsackie B virus. The characteristic feature is (in the course of a febrile illness) acute muscular pain, which can be very severe. The myalgia is usually sharp or stabbing and occurs in the muscles of the chest or abdomen on one or both sides. As breathing may make the pain worse, pleurisy is often suspected. The muscles in the affected areas may be superficially tender. Occasionally there is a pleural rub, but the lungs are usually clear on auscultation and on X-ray. Abdominal pain may mimic that of appendicitis. Fever and pain usually subside after a few days, but may last a couple of weeks, and relapses can occur.

VIRAL MENINGITIS

The main culprits are mumps and enteroviruses. More rarely measles, Epstein–Barr, rubella, herpes, chickenpox, or others are responsible. In addition to fever and headache with slight or moderate meningeal irritation, there may be a sore throat, myalgia, nausea, vomiting, and cervical or generalized lymphadenopathy. With some viruses a rash occurs.

The course of viral meningitis is usually benign with fever lasting about a week, but malaise may persist some time after this, particularly in older patients. The long-term prognosis is excellent.

Any infant in whom meningitis of any type is suspected must be referred for a lumbar puncture. If the GP feels that a not very ill older child with a viral infection has only mild signs of meningeal irritation and is not toxic, and is without clouding of consciousness or a haemorrhagic rash, he may decide to keep the child at home. He will usually need to visit twice a day until the meningeal irritation is subsiding. The danger of a missed bacterial meningitis is far greater than the trauma of lumbar puncture, and it is always uncomfortable for the GP to manage a child with meningeal signs at home. He should remember that prior antibiotics may have reduced the usually more severe clinical picture of bacterial meningitis and clouded the diagnosis.

In meningitis it is painful if the inflamed meninges are moved through flexion of the neck and muscles are contracted reflexly to prevent this. 'Neck stiffness' can be demonstrated in a number of ways but not, as is often incorrectly assumed, by how far the neck will bend when forcibly flexed. The doctor should flex the head of a supine child gently with a hand slipped under the occiput. When the head is slightly raised, do the shoulders stay put or lift up, as they do if neck stiffness is present? Alternatively, the co-operative child can be asked to bend his head forward in the sitting position. Does the chin easily reach the chest in a simple movement, or does he grimace and move his shoulders?

In babies there is no substitute for watching to see if the sitting baby bends his head downwards in response to having his tummy tickled or keys rattled in front of the umbilicus. In small infants, a bulging fontanelle from raised intracranial pressure or dopiness and irritability are more reliable signs of meningitis; neck stiffness may be absent at this age.

Having established that meningeal irritation is present, one has to weigh up whether a bacterial cause is possible. Bacterial meningitis is an important disease in general practice, both because it may lead to death or lasting brain damage (the avoidance of which depends on the speed of diagnosis) and also because it must be considered constantly in the differential diagnosis of any sick child who has no other obvious cause for his symptoms. The iller the child, the harder it is to assess the situation. Neck stiffness is always a potentially serious sign. Any hint of septicaemia, such as a purpuric skin rash or rapid development of toxaemia, should ring alarm bells. When bacterial meningitis is suspected, recent studies have confirmed that an injection of benzylpenicillin will lessen the chance of the child dying from the disease; 1200 mg over the age of ten, 600 mg for children aged 1–10 years, and 300 mg for younger infants (Begg 1992).

MALARIA

Has the family been abroad recently? It is an important question if a child presents with a fever without obvious cause. Malaria can develop within a year of a trip to a malaria area, even if prophylaxis has been taken. There are four species of malarial parasite. The most important of these is *Plasmodium falciparum*, which not only can kill the patient but also is often resistant to commonly used drugs. The annual number of cases of malaria in the UK increased from 1500 to 2300 between 1977 and 1991. Over half were caused by *Plasmodium falciparum* and 90 per cent of these were acquired in Africa. Those most commonly affected are immigrants returning from holidays with relatives, followed by businessmen, and then by tourists.

The usual incubation period is about 10 days from the time of the mosquito bite but it can be much longer. The use of antimalarials may delay the onset of symptoms. Primary attacks in a non-immune patient tend to have an abrupt onset, and follow a severe course unless treated. The temperature in children with *P. falciparum* infections may remain high, and there may not be the classical intermittent picture of other types of malaria. A child may have a fit, which is sometimes mistaken for a febrile convulsion, or merely lapse into a coma, and there is often a big spleen. The liver may also be enlarged. A child who is chronically unwell because of frequent attacks of malaria may fail to thrive or become lethargic and anaemic, developing a large spleen. To obtain a diagnostic smear, prick the child's finger and put the first drop of blood on one microscope slide and a second on another one. On the first slide spread a large drop into a circle about 1 cm in diameter. On the other spread a smaller drop to create a similar film; finally thoroughly dry the slides and send them to the laboratory with some blood collected into a bottle containing potassium EDTA.

Antimalarial prophylaxis is important before a visit to any area where malaria is endemic. It is particularly vital for all the family, including young children and pregnant mothers, who intend to visit an area where chloroquine resistant falciparum malaria occurs. It should be started a week before and continue until four to six weeks after departure from the area. Original inhabitants returning to an endemic malarial area after a year or two in Britain will also need to take prophylaxis.

Drugs are not a substitute for taking care to avoid anopheline mosquito bites. This insect is most active at dusk or during the night and children at risk must be protected by long sleeved clothes and long trousers. A mosquito net is essential; it should be checked for holes and the edges tucked under the mattress. A baby's cot can be screened with a net and impregnated with insecticide. Flying insects in the bedroom can be killed by a few sprays of insecticide shortly before bedtime. Burning mosquito coils may be helpful.

As drug resistance patterns vary regionally it is wise to obtain up-to-date advice on which ones to use from a Malarial Reference Centre listed in the BNF (for example, in London, tel. 0171 636 6099). The BNF also contains recommendations on malaria prophylaxis for different parts of the world.

TUBERCULOSIS

Tuberculosis (TB) remains a leading cause of death throughout the developing world. Recent evidence suggests that its incidence may be rising, which in part may be due to the increase in patients with AIDS. In the UK there has been an increase in notification of TB among migrants from the Indian subcontinent.

The infection is caused by *Mycobacterium tuberculosis* and is transmitted by droplets, usually from a household contact with open TB, such as a child-minder or a grandparent. Occasionally it may be caused by *Mycobacterium bovis* after drinking unpasteurized milk from affected cows. Inhaled tubercle bacilli settle and multiply at a peripheral site in the lung (usually subpleural) and this is accompanied by hilar lymphadenopathy to produce the primary complex. Most primary infections are asymptomatic; however, enlarged hilar lymph nodes may produce cough or a wheeze. Four to eight weeks after the infection, sensitivity to tuberculin develops, leading to a positive response on tuberculin testing. Rarely, the child may develop hypersensitivity reaction to the tubercle protein, causing fever, *erythema nodosum* (tender raised red lumps over the shins). Children with primary TB are not infectious.

Children under the age of three years are particularly susceptible to spread of infection to the lung and to extrapulmonary sites, including meninges, bones and joints, lymph nodes, kidneys, intestine and skin. This tends to occur within one year of the primary infection. Children with clinical disease may present with anorexia, weight loss, malaise, fever and cough. Those with miliary TB will have the classical 'snowstorm appearance' on the chest X-ray. They may have generalized lymphadenopathy, enlarged liver and spleen and choroidal tubercles on fundoscopy. Symptoms of early TB meningitis are non-specific and include fever, lethargy, headache, and irritability. If untreated, the affected child develops signs of meningeal irritation, cranial nerve palsies, convulsions, and coma.

Symptoms of TB are often non-specific and therefore diagnosis of TB requires a high index of suspicion. A strongly positive tuberculin test without any clinical or radiological signs will require chemoprophylaxis or treatment. The Mantoux test involves intradermal injection of 1 unit of 10 units/mL dilution of purified protein derivative (PPD) in 0.1 mL (1 in 10 000 dilution) on the upper third of the flexor aspect of the forearm. The reaction is read 48 to 72 hours after the injection, and is recorded as diameter of induration (and not erythema) in millimetres. A positive reaction consists of induration of at least 5 mm diameter. Such a response may occur following BCG or subclinical primary TB. A response of 15 mm or more should be considered as possible evidence of TB infection. A child in the possible incubation period may need testing on a weekly basis—a previous negative test may become spontaneously positive. The reaction to tuberculin test may be suppressed by immunocompromising diseases (including HIV), corticosteroid therapy, and viral infections. The Heaf or Tine tests are useful for screening programmes, for example in schools. An out-patient referral of the older child for collection of sputum, and admission of a toddler for collection of pooled early morning gastric aspirates for culture of the organism may be necessary. A chest X-ray should be obtained in a child with suspicion of TB or with a positive tuberculin test.

TB is a notifiable disease. This is important for tracing of contacts.

Choice of antituberculous treatment and its duration depend on the site and extent of disease. Children with overt pulmonary TB are treated with isoniazid and rifampicin for six to nine months and pyrazinamide for two months. Ethambutol (may cause visual disturbances) is not used until the child is old enough to have vision checked. Children with strongly positive tuberculin testing or who have been in contact with a case of smear positive TB and who have become tuberculin positive should be given isoniazid for six months, or isoniazid and rifampicin for three months. Isoniazid can lead to serious hepatotoxicity and the drug should be stopped promptly and the situation reviewed if clinical signs or symptoms of hepatitis develop. Mildly raised serum transaminases alone are not grounds for stopping the therapy. Rifampicin may cause orange discolouration of urine which is alarming but harmless, and coloured tears, which can damage contact lenses but are otherwise unimportant.

For BCG see p. 37.

ACQUIRED IMMUNE DEFICIENCY SYNDROME (AIDS)

AIDS is increasing among children as a result of perinatal transmission of the human immunodeficiency virus (HIV). About 15 per cent of infants born to infected mothers will become infected. Transmission of HIV via breast-milk has also been described. Tragically, some haemophiliac children have become infected from administration of blood products collected before the introduction of HIV screening procedures.

There may be a latent period of many years before symptoms of AIDS develop. Initial presentation may be with non-specific symptoms and signs, including generalized lymphadenopathy, enlarged liver and spleen, parotitis, chronic diarrhoea, developmental delay, or unexplained fevers. Later symptoms of AIDS include recurrent bacterial infections, infections with opportunistic organisms such as *Pneumocystis carinii* and candidiasis, dry cough, hypoxia, and dyspnoea on exertion due to chronic lymphoid interstitial pneumonitis, and HIV encephalopathy.

Perinatally acquired infections are difficult to diagnose in asymptomatic infants, as the maternally acquired antibody persists up the age of 18 months. Detection of the virus nucleic acid in blood by polymerase chain reaction amplification technique is sensitive and specific but not yet available in many centres.

Specific treatment with zidovudine may help to reduce the progression rate of AIDS, but no curative therapy is yet available. Thus, management of AIDS in children consists of treatment of secondary infections, immunoglobulin replacement therapy, nutritional and psychological support. The DoH has recommended that HIV positive children, with or without symptoms, can be given all the routine immunizations except BCG, because of the risk of dissemination of the BCG vaccine. It would be safer to give children with AIDS inactivated polio vaccine instead of live oral polio vaccine, because of the risk of developing vaccine-associated polio with the latter preparation. Breast-feeding by HIV positive mothers is contra-indicated, since breast-milk may carry the virus.

Fear of AIDS has caused an anxious attitude in schools towards children who are HIV positive. To date there is no evidence of a risk of spread from normal social contacts.

LYME DISEASE

Lyme disease is a chronic infection cased by the spirochaete *Borrelia burgdorferi* which is transmitted by the bite of an infected deer tick. Children playing in a tick infested forest (for example, the New Forest area in Hampshire) develop a characteristic rash consisting of red, slightly raised, expanding rings (*erythema migrans*) 2 to 30 days after the bite, at the site of the bite. About 50 per cent of children will develop recurrent attacks of arthritis affecting large joints one to four months after the infection, and 10 per cent will go on to develop chronic erosive arthritis. Neurological manifestations, including aseptic meningitis, encephalitis, Bell's palsy, or peripheral neuritis may develop in about 20 per cent. A self-limiting myocarditis may occur in some patients.

The diagnosis is usually made on clinical grounds as the causative agent is difficult to culture and serological tests are positive in only about 11 per cent of patients with early disease.

Treatment with oral amoxicillin or penicillin together with probenecid for two to three weeks is beneficial when started during the early (rash stage) of the illness. The same antibiotics can be used orally, but for longer duration, for arthritis. Neurological and cardiac complications require parenteral antibiotics. Prevention consists of avoidance of tick-infested areas, wearing protective clothing and using repellents.

Bibliography

Begg, N. (1992). Reducing mortality from meningococcal disease. *British Medical Journal*, **305**, 133–4.

Bender, C. E. (1967). The value of corticosteroids in the treatment of infectious mononucleosis. *Journal of the American Medical Association,* **199**, 529–31.

Best, J. M. and Banalvala, J. E. (1990). Congenital virus infections. *British Medical Journal,* **300**, 1151–2.

Bradley, D. (1993). Prophylaxis against malaria for travellers from the United Kingdom. On behalf of a meeting convened by the Malaria Reference Laboratory and the Ross Institute. *British Medical Journal,* **306**, 1247–52.

Clarke, S. (1992). Use of thermometers in general practice. *British Medical Journal*, **304**, 961–3

Controversy about chickenpox. (1992). *Lancet*, **340**, 639–40.

Cryan, B. and Wright, D. J. M. (1991). Lyme disease in pediatrics. *Archives of Disease in Childhood,* **66**, 1359–63.

DHSS. (1986). CMO (86) 1. (Discusses children at school and problems related to AIDS.)

Galbraith, N. S., Young, S. E. J., Pusey, J. J., Crombie, D. L., and Sparks, J. P. (1984). Mumps surveillance in England and Wales 1962–81. *Lancet,* **1**, 91–4.

Hanshaw, J. B., Dudgeon, J. A., and Marshall, W. C. (1985). *Viral diseases of the fetus and newborn. Major problems in clinical paediatrics,* Vol. 17, (2nd edn). Saunders, New York. (Very useful for advising pregnant women.)

Immunisation against infectious disease. (1992). HMSO, London.

Isaacs, D. (1992). Infections due to viruses and allied organisms. In *Forfar and Arneil's textbook of paediatrics* (ed. A. G. M. Campbell and N. McIntosh). Churchill Livingstone, London.

Krugman, S., Katz, S. L., Gershon, A. A., and Wilfert, C. (1992). *Infectious diseases of children*, (9th edn). Mosby, St. Louis. (An outstandingly accurate and helpful book.)

McIntosh, D. and Isaacs, D. (1993). Varicella zoster virus infection in pregnancy. *Archives of Disease in Childhood,* **68**, 1–2.

Management of childhood fever. (1991). *Lancet,* **338**, 1049.

Manson, M. M., Logan, W. P. D., and Loy, R. M. (1960). *Rubella and other virus infections during pregnancy.* Reports on Public Health and Medical Subjects, No. 101. HMSO, London.

Medical Research Council. (1977). Clinical trial of live measles vaccine given alone and live vaccine preceded by killed vaccine. *Lancet,* **ii**, 571–5.

Miller, E., Craddock-Watson, J. E., and Pollock, T. M. (1982). Consequences of confirmed maternal rubella at successive stages of pregnancy. *Lancet*, **2**, 781–4.

Morley, C. J., Hewson, P. H., Thornton, A. J., and Cole, T. J. (1992). Axillary and rectal temperature measurements in infants. *Archives of Disease in Childhood,* **67**, 122–5.

Morley, D. C. (1973). *Paediatric priorities in the developing world.* Butterworths, London.

Public health laboratory service working party on fifth disease. (1990). Prospective study of human parvovirus (B19) infection in pregnancy. *British Medical Journal*, **300**, 1166–70.

Smithells, R. W., Sheppard, S., and Holzel, H. (1990). Congenital rubella in Great Britain 1971–1988. *Health Trends*, **22**, 273–6.

Strang, J. R. and Pugh, E. J. (1992). Meningococcal infections: reducing the case fatality rate by giving penicillin before admission to hospital. *British Medical Journal,* **305**, 141–3.

Walker, E. (1986). Malarial prophylaxis. *Prescribers' Journal,* **26**(2), 39–45.

Warren, A. and Andiman, W. A. (1979). The Epstein–Barr virus and E–B virus infections in childhood. *Journal of Pediatrics,* **95**, 171–82.

11 Allergy and asthma

ALLERGY

Even though atopic disease in one form or another probably affects more than 10 per cent of the population, most GPs do not greet the suggestion that allergy may be the cause of a child's persistent catarrh, prolonged diarrhoea, or hyperactivity with much enthusiasm, and neither do we. It is a difficult hypothesis to prove, and treatment by, for example, dietary manipulation, is difficult to sustain, may be hazardous, and can lead to an obsessive attitude to the child's upbringing. However, allergy can sometimes be relevant to a wide range of diseases such as asthma, hay fever, eczema, perennial rhinitis, chronic conjunctivitis, urticaria, and failure to thrive with vomiting or diarrhoea.

The history may be helpful in identifying potential allergies. Did a definite allergic reaction (wheeze or urticarial rash) occur soon after contact with specific items? Do the child's symptoms occur at any particular time of the day or night? Are they seasonal? Has there been a recent family move or a new pet in the household? Did the diarrhoea begin when the baby was taken off the breast and given cows' milk? The relationship between diet and symptoms is seldom so clear, but there are sometimes foods which the family feels exacerbate the child's problem.

Physical examination may confirm an atopic picture with evidence of eczema or asthma. The child with allergic rhinitis may just be a bit sniffy or may have the full picture of a constantly runny, itchy nose, together with mouth breathing due to an obstructed nasal airway. In these cases, examination of the nose with an auroscope and speculum reveals a swollen mucous membrane. Constant nasal obstruction can also be due to large adenoids or to a deviated septum, or, more rarely, nasal polyps. In these situations the airway never clears completely; with allergic rhinitis it sometimes does.

Food allergy is an area of enormous controversy and its over-diagnosis may lead to the use of odd diets with poor nutritional value. When it does occur, it is usually temporary. Allergy and intolerance to cows' milk protein is a definite entity. According to David (1992), the diagnosis is more likely if allergic symptoms occur or become worse soon after the ingestion of cows' milk; there is a family history of cows' milk intolerance; there is the presence of severe atopic disease in an infant under 12 months of age, and if an allergic urticarial reaction occurs when cows' milk is spilled on non-eczema skin. Intolerance may cause infants to fail to thrive, with diarrhoea, vomiting, malabsorption and even gastrointestinal bleeding. The symptoms may be provoked by a varying amount of milk and are usually temporary, but in some children last a year or more. Referral is necessary if the diagnosis is a serious possibility. Other foods which are likely to cause reactions are various nuts, citrus fruit, wheat, fish, and shell fish. In some infants, these foods may cause obvious urticaria, a red flush, and 'colic'. Allergy to eggs is uncommon. When present, it occurs in the first few months of life and has usually disappeared by the time the child is three years old. Reactions can be quite striking, for example, a red flair around the mouth with swelling of the lips and tongue occurring shortly after ingestion of eggs.

Diagnostic tests are of limited value. There may be a raised eosinophil count. This also occurs in parasitic infections, drug reactions, and some infiltrative pulmonary diseases. Allergic skin tests and the measurement of IgE levels against specific antigens using the radio-allergosorbent (RAST) test are usually carried out in allergy clinics. They can be useful in confirming penicillin allergy or insect venom hypersensitivity (Warner 1985), but are of little use in planning management of an obviously atopic child as he will probably be positive to most antigens, including those whose exclusion gives no clinical benefit. Tests in commercial allergy clinics may be quite unreliable. In one study, such clinics failed to correctly diagnose fish allergy in blood and hair from nine subjects known to be allergic to fish. Multiple allergies were discovered in a group of healthy controls (Sethi *et al.* 1987).

It can be very difficult to satisfactorily manage children with chronic allergic problems. If the precipitating factors can be definitely identified and eliminated, this is ideal, although a child with a very positive skin test to the dander may be very reluctant to part with a family pet. He may prefer to continue sneezing and itching, even if he clearly improves when away for a few days from contact with the animal and the house in which it lives. Measures to reduce the house dust may be worthwhile, and are discussed later in the chapter.

General practitioners do not usually initiate complicated manipulations of diet. However, it is worth testing whether the elimination of a food suspected of causing symptoms for a month or so, results in an improvement in the patient's condition. In babies, various cows' milk substitutes on the market, such as the synthetic milk Pregestimil, or soya bean preparation such as Wysoy, can be useful, although some infants with milk protein intolerance develop soya protein intolerance also.

ANAPHYLAXIS

Anaphylaxis is a potentially life-threatening emergency, which may follow immunizations (adrenaline 1/1000 must always be available and the practice nurse trained in its use) or other injections, a wasp sting or ingestion of substances mentioned above. If old enough, the child may complain of feeling faint with an itchy skin and difficulty in breathing because of bronchospasm and/or swollen lips and tongue. He looks deathly pale and may be covered in an urticarial rash. His pulse may be weak and thready; shock and collapse may follow.

Lie the child with anaphylaxis on his side and raise the legs, give 1/1000 adrenaline (0.05 mL for children <1 year, 0.1 mL for one to two years, increasing by 0.1 mL per year to maximum dose of 0.5 mL) intramuscularly, and oxygen if available. Chlorpheniramine maleate (Piriton), 2.5–5 mg and hydrocortisone may be given intravenously. Nebulized bronchodilator (e.g. 2.5–5 mg of salbutamol) is given to relieve bronchospasm. Observation in hospital is advised. In severe cases the GP may need to start cardio-pulmonary resuscitation.

Peanut allergy

Peanut allergy is probably the most common cause of fatal food anaphylaxis, severe reactions occurring within a few minutes of ingestion. Patients (and their parents) with known allergy must carry preloaded adrenaline syringes, antihistamines, and medic-alert bracelets. Hidden sources of peanuts such as cakes, biscuits, and pastry need to be recognized and identified.

HAY FEVER

In hay fever the child's nose is blocked intermittently from May to September and he keeps sneezing. He is often unable to taste or smell properly. A profuse, watery rhinitis may soak the handkerchief, making it look as if it had been dipped in water. He may wheeze if severely affected. His eyes are itchy and red and become sore, sometimes with marked oedema of the conjunctiva (chemosis), particularly after he has rubbed them vigorously. The patient has become sensitized to wind-borne pollen, usually from grasses, but occasionally from trees, shrubs, flowers, or weeds. He overproduces immunoglobulin IgE. Contact between IgE and the antigen in the nose leads to degranulation of the mast cells with release of vasoactive amines:

Gary, aged four, was rushed into the surgery one June day looking grotesque with marked chemosis of both eyes. His mother said that he had been rubbing his eyes all day, but there were no other symptoms. By the next morning his eyes were back to normal. Over the next two years, he developed symptoms of classical hay fever.

It is not possible for the unfortunate patient to avoid all contact with pollen, but apart from drugs, symptoms may be improved by following this advice:

1. Sleep with the windows closed during June and July, and keep the windows closed if in a car.
2. Do not walk through long grass, and take extra prophylactic drugs before outings.
3. Get someone else to mow the lawn.

Non-sedating antihistamines such as terfenadine (Triludan), astemizole (Hist-amal) may be helpful and can be obtained without prescription. The latter may be more effective in hay fever but can cause a gain in weight. The metabolism of both may be inhibited by ketoconazole and erythromycin.

Sodium cromoglycate must be used several times a day, to be effective in preventing symptoms. It does not seem to be as useful in preventing rhinitis as asthma, but it can alleviate allergic eye symptoms. Local steroid eye drops are not recommended for hay fever.

Intranasal steroids, such as beclomethasone (two squirts up each nostril twice a day) often relieves allergic rhinitis. Treatment should be started before the hay fever season is fully established, but once the symptoms are under control (or on rainy days when the pollen count is low) it is often possible to reduce the dose. Children should be shown how to use the spray, which should be pointed away from the septum to reduce nasal irritation. There is no significant adrenal suppression from nasal steroids although there is possibly a risk of mucous-membrane atrophy in the nose if use is prolonged. Oral steroids are rarely prescribed for children with hay fever, but might be justified for a few days to cover an important examination (20 mg reducing to zero over four days). Although hyposensitization may reduce symptoms of severe hay fever, it is no longer recommended because of possible anaphylaxis. In fact, hyposensitization should probably be reserved for children with life-threatening allergy to wasp or bee sting.

In short, most children who have only nasal or ocular symptoms respond to a local preparation, whereas an antihistamine may be the best initial therapy when eyes, nose, and perhaps itchy palate are all involved.

ASTHMA

Asthma is a common condition, characterized by recurrent episodes of wheezing, cough, and breathlessness caused by variable obstruction to airflow, secondary to an inflammation of the airways and broncho-constriction. The bronchial lumen is narrowed causing air to be trapped in the lungs. The liability of the bronchi to undergo excessive changes of calibre is commonly referred to as hyperactivity, and the bronchi of most severely affected children hyperreact to a wide range of stimuli. The narrowing of the bronchial lumen is caused partly by constriction of bronchial muscle and partly by oedema of the mucous membranes and by excess secretions. As muscle constriction may not be the main problem in an individual attack, bronchodilator drugs acting on smooth muscle may have only an incomplete effect. Asthma is likely to originate from a mixture of environmental and genetic factors. If one parent has asthma, the child is more than twice as likely to develop the disease as offspring of non-asthmatic parents (Dold *et al.* 1992).

Childhood asthma affects about 10 per cent of children in the UK (Burney *et al.* 1990), and it appears to be getting more common world-wide, resulting in a doubling of admissions to hospital between 1977 and 1990. This probably reflects both a definite, but unexplained, increase in prevalence and severity and changes in the way in which doctors and parents label and deal with a wheezy child. However, those affected in 1991 had less time off school and their parents a less restricted social life than in previous years. Perhaps this reflects improved medical management and a more confident parental attitude (Anderson *et al.* 1994).

The natural history of asthma is becoming more clearly understood. In an Australian study, Jenkins *et al.* (1994) reported that three-quarters of children who had asthma at the age of seven had no symptoms at the age of 30. Important risk factors for continuation of symptoms into adulthood include history of eczema, a parent with asthma, and first attack after the age of two years. Not surprisingly, those children with severe asthma are less likely to grow out of their disease. However, one cannot necessarily assume that the natural history in children who are currently asthmatic will be the same.

Asthma ranges in severity from an occasional episode of infection-provoked wheezing through severe intermittent classical episodes in a child well at other times, to the child who is permanently disabled by airways obstruction. Wheeze may not be the presenting symptom and asthma should be suspected in children who have a persistent nocturnal cough, repeated 'respiratory infections', or excess shortness of breath or cough during exercise, with poor performance in, or dislike of games. There may also be chest deformity (Harrison's sulcus) and, in severe cases, stunting of growth and delayed puberty.

Other conditions besides asthma and respiratory infections can cause wheezing. The child with his first attack of asthma may have inhaled a foreign body:

Susan, aged four years, had been wheezing for a day by the time she was seen. She appeared to have a moderately severe attack of asthma, but her mother told the doctor that she had been playing with her younger brother the day before, throwing peanuts at each other. She had inhaled one, and symptoms subsided after it had been removed by bronchoscopy.

Cystic fibrosis may be associated with recurrent attacks of wheeziness, poor growth associated with excessive appetite or with greasy stools, finger clubbing, and fine crepitations on auscultation of the chest. In babies, cardiac failure is another rare possibility, as is gastro-oesophageal reflux leading to low-grade inhalation of gastric contents.

The GP is sometimes reluctant to diagnose asthma in a child who has had several episodes of wheeziness because of the anxiety the word may provoke in parents. This is a mistake, as asthmatic children labelled as having 'recurrent bronchitis' will often be prescribed ineffective antibiotics instead of more appropriate therapy. Asthma is still a disease which, in its most severe form, may lead to stunting of growth and even to sudden and unexpected death. In a detailed analysis of the deaths of 90 patients over the age of 15 Johnson *et al.* (1984) concluded that the main cause of fatal delay in starting effective treatment, was that the patient, relative, or doctor did not realize how severe the attack was. Carswell (1985), describing the deaths of 30 asthmatic children, concluded that inadequate treatment with steroids contributed to the fatal outcome. Most childhood asthmatic deaths are in adolescents and especially in those who get low peak flows in the early morning hours, often waking struggling for breath at 3–6 a.m. This is more dangerous when compounded by a teenager's naturally rebellious feelings about illness management, which may make them play down the history and be reluctant to take any treatment which involves them taking their inhalers about with them. There is documented increase in emotional disturbance in children who have severe asthma at 14 years, but this may often be the result of, rather than the cause of, their symptoms. The commonest reason for failure to control asthma is ineffective use of the available drugs. This may be the doctor's or parent's fault, but even a well-instructed child may decide through embarrassment not to use his inhaler at school.

Assessment

When a GP takes over the care of a patient with asthma, or makes the diagnosis for the first time, he should use the opportunity to make a full assessment of its severity. The aim is to decide not only on the most appropriate therapy but also to begin to build up a relationship with the family and to give them the confidence necessary to monitor their child's asthma (for example, by peak flow measurements), to alter treatment in relation to severity of the disease, and when to seek medical help.

The initial assessment must establish the following:

1. Frequency and severity of attacks. How severe was the worst attack to date, and has the child needed admission to hospital? How does the family manage a typical attack?
2. Is the child using an appropriate inhaler correctly? How often does the child have to use the 'reliever' inhaler, and at what time of the day or night?
3. Degree of social handicap; amount of time off school.
4. Is there a past history of atopic disease or a family history of atopy?
5. What is the child like between attacks?
6. Does he get nocturnal or exercise induced wheezing or cough?
7. What provokes an asthmatic attack; is there evidence of a strong allergic component? Is his bedroom dusty? Does he have feather filling in his pillow or duvet? What is the number of teddy bears, which harbour dust and house-dust mites?
8. Is there evidence to support an alternative diagnosis to asthma?
9. Does a parent smoke; does this make the child's asthma worse?

During the interview the doctor will try to make an assessment of the relationships within the family—does the mother allow her nine-year-old child to speak for himself? If a child is wheezing, how concerned does the mother appear to be?

The following basic data are also required for the moderately or severely affected child:

1. Height and weight, recorded on a centile chart. A child who is very underweight for his height or who is very short may have worse asthma than was thought.

2. Chest X-ray; the occasional unexpected abnormality will be revealed.

3. Peak expiratory flow rate. Children of four or five and over should be able to use a peak flow meter, allowing comparison with the value predicted for a child of the same height (p. 322.)

If the peak flow rate is low for the child's size, it can be remeasured 10 minutes after the inhalation of a bronchodilator. In childhood asthma there is usually improvement within this time. Conversely, if there is a history of cough or wheeze only during exercise, it is occasionally helpful to record the peak flow and listen to the chest before and 5 and 10 minutes after the child has run about 200 yards.

When the child is examined, it should be noted whether his chest has the configuration of a severe asthmatic (the ribs more horizontal than normal with the shoulders moved up towards the ears and with a Harrison's sulcus visible where the attachment of the diaphragm has pulled the ribs in). It is important to record whether his chest contains a lot of wheeze and whether peak flow is reduced at a time when he and his parents consider he is well. Wheeze is not always present, even in severe attacks. This important fact is one reason why peak flow measurements are needed. A non-wheezy chest is compatible with even a life-threatening attack of asthma.

Drug treatment

Attention to detail is the key to asthma drug therapy. If a drug is not working the first step is to check inhaler technique and whether dose is adequate rather than to change the drug.The prescription should be accompanied by careful explanation (which often includes written instructions) on how to use the drugs given and how each one can help. The patient and his family must realize which drugs should be used prophylactically, and which should be used to relieve symptoms. There are some useful booklets and videos for parents and children produced in various languages by the National Asthma Campaign (p. 330).

Prophylactic drugs such as cromoglycate and inhaled steroids are not effective in relieving an acute attack. If the child is wheezy their introduction is more successful if one or two doses of inhaled bronchodilator are given just before the cromoglycate or steroid. A chronically wheezy child often responds to oral prednisolone (2 mg/kg—maximum dose 40 mg/day) given for five days or less.

Dried powder inhalers (Table 11.2) are best for convenience and effectiveness and can be used by most well taught children over the age of four years.

Table 11.1 Anti-asthma drugs

β-agonists
Salbutamol, terbutaline. Effective during bronchospasm. Action is rapid especially if inhaled. (Salmeterol is a long-acting bronchodilator which is useful in severe or nocturnal or exercise-induced asthma. It is only to be used as an adjunct to prophylactic cromoglycate or steroids.)

Slow-release xanthines
Prescribed decreasingly; sometimes useful for children too young for inhalers, for those inadequately controlled on inhaled steroids, and for late night-time wheezing. They have a narrow therapeutic range, and monitoring of blood and saliva levels is recommended. Side-effects such as gastro-intestinal upsets or sleep disturbance occur in up to one-third of patients.

Sodium cromoglycate
Prophylactic only. Very low toxicity. Effective in 60 per cent of children but has to be used at least three, preferably four times a day.

Steroids

SYSTEMIC
Oral prednisolone. Effective during bronchospasm. Necessary for acute attacks of asthma that do not respond rapidly to inhaled bronchodilators. Maximum effect about five hours after administration and lasts about twenty hours. Give as single morning dose (2 mg/kg body weight—maximum dose 40 mg daily). If used long-term, any steroid side-effects may occur, poor growth the most important. Maintenance oral steroids not initiated in primary care.

INHALED
Beclomethasone, fluticasone, or budesonide. Prophylactic only; very effective. Most inhalers deposit only 10 per cent in the lungs. Large volume spacers may do better and reduce side-effects because less is deposited in the mouth and pharynx, causing candidiasis and hoarseness from vocal chord involvement. Risk may be reduced if mouth rinsed.

Dummies are available from drug firms and one type of device may suit a particular child better than another. In an acute attack a metered-dose inhaler (MDI) with a spacer is needed to give effective therapy because in that situation the powder cannot be sucked in effectively. Every child subject to acute asthmatic attacks should have a spacer and metered-dose inhaler available for use in an emergency. For young babies, a spacer and mask can be used with a metered-dose inhaler (a polystyrene cup is an alternative, the mouth-piece of the canister being pushed through the base and the aerosol trickled past the child's face). The dose of bronchodilator (for example, salbutamol) delivered in a single puff from a metered-dose inhaler is tiny—a twelfth or less of a single dose using a powered nebulizer—so the doctor need have no fears if several puffs are needed.

Theoretically antibiotics do not have a place in asthma but, if the wheezy child has had symptoms which may have an infectious basis, such as a purulent nasal discharge with fever, many GPs may give a course of amoxycillin.

Table 11.2 Inhalation delivery systems for children

Age (years)	Inhalation delivery system
<2	Powered nebulizer Valved large volume spacer and face mask (McCarthy). Use with MDI; hold spacer vertical to keep valve open Polystyrene cup and MDI allow aerosol to drift onto face.
2–4	Valved large volume spacer: Nebuhaler (Astra). Can also be used with Intal MDI. Volumatic (Allen & Hanburys). Valved spacers used with MDI; valve opens on inspiration.
5–8	Powder inhalers: Spinhaler (Fisons). Use cromoglycate capsules. Rotahaler (Allen & Hanburys). Salbutamol and beclomethasone capsules. Diskhaler (Allen & Hanburys). Salbutamol, beclomethasone and fluticasone discs. Accuhaler (Allen & Hanburys). Salbutamol, beclomethasone and fluticasone. Turbohaler (Astra). Powder flavourless; good if taste a problem.
>8	MDI with large volume valved spacer. Inconvenient at school; good for emergencies. Powder inhalers: Autohaler (Riker; 3M Breath activated MDI) MDI *with training*

Source: adapted from *Archives of Disease in Childhood* (1992), **67**, 240–8.

Home use of nebulizers

The use of home nebulizers to administer bronchodilator drugs is controversial, because of the reports of their use being followed by unexpected deaths. They are dangerous if the family cannot be relied upon to monitor response to treatment carefully, or to contact the practice promptly if either there is no response to the initial nebulizer drug, or if temporary improvement is not sustained after one further dose two to four hours after the first. The main danger is failing to realize that an initial brisk improvement may be followed some hours later by dangerous recurrence of bronchospasm. Nebulizers are invaluable for delivering prophylactic drugs (that is, cromoglycate or budesonide) to young children who are unable to use a large volume spacer with an MDI. As with inhalers they need to have their use demonstrated; they also need regular cleaning. In older children, a nebulizer should only be used with peak flow measurements to check if perceived improvement is genuine. Dose of salbutamol is 2.5 mg which can be increased to 5 mg for the very wheezy older child. Spacers are often as effective as nebulizers in an emergency, being cheap, available on prescription and easily carried in the GP's car. One puff of the bronchodilator

Table 11.3 General practice asthma management plan

Asthma severity	Definition	Treatment
Mild	Symptoms do not interfere with sleep, exercise, or schooling and respond to bronchodilators inhaled once a day or less frequently. Very infrequent acute attacks.	Inhaled bronchodilators when necessary.
Moderate	Discrete attacks occurring once a month or/and more chronic asthma which interferes with lifestyle to some extent.	Inhaled bronchodilators plus cromoglycate 3 or 4 times a day, as dry powder (20 mg) or via MDI + spacer (10 mg). If no substantial improvement after 6 weeks replace this by inhaled steroids 50–100 micrograms twice daily, gradually increasing the dose depending on child's age and size.
Severe	Asthma more severe than the above.	Inhaled bronchodilators plus inhaled steroids morning and evening via a spacer to reduce the risk of side-effects, to a maximum of 400 micrograms twice daily. If asthma not controlled by this: add long acting β agonists (e.g. salmeterol) or slow release xanthines and *consider referral.*
Stepping down	At each stage consider reducing treatment if improvement is sustained.	

Children with moderate/severe asthma attacks: they may initially need, to bring the wheeziness under rapid control, a short course of prednisolone (2 mg/kg/day—maximum 40 mg by about 8 years for a maximum of 5 days; no need to taper dose unless given longer).

(to a maximum of 20) is delivered into the device every few seconds until the patient improves (Keeley 1992).

Management planning

Management plans are based on the doctor having a stepwise approach to treatment. Our 'General Practice' version, shown in Table 11.3, is in keeping with the excellent and more detailed guidelines of the British Thoracic Society (1993). Most families cope with the condition well, especially if given clear instructions about what action to take at different stages of an attack. It must be made clear to the parents that they are the 'front-line doctors'.

Peak flow meters

Peak flow meters are only useful as part of an agreed plan of management. It is unrealistic to expect children to monitor their peak flow when they are perfectly well and adolescents can manipulate their readings up and down by various tricks such as 'pea shooting', or by fabricating them! Twice daily readings recorded on a diary may confirm a deteriorating situation, enabling the child to increase prophylactic medication before an acute attack develops. Clear instructions are essential. For example: 'Double the dose of inhaled steroids if the peak flow drops to 60–80 per cent of usual value. Seek medical help rapidly if there is no improvement in symptoms and/or peak flow is less than 60 per cent of the usual value.' Many children with asthma may show up to 20 per cent diurnal variation in their peak flow even if they are not suffering from an acute attack.

The practice asthma clinic

Many practices have established asthma clinics, often run by the nurse backed-up by a named partner. The nurse will need additional training in the management of asthma in children and will have a major commitment to the key task—patient and parent education. A well run clinic will have a couple of nebulizers available; a wide range of inhaler device systems for the child to try; clear, preferably customized, guidelines for patients and an unambiguous description of the circumstances when the nurse should seek doctor advice; adequate time for explanation and a system for following non-attenders. Liaison with school may help to dispel teachers' fears and encourage co-operation. Children taking cromoglycate or steroids should be reviewed every six months. For less well controlled children the frequency of review will depend on the severity of the symptoms and the peak flow reading. A change in therapy should lead to an early reassessment. Poor control does not necessarily mean more medication—perhaps the wheeziness can be explained by a recent series of upper respiratory tract infections, new smoking by others at home or by the teenage patient, or a Christmas present of a kitten.

Some problem areas

The under two-year-old

Young infants may wheeze for a few days with every cold. As neither bronchodilators nor steroids are very effective at this age the main questions are, when should the child need admission to hospital, when should he be reviewed and is the diagnosis correct?

A cheerful older baby taking his feeds relatively well and whose sleep is not disturbed by respiratory symptoms can reasonably be observed at home even if breathing is noisy, perhaps at 50 breaths per minute and associated with some rib recession. A repeat consultation 24 hours later is advisable. One needs to err on the side of caution for a baby with a first attack of bronchospasm or with an infant under three or four months; is the diagnosis really bronchiolitis or pneumonia? Some doctors may try oral salbutamol but there is not much point in persisting unless there is a clear improvement. For the young child more seriously affected than this, and over one-year-old, β agonist with a home nebulizer or valved spacer held vertically with a face mask may give significant relief. Prophylactic inhaled budesonide (Pulmicort), after consultation with a paediatrician, appears to benefit some.

Asthma presenting as a cough (p. 196)

A chronic nocturnal cough is a well known presentation of asthma. It may be reasonable on occasions to treat a chronic cough in a well child with β agonist. Prophylactic medication should only be instituted following peak flow evidence of reversible airways obstruction.

The acute attack

Parents should know when to consult the GP—primarily when the asthma does not respond to the child's standard therapy. A previously under-treated patient may well respond to bronchodilator delivered by a metered-dose inhaler into a spacer. If this fails, or the child is too young to cope, nebulized salbutamol may be very effective. Unfortunately, the patient may deteriorate after initial improvement. Unless there is dramatic and sustained relief from bronchodilators prednisolone 30–40 mg by mouth or hydrocortisone 100 mg i.m. or i.v. must also be given. Hospital admission will be necessary if the child is deteriorating despite this therapy, if there is unusual agitation—an early and undervalued sign of hypoxia—cyanosis, gross tachycardia at rest, parental incompetence, or difficulty in offering continued medical supervision. A PEFR less than 40 per cent of normal value, a silent chest, cyanosis, exhaustion, confusion, and bradycardia are signs of a life-threatening situation. As mentioned before, parents of a child with severe asthma should be told that severe and dangerous attacks, while rare, are a remote possibility. If their child ever becomes so breathless that he cannot talk, or walk across the room, or goes blue, they should get help at once.

Allergic factors

The number of children with asthma admitted to hospitals in inner city areas increases on windless summer days. This is presumably because of a rise in the number of trapped pollen particles in polluted particles. Avoidance of allergens and hypo-sensitization have proved somewhat disappointing in the management of asthma and it is necessary to select, from the large number of asthmatics, those few with a strong clinical history of an allergic component to their symptoms. In them, a more detailed attention to immunological factors may be worthwhile.

Allergies demonstrated by skin tests do not always reflect bronchial allergy but if there is a clear history of wheezing being provoked by a particular exposure, such as to an animal, dust, aspirin, pollens, or certain foods, it may be possible to reduce the degree of exposure. However, this does not, in our experience, have much effect in reducing the number of asthmatic attacks.

A lot of attention has been paid to the role of the house-dust mite, particularly in provoking asthma or wheezing and coughing in dusty circumstances. Unfortunately, this mite is present in most houses, but the following measures will reduce the number the child inhales:

1. Regular vacuum cleaning in the morning to allow residual dust to settle by bed time.
2. Regular damp dusting.
3. Frequent washing of bedding.
4. Mattresses made of synthetic material rather than fibre of animal origin.
5. Plastic covers round mattresses and pillows.
6. Avoidance of a down duvet.

Indications for referral for specialist opinion

1. Doubt about diagnosis.
2. Failure to respond to treatment with moderate doses of inhaled steroids (for example, >400 micrograms twice daily of beclomethasone).
3. Frequent need for courses of oral steroids, or long-term steroid treatment is being considered.
4. If the GP considers that a hospital referral will encourage patient compliance.
5. Children who have attacks of sudden very severe asthma. They should be able to self-refer to hospital.

Some of these patients can be discharged back to their GP once their asthma is well controlled. For others shared care is appropriate.

Audit

The care of children with asthma is a very good area for audit: do the number of wheezy children approach the expected 10 per cent of the under-15-years practice population? Are children who receive a repeat prescription for a bronchodilator more often than every two months also on prophylactic medication, and is their asthma checked at regular intervals? Are the young people using age-appropriate inhalation devices? What proportion of asthmatic children fail to attend their follow-up appointment?

Finally, to end on a positive note, Ross *et al.* (1992) followed-up a cohort of people who had been diagnosed as suffering from asthma or wheeziness in the early 1960s. They concluded that childhood wheeze did not adversely affect educational attainment, employment prospects, housing or social class, 25 years later.

Bibliography

Anderson, H. R. (1989). Increase in hospital admissions for childhood asthma: trends in referral, severity, and readmission from 1970 to 1985 in a health region of the United Kingdom. *Thorax,* **44**, 614–9.

Anderson, H. R., Butland, B. K., and Strachan, D. P. (1994). Trends in prevalence and severity of childhood asthma. *British Medical Journal*, **308**, 1600–4.

Asthma. (1992). A follow up statement from an International Paediatric Asthma Consensus Group. A special report by the Steering Committee. *Archives of Disease in Childhood*, **67**, 240–8.

Burney, P. G. J., Chinn, S., and Rona, R. J. (1990). Has the prevalence of asthma increased in children. Evidence from the National Study of Health and Growth 1973–1986. *British Medical Journal*, **300**, 1306–10.

Carswell, F. (1985). Thirty deaths from asthma. *Archives of Disease in Childhood*, **60**, 25–8.

Connolly, K. (1992). Inhaled corticosteroids in the management of asthma. *Prescribers' Journal,* **32**, 99–106.

David, T. J. (1992). Allergic disorders In *Forfar and Arneil's textbook of paediatrics*, (ed. A. G. M. Campbell and N. McIntosh), (4th edn). Churchill Livingstone, London.

Dold, S., Wjst, M. *et al.* (1992). Genetic risk for asthma, allergic rhinitis, and atopic dermatitis. *Archives of Disease in Childhood*, **67**, 1018–22.

Guidelines on the management of asthma. Statement by the British Thoracic Society *et al.* (1993). *Thorax,* **48** (2 Suppl), S1–24.

Hetzel, M. and Modell, M. (1992). Asthma. In *Clinical guidelines—report of a local initiative*, (ed. A. Haines and B. Hurwitz). R.C.G.P., London.

Jenkins, M. A., Hopper, J. L., Bowes, G. *et al.* (1994). Factors in childhood as predictors of asthma in adult life. *British Medical Journal*, **309**, 90–3.

Johnson, A. J., Nunn, A. J., Somner, A. R. *et al.* (1984). Circumstances of death from asthma. *British Medical Journal*, **288**, 1870–2.

Keeley, D. (1992). Large volume plastic spacers in asthma. *British Medical Journal*, **305**, 598–9.

Luyt, D. K., Burton P. R., and Simpson, H. (1993). Epidemiological study of wheeze, doctor diagnosed asthma, and cough in preschool children in Leicestershire. *British Medical Journal,* **306**, 1386–90.

McKenzie, S. (1994). Cough—but is it asthma? *Archives of Disease in Childhood,* **70**, 1–2.

Ninan, T. K. and Russell, G. (1992). Respiratory symptoms and atopy in Aberdeen schoolchildren: evidence from two surveys 25 years apart. *British Medical Journal,* **304**, 873–5.

Noble, V., Ruggins, N. R., Everard, M. L., and Milner, A. D. (1992). Inhaled budesonide for chronic wheezing under 18 months of age. *Archives of Disease in Childhood,* **67**, 285–8.

Ross, S., Godden, D., McMurray, D., Douglas, A., Oldman, D., Friend, J. *et al.* (1992). Social effects of wheeze in childhood: a 25 year follow up. *British Medical Journal,* **305**, 545–8.

Sethi, T. J., Lessof, M. H., Kemeny, D. M. *et al.* (1987). How reliable are commercial allergy tests? *Lancet,* **i**, 92–4.

Storr, J., Barrell, E., Barry, W., Lenney, W., and Hatcher, G. (1987). Effect of a single oral dose of prednisolone in acute childhood asthma. *Lancet,* **i**, 879–82.

Strachan, D. P. and Anderson, H. R. (1992). Trends in hospital admission rates for asthma in children. *British Medical Journal,* **304**, 819–20.

Strachan, D. P., Anderson, H. R., Limb, E. S. *et al.* (1994). A national survey of asthma prevalence, severity, and treatment in Great Britain. *Archives of Disease in Childhood,* **70**, 1741–78.

Warner, J. O. (1985). Allergies in childhood. In *Progress in child health,* Vol 2, (ed. J.A. MacFarlane). Churchill Livingstone, London.

12 Other respiratory disorders

Respiratory disease and otitis media account for 40 per cent of consultations by children under five years (Morbidity statistics from general practice 1986). This is not surprising considering that, on average, children have 12 acute respiratory infections in their first two years of life.

Parental smoking is important. In a large British study involving 13 000 children under five years, maternal smoking during pregnancy was associated with a significantly increased risk of the child being admitted to hospital with a lower respiratory tract infection. 'Bronchitis' was most likely in children of mothers who smoked, surprisingly even if this was only in the antenatal period. Paternal smoking did not have a significant influence on the amount of serious respiratory disease.

Most respiratory pathogens can, on occasion, cause any one of the respiratory infections, ranging from mild rhinitis to fulminating pneumonia; thus, a baby may catch bronchiolitis from a neighbour or older sibling, who has only a cold due to respiratory syncytial virus (RSV). Certain organisms are, however, particularly associated with certain syndromes (Table 12.1). Ninety per cent of infections are viral and are unlikely to be helped by antibiotics. Non-viral infections are commonly caused by a limited range of pathogens: *Haemophilus influenzae, Streptococcus pneumoniae, Streptococcus pyogenes*, mycoplasma, and one or two others. In planning antibacterial treatment, their sensitivities should always be in the forefront of one's mind. Most of them are sensitive to erythromycin—a rather under-used antibiotic, relatively free of side-effects.

Recurrent or persistent respiratory symptoms are frequent reasons for consultations: 'The nose is always running'; 'he always has a cough'; 'always chesty'. Frequently, such children are atopic (Chapter 11). Sometimes the environment is to blame. Children from poor families living in damp, mouldy housing are more likely to suffer from these infections (Platt *et al.* 1989). Sometimes repeated infections in a child are due to cross-infection in a day-nursery or from an extended family. Occasionally, structural nasal obstruction, a swallowing problem, a respiratory tract foreign body, or, in a generally poorly child, immunodeficiency or cystic fibrosis may be the cause.

Table 12.1 Important respiratory pathogens

Disease	Viruses	Other pathogens
Colds and rhinitis	Rhino (most important) RSV, adeno parainfluenza, others	
Febrile naso-pharyngitis (in infants under 6 months)		*Strep. pyogenes* *Strep. pneumoniae*
Otitis media	RSV, influenza rhino, others	*Strep. pneumoniae* *Haemophilus influenzae* *Strep. pyogenes* *M. catarrhalis* *Staph. aureus*
Acute tonsillitis with exudate	Adeno, E–BV	*Strep. pyogenes* *C. diphtheriae*
Acute tonsillitis with vesicles or ulcers	Coxsackie group A, herpes simplex	
Croup	Parainfluenza (most important) RSV, adeno, and others	*H. influenzae* type B (epiglottitis)
Bronchiolitis	RSV (most important), parainfluenza and others	
Pneumonia	RSV, parainfluenza, adeno-, influenza, varicella-zoster	*Strep. pneumoniae* *Strep. pyogenes* *Haemophilus influenzae* Mycoplasma *Staph. aureus* Chlamydia *Pneumocystis carinii*, legionella
Influenza-like illness	Influenza parainfluenza adenovirus	

E-BV = Epstein–Barr virus; RSV = respiratory syncytial virus. Modified from Krugman *et al.* (1992).

COLDS

Most are minor and self-limiting after an incubation period of two or three days, with a period of infectivity lasting one or two days after the onset of symptoms. Although GPs accept that these are caused by viruses, many infected children receive antibiotics, even if not clinically indicated. This is partly because of a wish (often in the context of parental pressure) to play for safety, and partly from a feeling that if there should be a deterioration in the child's condition, this could have been prevented if antibiotics had been given. Confidence that antibiotics can prevent a disaster may, however, be misplaced. Dehydration from poor feeding or even unexplained apnoea leading to a cot death can follow from a cold, and are not prevented by antibiotics. A follow-up consultation may be of more real value than a prescription. Stott (1979) showed that the widely differing prescribing habits of GPs did not correlate with clinical outcome. He suggested that a mother will be given more confidence in dealing with the child's cold if she is warned at the beginning that a cough may continue for up to two weeks and that short-lived episodes of diarrhoea and vomiting may be associated with respiratory symptoms. A cold in infants causes troublesome nasal obstruction, interfering with their ability to suck. The nostrils can be cleaned before feeds with a moist cotton bud. It is particularly important to pay careful attention to the fluid intake of these babies.

Babies admitted to hospital with pneumonia have usually had a preceding cold so, despite the common and trivial nature of most colds, parents should usually be warned that apathy, prolonged irritability, consistently poor feeding, and a respiratory rate that remains high (over 50 or so per minute) when the baby is at rest are reasons for a further consultation.

Infection from a cold may spread in various directions, notably up the Eustachian tube to the middle-ear or, in older children, to the sinuses. In infants, dull, slightly pink ear-drums are an almost uniform feature of the common cold, regardless of whether full-scale acute otitis media subsequently develops or not. Pharyngitis, laryngitis, tracheitis, or pneumonia can occur if infection spreads down the respiratory tract. Not all runny noses are colds. In allergic rhinitis, the child does not become feverish nor the nasal discharge purulent. There are usually other signs of allergy—continual sneezing, itchy nose, and itchy eyes.

ACUTE SINUSITIS

When a child whose sinuses have developed (maxillary and ethmoid sinuses first, frontal and sphenoidal in later childhood) has a cold, they are usually involved to some extent. Often the symptoms are mild, difficult to distinguish from those of a nasty cold. More severe infection of the sinuses appears to be uncommon in children. If it does develop, they become feverish, with facial pain and tenderness over the affected sinus. Amoxycillin is an appropriate antibiotic in most cases. A couple of days of ephedrine nose drops may help with draining. Ethmoid sinusitis may produce an alarming periorbital swelling and even proptosis—an indication for admission because of the remote risk of spread within the skull.

PHARYNGITIS AND TONSILLITIS

Sore throat is part of many syndromes produced by respiratory viruses; occasionally throat symptoms predominate. The normal pharynx can be mildly redder than the surrounding tissue, but this does not necessarily indicate that pharyngitis is the cause of a child's fever. Even though a GP will often say that a mildly unwell child has a red throat in an attempt to reassure the parent with a label, he must not delude himself and miss a more important diagnosis, such as a urinary tract infection. If the child is too young to say his throat is sore, it is difficult to be sure of the diagnosis in the absence of an exudate, or of marked cervical lymphadenopathy with a very red throat.

Two-thirds of sore throats have a viral origin, usually one of the many respiratory viruses. Occasionally, in older children, glandular fever is responsible and may cause a rather prominent confluent exudate. Although diphtheria can still very rarely be seen in an unimmunized, recently arrived, refugee, *Streptococcus pyogenes* is the only significant bacterial cause in Britain today. It can be cultured in about a quarter of children with a sore throat and is penicillin-sensitive. If the child is allergic to penicillin, erythromycin is an alternative. Amoxycillin is liable to cause a rash if the child turns out to be suffering from glandular fever—therefore penicillin-V is better. It is very difficult to decide on clinical grounds whether an infection is likely to be streptococcal or viral. The child over two years old who has a marked sore throat with intense redness, swelling, or an exudate, with perhaps palatal petechiae and tender enlarged cervical nodes, is more likely to have a β-haemolytic streptococcal infection than the infant or child whose predominant symptoms are cough or hoarseness. Of 44 children with a diagnosis of a streptococcal pharyngitis made using such clinical criteria, those treated with oral penicillin recovered more quickly than those on placebo, but both groups were much better within three days (Krober *et al.* 1985).

Scarlet fever is caused by an erythrogenic-toxin-producing strain of *Strep. pyogenes*, the incubation period being two to four days. The typical rash consists of fine erythematous macules appearing first on the trunk and limbs. The face is flushed, often with a pale area around the mouth. The classic 'strawberry' or raw red 'raspberry' tongue is sometimes seen. The rash is of no importance in itself except as an indicator of streptococcal infection and the GP will often have difficulty in deciding whether a child with a rash and sore throat has a viral or streptococcal illness or Kawasaki's syndrome (p. 14), which is important because it requires specific therapy. In scarlet fever one or two weeks after the onset of the rash the skin (particularly on the hands and feet) sometimes begins to desquamate. This may be a useful diagnostic clue in patients first seen after the acute illness. Scarlet fever may be very mild with minimal sore throat and a fine macular rash:

Mrs O'Connor had four children: one presented with a fine macular rash but without a sore throat, a second had the same rash with a sore throat from which *Strep. pyogenes* was isolated, and a third had a rip-roaring tonsillitis.

An oral dose of penicillin-V—125 mg four times daily for small children, 250–500 mg four times daily for older children and teenagers—seems to be satisfactory for most bacterial sore throats. There is evidence that the organisms are only reliably eradicated by continuing for a full 10 days, or by a single intramuscular injection of a long-acting penicillin. In practice only a five-day oral course is usually given, perhaps because GPs know that streptococcal complications are rare in Britain today and parents are unlikely to continue treatment for many days after a child has recovered.

Parenteral penicillin may be a good idea for the rare child with tonsillitis and marked peritonsillar oedema, who has difficulty in swallowing even saliva, and who talks as if he has a large object in his mouth—which is indeed the case. If such a patient does not improve rapidly, referral is indicated. This may also be necessary for the toxic child with a red, hot, tender, indurated, well demarcated area of erysipelas, usually caused by β-haemolytic streptococcus, occasionally by *Staph. aureus*. If there is any doubt of the causative organism, or if the lesion could possibly be the more deep-seated cellulitis, flucloxacillin should be given with penicillin.

Acute glomerulonephritis with facial oedema, oliguria, haematuria, and hypertension, rheumatic fever with joint pain and swelling and perhaps carditis, and Sydenham's chorea with gross clumsiness of small movements may all follow within a few weeks of a streptococcal infection. These are very rare in Britain today.

ACUTE OTITIS MEDIA

There are many grey areas around otitis media: uncertainties about the diagnostic criteria, about the natural history of middle-ear effusions in young children, and confusion concerning the efficacy of antibiotics or of surgical intervention—a fertile area for GP research. Infants and young children are very prone to middle-ear inflammation, usually following a cold. Most children have had at least one attack by the age of three years, up to half have had three or more attacks (Klein 1992).

A typical case is not difficult to diagnose. The older child usually complains of earache a few days after a cold has started. In addition, he usually shows signs of a conductive deafness in the affected ear, or may complain of distortion of sound. There is often a fever. Fever and pain will remit after an analgesic, only to recur after its effects have worn off. A well child whose earache disappears permanently after a single dose of analgesic almost certainly does not have acute bacterial otitis media, and does not need antibiotics. He may have a serous effusion in the middle-ear, secondary to blockage of the Eustachian tube. Young children with acute otitis media are not invariably feverish. Infants may be irritable and restless, often with bouts of inconsolable crying. They may sleep badly at night and pull at the affected ear; not very helpful because well infants often perform the same manoeuvre.

If the child is seen at the onset of symptoms, the affected tympanic membrane may only be slightly redder than the other side, the redness being confined mainly to the rim or only to part of the drum. By the next day, the drum is often bright red, bulging or crinkly. Abnormal whiteness of the drum may be due either to scarring from previous infection or to the presence of pus. It is not unusual for the drum to perforate and discharge, and most such drums heal rapidly. Unfortunately, the common belief that heat from acute otitis media will melt wax and render an inflamed drum visible is false. In one study, mechanical removal of wax was necessary to allow visualization of the drum in about 30 per cent of 279 children with acute otitis media (Schwartz *et al.* 1983). This was most frequently necessary in infants. Paradoxically, because the canal is straight in a baby, it is sometimes easier to see the tympanic membrane using a bigger speculum rather than a tiny one. There is no need to insert it into the baby's external auditory meatus.

Several considerations can confuse the differential diagnosis, including the fact that the ear-drums of a cheerful, well infant may be dull and lack a well-defined light reflex. This appearance will also follow an episode of acute inflammation and the drum may take several weeks to regain its previous pristine hue. Crying of itself makes the drum pink, and the cause of the child's discomfort may then often be wrongly assumed to be otitis media. Ingvarsson (1982) looked at 171 children under 15 who were seen at an ENT department because of earache and suspected acute otitis media. The younger the child, the more difficult it was to be certain, and 39 per cent of children under two years of age thought to have earache had a normal drum. It is often impossible in primary care conditions to visualize the ear-drum of an infant. If this is the case, a diagnosis of otitis media can only be made with reasonable certainty if there is fever and otorrhoea, and then only if the discharge is not coming from the external auditory meatus. Another possible diagnosis is myringitis bullosa, in which earache is associated with the presence of vesicles on the tympanic membrane. The organisms involved are usually mycoplasma.

Red ear drums are associated with many viral infections, and we are more inclined to wait and see than a few years ago (Bollag and Bollag-Albrecht 1991), and not prescribe antibiotics just because the patient has a dull, smooth, red ear-drum with a cold. The following factors suggest that antibiotics are necessary in a child with a red tympanic membrane:

1. An infant with a cold who is miserable and irritable, with a history of bouts of screaming and of pulling at his ear-lobe in an unaccustomed manner—assuming that there is no suspicion of meningitis or any other condition as the cause.

2. A history of severe or persistent earache associated with a fever.
3. An associated purulent nasal discharge and perhaps fruity cough which does not resolve in a few days.
4. Marked difference in appearance of the two drums in a child who is unwell.
5. An ear discharging pus, unless it is clearly coming from the auditory meatus alone.

When unfortunate children with otitis media have had tympanocenteses, pathogenic bacteria have been isolated in the majority of cases. The most common bacterial isolates in young children are the pneumococcus. *H. influenzae, Strep. pyogenes* and *Staph. aureus* are less common. In older children, *H. influenzae* is rather less frequent. Amoxycillin will be effective for most of these. Co-amoxiclav (which may cause diarrhoea) or erythromycin are alternatives.

In the first day or so of the illness, the child's earache can be eased by paracetamol while waiting for the antibiotic to take effect. Nasal decongestants and antihistamines have not usually been shown to be beneficial. It is doubtful whether an older child with otitis media needs more than a few days of antibiotics. Bain *et al.* (1985) found no difference in the time taken for symptoms and signs to resolve, in 243 children over three treated with a seven-day course of amoxycillin 125 mg three times a day, compared to a two-day course of a higher dosage, 750 mg twice a day. A group of 185 of these children were followed for a year and there was no appreciable difference in subsequent hearing loss or recurrence rate.

The ideal treatment still appears to be uncertain, especially as recurrences are common after one attack. Children's ears seem particularly vulnerable for about two months after an acute infection, and parents should be warned that their child may well get another attack during this time if he gets a new cold.

A number of studies suggest that several months of chemoprophylaxis with a daily dose of amoxycillin (20 mg/kg) may reduce the frequency of fresh episodes. This treatment is suggested for children who have had either three documented episodes of infection in the previous six months or four in the previous twelve months (Klein 1992).

How often should the GP see a child with an acute otitis media? If the fever or earache have not resolved after 48–72 hours of treatment, a different antibiotic may be needed. Even if the child improves quickly, he should be seen again a week later to make sure that the ears look as if they are on the mend. A further consultation three or four weeks later is advisable for those children whose eardrums still look significantly abnormal. If the doctor has access to audiometry, he can arrange for the older child's hearing to be tested if the drums do not look quite right two or three months after an acute infection.

GLUE EAR (OTITIS MEDIA WITH EFFUSION)

When children first show signs of difficulty in hearing, parents are prone to attribute this to inattention, and so, by the time they bring the child to the GP because they fear he is deaf, they are usually right. Deafness in childhood is usually due to otitis media with effusion (OME), or glue ear. This is particularly likely if the deafness appears to fluctuate and to be more noticeable after an upper respiratory tract infection. It may be possible to get an audiogram or a measurement of drum mobility by the quick and easy test of impedance tympanometry to confirm the diagnosis. These are available in ENT departments or in some districts in child health clinics. Otherwise, the GP will have to make do with cruder surgery tests of hearing and examination of the tympanic membrane.

The aetiology of glue ear is uncertain, but is probably related to obstruction of the Eustachian tube through infection, adenoidal obstruction, or allergic rhinitis. Chronic middle-ear effusion can also follow acute otitis media. Some children with glue ear have a history of episodes of earache associated with fever, while others present with difficulty in hearing; a third group have had episodes of quickly resolving earache unassociated with fever. The allergic, sniffing, 'catarrhal' child may suffer from chronic middle-ear effusion, and these children will often have a clear, watery, nasal discharge as compared with the thick, yellow discharge of a child after a cold. Asymptomatic middle-ear effusions in babies seen because they fail their eight month screening test of hearing are also common.

The tympanic membrane presents a variable appearance and may be retracted. Its shiny, grey–pink appearance is usually lost and it appears paler, less smooth and opaque. There may be visible bubbles or fluid levels. Tuning fork tests may be useful in the older child to confirm that there is a conductive deafness.

Glue ear appears to be commonest in preschool children (Zielhuis *et al*. 1990), with 15–20 per cent of children aged one to five years affected at any one time. Its natural history in the individual child is not predictable. About 50 per cent of glue ears will resolve spontaneously within three months, and 95 per cent within a year (Effective Health Care 1992). Recurrences are common. It is uncertain whether there is any significant link between glue ear and persistently disabling loss of hearing. There is no convincing evidence from randomized trials that nose drops, oral decongestants or even antibiotics, encourage the fluid to disperse (*Lancet* 1992).

Surgical treatment consists of insertion of grommets into the tympanic membrane to ventilate the middle-ear, after myringotomy and aspiration of the exudate, perhaps together with adenoidectomy, which may possibly improve the outcome. Grommets tend to remain in place for an average of about six months before being spontaneously extruded, but they may remain *in situ* only for days, or at the other extreme, for a year or more. Children with grommets may continue to swim. Prolonged immersion of the ears in soapy bath water, which may contain large numbers of bacteria, may be a greater menace than the swimming pool. If an attack of acute otitis media takes place while the grommets are *in situ*, as shown by a purulent discharge or persistent earache with fever, the appropriate antibiotic will still be needed.

Each year 4.7 in 1000 children under the age of 15 have surgical treatment for glue ear—like tonsillectomy before it, the rate is higher for children from social class 1 than social class 5. Any long-term benefits are not proven. According to one analysis of many randomized controlled trials, the insertion of grommets and/or adenoidectomy resulted in a mean hearing improvement of about 12dBs after six months, falling to about 5dBs after a year (Effective Health Care 1992). In addition, we do not know which children are likely to benefit, and it has been suggested that hearing aids may be an alternative to surgery (*Lancet* 1992). A reduction in parental smoking may hasten the resolution of the middle-ear effusion. Surgery is not always entirely successful. Some children develop discharge in ears after the grommets have been inserted and, as glue ear often recurs after surgical treatment, they may need to be reinserted. There is no evidence grommets prevent chronic suppurative otitis media. Sclerotic patches of uncertain long-term significance may develop on the ear-drum after the grommets have fallen out.

'The lack of any scientific evidence for the long-term value of this treatment, and the discomfort of being party to a soaring surgical rate' (Black 1985) makes us hesitate to refer children too enthusiastically for sugical treatment for their glue ears.

Action?

When glue ear is first diagnosed, time and no drugs is often the most appropriate management. The GP is best advised to keep his itchy fingers off the prescription pad, while arranging to see the child again in 12 weeks or so, preferably with an audiogram in those children old enough (about three to four years of age) to co-operate. We consider referral of a child (with both ears affected) whose hearing does not return to within 20dB of normal over four to six months. Earlier referral is indicated for severely deaf children (loss of greater than 30 decibels in each ear), those who may have other diagnoses, and those with an additional handicap or speech delay. A child on the surgical waiting list should have audiometry repeated just before the operation—the glue ear may have resolved.

Referral of other children with ear problems for consideration of adenoidectomy is also sometimes needed. We refer those children in whom we never see a normal drum between attacks of earache, and those who seem to be getting acute otitis media more than three or four times a year, especially if they have not responded to a prolonged course of antibiotics, together with the occasional child with grommets already *in situ* who is getting repeated attacks of suppurative otitis media.

OTITIS EXTERNA

It is sometimes difficult to be certain whether a child with a meatus filled with purulent secretions has otitis media or otitis externa. The former is more likely if there was a preceding cold or a pain relieved suddenly, presumably as the drum burst. Otitis media is certain if a tympanic perforation can be seen or if the pus moves when the patient coughs. In infants, the cause of a discharging ear is almost certain to be otitis media, which should be treated with oral antibiotics.

Otitis externa ranges in severity from a mild redness of the canal to swelling so severe and tender that proper examination is impossible. Severe otitis externa appears to be commoner in older children and teenagers. Discomfort is increased when the pinna is moved, a speculum inserted, or the tragus pressed. A boil in the external auditory meatus will also make insertion of a speculum acutely painful and can be seen as a local swelling with, perhaps, a pussy discharge. This diagnosis must be distinguished from the rare, and serious, mastoiditis, in which tenderness and swelling is maximal behind the pinna, which may be pushed forward. A foreign body may cause unilateral discharge.

Mild or moderate otitis externa can be treated with ear drops containing an anti-infective preparation, usually with a corticosteroid such as Locorten-vioform. If the meatus is full of secretion, gentle cleaning with a probe is necessary before applying the drops, which will otherwise just lie on top of the discharge—the toilet perhaps being repeated on several occasions. Prolonged use of antibacterial corticosteroid drops may lead to a secondary fungal infection.

Skin lines the external auditory meatus, and otitis externa may thus be an extension of eczema of the pinna. It can, if mild, be treated with hydrocortisone cream.

TONSILLECTOMY AND ADENOIDECTOMY

Non-aural indications for adenoidectomy, tonsillectomy, or both, are either marked airways obstruction or recurrent tonsillitis. Severe airways obstruction is fairly easy to evaluate. Its important complication is obstructive sleep apnoea. This occurs when obstruction of the airway is so severe that snoring and restless sleep is associated with episodes of apnoea between the snores. This can occasionally lead to day-time somnolence, associated with poor school performance, and, rarely, to pulmonary hypertension (loud second sound and parasternal heave). The symptoms of airways obstruction are obviously more evident during a respiratory infection. The child who can never breathe through the nose and also snores so much at night that he continually disturbs his parents may need referral, even when sleep apnoea has not been noted. The rare child who gets obstruction of the airways from enormous tonsils when he has tonsillitis also needs referral.

It is more difficult to decide whether to refer the much more common problem of the child who has recurrent attacks of tonsillitis, causing a lot of time off school. The usual criterion is the severity and frequency of tonsillitis, normally as reported by the mother. This factor is very difficult to assess objectively, so it is often the parents who, in reality, make the decision whether their child's tonsils and adenoids are removed. Though many parents are able to give an objective description of their child's infection, others exaggerate the incidence and severity of previous infections and attribute other symptoms incorrectly to the tonsils. Incidentally, this last point is one reason why any child with 'recurrent tonsillitis' should have his urine cultured. His recurrent fevers may really be due to urinary tract infection.

Three approaches to the child's recurrent sore throats are possible, First, encouraging the mother to play down the symptoms and get the child back to school as soon as possible after an attack; secondly, a trial of oral penicillin for a few months in low dosage (125 mg twice daily) and, finally, ENT referral for possible tonsillectomy. When the child has been off school more than three or four times a year for two years with attacks of tonsillitis, the moment has perhaps come when the morbidity and very rare mortality from tonsillectomy is outweighed by the bother of the recurrent sore throat. Although many children who have had their tonsils out subsequently appear to the GP to have less trouble with their throats, it is difficult to be certain whether this is because they have genuinely improved, or merely because the family have put their money on surgery and wish to back up the results.

PERSISTENT COUGH

A child is often brought to the GP with the single complaint of a persistent cough in the unimmunized child. It may be pertussis. Cough may also last for several weeks after a cold especially if the parents smoke heavily. Persistent cough, even without a wheeze, will often be asthma. A wheezy cough, especially if episodic, or worse at night, or after exercise, makes asthma even more likely. A family history, or a story of wheezing by the child on other occasions, supports the diagnosis, which becomes definite if a diminished peak flow is present at night, or after exercise, and improves when the child inhales a bronchodilator. Some children, otherwise well, seem to cough for months without a clear diagnosis ever being established. It is often sensible to see if anti-asthma treatment is helpful.

If the child is asked to cough a few times, it will become evident whether he has a 'dry', a 'wet' or wheezy cough. Dry coughs are usually unimportant. A cough that remains wet or fruity after one or two coughs is much more likely to indicate lung disease and an X-ray may be indicated, especially if the child is mildly unwell or does not improve after treatment with antibiotics. This may show a patch of consolidation or collapse, resolving after further antibiotics and physiotherapy. Rarely, it may suggest cystic fibrosis or other serious lung pathology, or perhaps show the effects of an inhaled foreign body.

The child who produces several short, dry coughs may have a 'tic'. The coughing adolescent may have recently started smoking. Some parents become anxious that their child's cough may indicate a serious disease such as TB or chronic bronchitis 'like Grandad' and it is often useful to ask them if there is any particular disease they are worried about. Rarely, a coughing Grandad will have genuinely given TB to the child. The upset caused by a child's persistent cough may be the key that is used to lead on to a discussion of the family's cramped housing conditions.

In general, if the child is well and his chest clear, his parents can be reassured—the child will not damage his lungs, can go to school, and is not going to harm himself by vigorous coughing at night.

INFLUENZA

Outside an epidemic, and in the younger child, it is often impossible to distinguish flu from infections caused by other viruses. In Britain, epidemics occur around Christmas or in the early months of the year. The incubation period is usually one to three days and the patient is infectious for about four or five days after the onset of symptoms. Influenza varies in intensity. After appearance of a new serotype the highest incidence of the disease is in children 5–14 years old, with an attack rate of up to 50 per cent. This rate drops to about 15 per cent in subsequent outbreaks caused by a variant of the same subtype (Cherry 1983).

Classically, the onset is abrupt and older children have symptoms of an upper respiratory tract infection with a high fever, malaise, a headache with painful movements of the eyes, general muscular aches and pains, and a sore throat. There is usually a cough, the child may vomit or have occasional diarrhoea. After two or three days the temperature subsides, but the cough and general debility continue for another week or so. The great danger is that an inaccurate 'phone diagnosis of influenza will be made when a parent describes the symptoms of a febrile, sick child. Babies and toddlers who are feverish and toxic need to be seen promptly, as does any chronically sick child who is in addition acutely unwell. Older children who are not reported as particularly unwell will need to be examined if their condition has not improved after 48 hours, or if they develop earache, wheeziness, shortness of breath, or a severe headache. Secondary bacterial infection of the middle-ear, chest, or sinuses are the commonest complications, and febrile convulsions are a risk for the younger child. Very rarely, pneumonia or CNS or cardiac complications occur.

Rest, fluids, and paracetamol are the mainstays of treatment for uncomplicated infection. For vaccination, see p. 38. Hanshaw *et al.* (1985) conclude that a causal relationship between maternal influenza and congenital malformations 'is at present not proven'.

BRONCHITIS AND TRACHEITIS

Mild bronchitis and tracheitis are common in children with respiratory viral infections. After a cold, their cough becomes more persistent, often with retrosternal soreness and perhaps slight wheeziness. An obvious difference from adults is that the child swallows his sputum.

On auscultation there may be scattered coarse crackles and low-pitched rhonchi; widespread, high-pitched rhonchi are more likely to mean that the child has asthma or bronchiolitis. Antibiotics are usually given if there is no asthmatic history, especially if the child is toxic, or if there are widespread adventitia or a localized area of crepitations.

Chronic bronchitis is not an acceptable childhood diagnosis and, if a child has repeated attacks of 'bronchitis', asthma becomes almost certain. This diagnosis is less definite if the child has only had one or two episodes of observed wheeze after a cold, especially if the noises come from high up in the respiratory tract.

The group of children who wheeze recurrently with respiratory infections may have other evidence of asthma, such as exercise-provoked wheezing or nocturnal cough. Therefore, for these, a bronchodilator, which may not work in infants, is more appropriate than an antibiotic. The rare recurrent 'bronchitic' who does not have asthma may have serious lung disease or an inhaled foreign body.

CROUP AND EPIGLOTTITIS

The word croup is used to describe the symptoms of laryngeal inflammation: hoarseness, barking cough, and inspiratory stridor. It is usually caused by a viral infection of the larynx and trachea, sometimes extending to affect the bronchi and bronchioles. The child's breathing may be considerably impaired by inflammatory oedema, and the small but real risk of respiratory obstruction is the main worry. The parainfluenza virus appears to be the principal agent, usually affecting children between the ages of six months and four years. Though the majority will recover at home, about 3 per cent of patients admitted to hospital will need endotracheal intubation. Croup, perhaps in an asthmatic, may be recurrent in an individual child or family. Other causes of acute laryngeal obstruction in children are laryngeal malformations, acute epiglottitis, and foreign bodies.

The child with croup will often have had a cold with a slight cough for a day or two before the symptoms start. Croup is a common cause for a night call. The diagnosis can be confirmed if the parent holds the telephone to the child. The usual story is that the child has awakened during the early hours with a harsh, barking cough and hoarseness, alarming to both child and parents. If he is only mildly affected, crowing inspiratory stridor with some subcostal recession is apparent only when he is upset or hyperventilates. The following factors indicate that hospital admission is necessary:

1. Airway obstruction at rest, as indicated by subcostal and intercostal recession and use of the accessory muscles of respiration.
2. Other signs of inadequate ventilation: increasing tachycardia and tachypnoea, restlessness, eventual cyanosis. Unfortunately, the child who is dangerously ill and becoming exhausted may cease breathing violently, so that stridor and rib

recession become less obvious. There is a rising pulse rate, diminished breath sounds on auscultation and increasing lethargy. Hypoxic restlessness can be mistaken for irritability in the toddler.

3. Any suggestion that acute epiglottitis or an inhaled foreign body rather than viral croup is responsible for the clinical picture.

A foreign body should be suspected if the onset of stridor is sudden, perhaps with an episode of choking and severe coughing and no sign of respiratory tract infection. Diphtheria should not be completely forgotten in the unimmunized child.

If the child has simple croup and is managed at home, as most will be, the parents must be warned about the signs of increasing respiratory obstruction which should lead to their recalling the doctor. Although moisture sometimes appears to be helpful in relieving stridor, objective evidence to support its use is lacking. We still advise parents to sit in the bathroom with a hot shower running, the child on their lap, being read a story. Hot kettles belching out steam are not a good idea. They have lead to a number of admissions for scalds and make the wallpaper fall off! An unhappy child is more likely to have respiratory distress than one allowed to go back quietly to sleep, but sedatives should not be used. Recent evidence (Doull 1995) suggests that mild to moderate croup is helped by 2 mg of nebulized budesonide. Antibiotics should only be given to children with evidence of secondary bacterial infection such as acute otitis media. The child usually gets better in one to three days. Stridor may recur with diminishing severity for a night or two as the child improves even though day-time symptoms have completely resolved.

Acute epiglottitis, hopefully a rapidly disappearing disease thanks to immunization, is one of the most frightening paediatric emergencies. It occurs most commonly in children under five and is usually caused by *H. influenzae* type B. There is associated bacteraemia and the child is toxic and looks very ill. He has a high fever and marked tachycardia. The illness usually progresses rapidly and over a few hours there is increasing difficulty in breathing with a lower-pitched inspiratory stridor than in children with ordinary croup. The child will have a very sore throat with difficulty in swallowing; drooling is a key physical sign. The severity of the obstruction can be judged not by the loudness of the inspiratory noise which is characteristically often muffled and gurgling, different from the barking cough of croup, but by the extent of in-drawing of the thoracic cage and sternum on inspiration and by signs of toxicity and hypoxia—agitation and cyanosis. The throat should not be examined because use of a tongue depressor may precipitate fatal respiratory obstruction. No child with persistent inspiratory stridor at rest should have his throat examined at home. The GP must not risk making the child cry by vigorous examination or injecting ampicillin (unless admission will be very long delayed). The child should sit on the parent's lap in the ambulance—lying down increases the risk of respiratory obstruction. Intubation is the treatment of choice, but may be difficult.

BRONCHIOLITIS

An unwell, breathless, wheezing, coughing, young baby very probably has bronchiolitis, the commonest lower respiratory tract infection of infants. Epidemics occur during the winter and are caused mainly by the respiratory syncytial virus. If the service is available, this viral cause can be confirmed within a couple of hours on a pharyngeal aspirate using a fluorescent antibody test.

In bronchiolitis, there is gradual development of respiratory distress, usually after a cold. Over a couple of days, the infant becomes more wheezy and dyspnoeic with an irritating cough. Even if he is not very toxic, there may be difficulty in feeding because the rapid respiratory rate (60–80 per minute) does not permit time for sucking and swallowing. There is subcostal and intercostal recession. Hyperinflation of the lungs pushes down the liver and distends the chest. On auscultation, there is an expiratory wheeze and there are also often widespread fine inspiratory crepitations. A baby with the clinical picture just described will need to be admitted to hospital, where he will be given additional oxygen if he is hypoxic, and tube feeds to maintain adequate hydration. It is also important to refer the child with pre-existing heart or lung disease, who may be given the inhaled antiviral ribavarin in hospital (£200 a vial).

If an infant with a milder version of the disease is looked after at home he will often need to be seen twice every 24 hours until he starts improving. A rising respiratory rate, or irregular respirations and episodes of apnoea, or increasing difficulty in feeding are indications for admission, and he should certainly be in hospital if he begins to look blue. Bronchodilators have not been shown to have beneficial effects (Wang *et al.* 1992). Though the same applies to antibiotics, it is probably unrealistic to expect the GP managing a patient at home not to give amoxycillin. The majority of infants recover within a week or so, although a few may continue to cough and may be a bit breathless for longer.

There have been several studies which indicate that children who have suffered from severe bronchiolitis in babyhood are at an increased risk of developing asthma. Murray *et al.* (1992) reassessed 73 children five-and-a-half years after their original severe infection; 31 reported episodes of wheezing in the previous year, compared to only 11 of the control group. Maternal smoking was associated with an increased incidence of wheezing. Asthma is probably a less common sequel to mild bronchiolitis (Twiggs *et al.* 1981). It is however always difficult to be sure that any association is causal. It may be that children predisposed to asthma are more likely to get bronchiolitis from RSV infection than just a cold.

Several other conditions should be thought of when making a provisional diagnosis of bronchiolitis. One is pneumonia (see below). The generally poorly, underweight baby may have an underlying chest condition, for example, cystic fibrosis. Another possibility in the neonate with persistent chestiness and a sticky eye is chlamydia. Heart disease will usually be associated with a strikingly palpable heart beat, breathlessness, and a large liver.

PERTUSSIS

This highly infectious, debilitating, tedious illness is caused by *Bordetella pertussis*, a small, non-motile, gram-negative rod. Adenovirus infection may cause a similar picture. Whooping cough is most dangerous in babies under six months of age. A full course of immunization provides over 80 per cent protection, and notifications of whooping cough have fallen from over 65 000 in 1978 to 5300 in 1991, with no deaths reported. This is certain to be an underestimate, because immunized children presenting with atypical disease will not be recognized as suffering from whooping cough. There appears to be no transfer of maternal immunity, and infants are susceptible from birth.

The incubation period is usually 7–13 days, occasionally longer, and the unmodified illness may run a very protracted course. It can last two or three months or even longer in some children, who develop paroxysms again every time they get a cold. There is an initial 'catarrhal' state, during which the child is most infectious, usually indistinguishable from a cold with a rather persistent cough. During the second week the cough becomes still more persistent, and gradually the typical paroxysms develop. Repeated spasms of coughing often, but not always, end in an inspiratory whoop. A whoop is not necessary for the diagnosis and is often absent in infants. The parent's complaint may be of vomiting which has been induced by the cough, rather than of the cough itself.

The number of coughing paroxysms per day vary from a handful to 50 or more. All children find the spasms exhausting, and young ones may become frightened, needing a lot of comfort and careful nursing. They soon learn to try and avoid factors such as crumbly food, sudden cold air, and parental cigarette smoke that provoke the cough. Most children are well between attacks. The number and severity of the coughing fits gradually decrease after some weeks, and the child is left with a more ordinary sounding cough that may linger for a while.

Babies are particularly likely to develop apnoea after a paroxysm—frightening to both parent and doctor. Most babies under six months should be treated in hospital. Though a fatal outcome is now very uncommon there is a danger of apnoea, and of malnutrition and dehydration from recurrent vomiting.

Whooping cough is an exhausting disease for the patient and family, and a nightmare if more than one child is affected. Admission of an older child to hospital may be fully justified to allow the parents to rest at night and to restore family morale. Bronchopneumonia may result from secondary bacterial infection. The child who becomes unwell and breathless will need a chest X-ray to detect any consolidation or collapse needing treatment with antibiotics and physiotherapy. The mechanical effects of the paroxysms may cause epistaxes, conjunctival haemorrhages, and, rarely, a catastrophic cerebral haemorrhage.

If good bacteriological services are available, *B. pertussis* can usually be grown from a pernasal swab in the earlier stages of the illness. A high white-cell count with a lymphocytosis strongly supports the diagnosis.

The crux of good management is nursing care, and the district nurse or community paediatric nurse can give the family helpful advice, for example, re-feeding may be necessary after each vomit. Antibiotics do not alter the clinical course once the paroxysmal stage has begun, but a 10-day course of erythromycin may be effective in eliminating the organism and therefore in reducing the infectivity of the patient to others. If given to a sibling under six months of age (20 mg/kg per day) it may prevent him catching the illness at an age when he is most likely to get a dangerous attack.

PNEUMONIA

Many different bacteria and viruses give rise to pneumonia. The clinical picture ranges from a severely ill, toxic, breathless infant to a mildly unwell older child who has had a cough for a couple of weeks, usually with a raised respiratory rate, but occasionally with little or no sign of respiratory distress. In the latter, pneumonia is often not suspected until an X-ray shows consolidation.

The acutely unwell infant with pneumonia will often have suffered from a cold during the preceding few days, subsequently becoming toxic with rapid respiration, a more frequent cough, and often a high temperature. The infant will refuse to feed, may vomit, or may become irritable or drowsy. He will be less wheezy than the baby with bronchiolitis, though differentiation may not be easy. The diagnosis cannot always be confirmed on auscultation as the chest may sound clear. The younger the child the less likely there are to be localizing chest signs. The crucial diagnostic pointer in a baby is a raised respiratory rate. In older children there will usually be an audible patch of crackles, in addition to cough and tachypnoea.

The child with a fever for other reasons may pose a diagnostic problem if he has a raised respiratory rate, perhaps because of a combination of fever and the ketoacidosis of fasting. It may be necessary for the GP to request an X-ray to clarify the situation. In pneumonia the rate will, at least in a baby, usually be persistently over 50 to 60. Aspiration of milk or vomit in a sick infant may cause a pneumonic picture and, in the older child, a peanut which has gone down the wrong way may also be missed, unless specifically asked about. There are other reasons for breathlessness, discussed on p. 12.

Pneumococcal pneumonia may cause an illness in older children, with an abrupt onset without an associated cold, but perhaps with herpes, a high fever, a somewhat grunting pattern of respiration, flaring nostrils, and, occasionally, acute abdominal instead of pleuritic pain. A stiff neck is a possibility if consolidation involves the upper lobe. Children with sickle cell disease, HIV infection, nephrotic syndrome, and other chronic diseases of the heart or lung are all at increased risk of infection with *Strep. pneumoniae*. Mycoplasma is an important cause of pneumonia in older children and young adults. This is associated with a more indolent course, presenting with a fever, cough and sore throat. Chest signs and X-ray appearance are very variable. Occasionally, mycoplasma infection is associated with *erythema multiforme*, other rashes, and various neurological complications such as meningoencephalitis. A variety of rare underlying disorders, such as hypogammaglobulinaemia, cystic fibrosis, anatomical malformations of the lung, and primary tuberculosis, may also present with apparent pneumonia. Their exclusion is the main reason for making sure that the chest X-ray has returned to normal three or four weeks after the illness. Missed asthma is much commoner than any of them.

If a previously healthy child is pink and has a respiratory rate at rest of less than about 60, he generally need not be sent into hospital unless there is failure to improve within 24–48 hours (provided, of course, that the home circumstances are satisfactory and that the parents can be relied upon to give the prescribed treatment and contact the doctor if the child's condition should deteriorate). The younger the baby, the lower the threshold for admission, and most infants under six months will probably need to be in hospital. Sufficient fluids are important if a baby managed at home is not to become dehydrated.

Most bacterial pneumonias in children over the age of about two are caused by the pneumococcus, others by *H. influenzae*. Under that age infection is more likely to be due to other organisms. Bearing this in mind, we treat infants and preschool children with amoxycillin or co-amoxiclav. The intramuscular route may be needed for a child who is vomiting, or if the parents cannot be relied upon to give oral antibiotics regularly. Penicillin (or erythromycin) are good choices for older children with an acute onset of pneumonia, possibly starting with an intramuscular dose in a toxic child. Co-amoxiclav may again be appropriate for more obvious secondary infection in older children. Erythromycin is the correct choice for possible mycoplasma pneumonia. In children who have underlying disease such as cystic fibrosis, or in babies who are particularly severely ill, flucloxacillin will also be necessary to cover the risk of staphylococcal infection. This is a rare cause of severe pneumonia in babies in whom the chest X-ray may show abscesses, cysts, or empyema. They should be in hospital.

Bibliography

Anonymous. (1992). Glue ear guidelines: time to act on the evidence. *Lancet,* **340**, 1324–5.

Bain, J., Murphy, E., and Ross, F. (1985). Acute otitis media: clinical course among children who received a short course of high dose antibiotic. *British Medical Journal*, **291**, 1243–6.

Black, N. A. (1985). Surgery for glue ear—the determinants of an epidemic. In *Progress in child health*, Vol. 2, (ed. J. A. MacFarlane). Churchill Livingstone, London.

Bollag, U. and Bollag-Albrecht, E. (1991). Recommendations derived from practice audit for the treatment of acute otitis media. *Lancet,* **338**, 96–99.

Cherry, J. D. (1983). Influenza viral infections. In *Nelson text book of paediatrics*, (12th edn), (ed. R. E. Behrman and V.C. Vaughan), pp. 772–6. Saunders, Philadelphia.

de Melker, R. A. (1993). Treating persistent glue ear in children. *British Medical Journal*, **306**, 5–6.

Doull, J. (1995). Corticosteroids in the management of croup. *British Medical Journal*, **311**, 1244.

Effective Health Care. (1992). The treatment of persistent glue ear in children. Bulletin No 4. University of Leeds.

Hanshaw, J. B., Dudgeon, J. A., and Marshall, W. C. (1985). *Viral diseases of the fetus and newborn. Major problems in clinical paediatrics*, Vol. 17, (2nd edn). Saunders, New York.

Ingvarsson, L. (1982). Acute otalgia in children—findings and diagnosis. *Acta Paediatrica Scandinavica*, **71**, 705–10.

Klein, J. O. (1992). In *Infectious diseases of children*, (9th edn), (ed. S. Krugman *et al.*). Mosby, St. Louis.

Krober, M. S., Bass, J. W., and Michels, G. N. (1985). Streptococcal pharyngitis. Placebo-controlled double-blind evaluation of clinical response to penicillin therapy. *Journal of the American Medical Association*, **253**, 1271–4.

Krugman, S., Katz, S. L., Gershon, A. A., and Wilfert, C. M. (1992). *Infectious diseases of children*, (9th edn). Mosby, St. Louis.

Morbidity statistics from general practice. (1986). Third National Study, 1981–1982. Royal College of General Practitioners, Office of Population Censuses and Studies, Department of Health and Social Security. HMSO, London.

Murray, M., Webb M. S. C., O'Callaghan, C. *et al.* (1992). Respiratory status and allergy after bronchiolitis. *Archives of Disease in Childhood*, **67**, 482–7.

Platt, S. D., Martin, C. J., Hunt, F. M., and Lewis C. W. (1989). Damp housing, mould and symptomatic health state. *British Medical Journal*, **298**, 1673–8.

Pringle, M. B. (1992). Swimming with grommets. *British Medical Journal*, **304**, 198.

Schwartz, R. H., Rodriguez, W. J., McAveney, W., and Grundfast, K. M. (1983). Cerumen removal. How necessary is it to diagnose acute otitis media? *American Journal of Diseases of Children*, **137**, 1064–5.

Stott, N. C. H. (1979). Management and outcome of winter upper respiratory tract infections in children aged 0–9 years. *British Medical Journal*, **i**, 29–31.

Taylor, B. and Wadsworth, J. (1987). Maternal smoking during pregnancy and lower respiratory tract illness in early life. *Archives of Disease in Childhood*, **62**, 786–91.

Tibballs, J., Shann, F. A., and Landau, L. I. (1992). Placebo-controlled trial of prednisolone in children intubated for croup. *Lancet*, **340**, 745–7.

Twiggs, J. T., Larson, L. A., O'Connell, E. J., and Ilstrup, D. M. (1981). Respiratory syncytial virus infection. Ten year follow up. *Clinical Paediatrics*, **20**, 187–90.

Wang, E. L. W., Milner, R., Allen, U., and Maj, H. (1992). Bronchodilators for treatment of mild bronchiolitis: a factorial randomised trial. *Archives of Disease in Childhood*, **67**, 289–93.

Zielhuis, G. A., Rach, G. H., Bosch, A. V., and Brock, P. V. (1990). The prevalence of otitis media with effusion: a critical review of the literature. *Clinical Otolaryngology*, **15**, 283–8.

13 The gut

When faced with diarrhoea and vomiting, especially in an infant, the GP's initial tasks are to decide whether gastro-enteritis is indeed the diagnosis and to assess the state of hydration. The latter is the most important factor in deciding whether the child with gastro-enteritis should be treated at home or in hospital.

DIARRHOEA

Several conditions can be confused with gastro-enteritis. First, normality. Diarrhoea is usually defined as the too frequent passage of too fluid stools, but the stools of breast-fed babies are not formed, may be frequent, explosive, and sometimes contain mucus—however, true gastro-enteritis is rare in fully breast-fed babies. Parents often seem to worry unnecessarily if the colour of the faeces deviates from the standard brown. A green colour is not important, although a jet-black or red stool is another matter.

Diarrhoea may be a sign of infection away from the abdomen, although perhaps less often than is described in older textbooks. Diarrhoea attributed, for example, to otitis media, may be associated with the presence of rotavirus in the stools.

Acute abdominal disease, notably pelvic appendicitis, may present with loose stools; this is also true of intussusception. Children who are taking antibiotics, such as amoxycillin, often have mild diarrhoea. In addition, it is not uncommon to find perfectly well toddlers who produce frequent, loose motions, and this is discussed on p. 211.

Bloody diarrhoea is not infrequent in bacterial enteritis caused by campylobacter, shigella or sometimes salmonella. It is also occasionally seen with intussusception and, in very preterm babies with necrotizing enterocolitis. In this condition gas is seen in the bowel wall on X-ray, the abdomen is distended, and perforation or stricture formation are common. This is a very serious condition which very rarely presents after discharge from hospital. Blood in the stools of breast-fed babies may mean vitamin K deficient haemorrhagic disease (p. 259).

VOMITING

Minor vomiting is common and young children vomit very easily for a variety of reasons. For example, many with a respiratory infection do so as a result of coughing, or swallowing mucus. Vomiting with diarrhoea usually means gastro-enteritis, but a short-lived attack of repeated vomiting without diarrhoea is also common and often viral in origin. Sudden onset of vomiting in an ill baby or child who does not have either of the above may be the presentation of urinary tract infection, meningitis, an acute abdomen, a metabolic defect or other serious illness. Vomiting, especially bile-stained, may be the first sign of intestinal obstruction (p. 277).

Chronic vomiting is also fairly common and, like loose motions, need not have pathological significance. Many babies bring up a small amount of milk with their feeds, and any free-floating maternal anxiety may present to the GP in the guise of a vomiting baby. Sometimes checking that the bottle feed is correctly diluted, at a reasonable temperature, and not being forced upon the baby in large volumes as the only response to crying, may resolve the situation.

Normal 'possetting' merges clinically with the commonly seen symptoms of **gastro-oesophageal reflux** in which milk is regurgitated after feeds. The great majority do very well and grow out of the symptom after a few months. In severe cases, large volumes of milk may be lost, weight gain is poor, and, extremely rarely, pneumonia or oesophageal stricture occur. Referral is needed if the baby has obvious discomfort from acid oesophagitis on swallowing, if weight gain is falling across centiles, if there is chestiness, raising the possibility of inhaled gastric juice, or pallor because of the anaemia of oesophageal bleeding. There is a possible relationship between recurrent reflux and recurrent apnoea. Infants suffering from cerebral palsy are particularly likely to develop troublesome reflux because of disturbance of the swallowing mechanism.

Fortunately, complications are rare. For the great majority, mildly affected, reassurance of the parents and, perhaps, the early introduction of solids from about three months of age, suffice. Doubt has been cast on the value of the traditional advice to nurse the baby in an upright position but babies with more troublesome regurgitation may be helped by Gaviscon Infant, or by thickening agents such as Nestargel or Carobel. The family may have to put up with several months of tedious vomiting before significant improvement occurs.

Some babies with this picture may not have a hiatus hernia but may be allergic to a dietary component such as cows' milk protein or eggs (p. 171). A careful dietary history relating the introduction of new foods to the onset of symptoms may provide the clue, as can associated eczema, wheezing, other rashes, and diarrhoea. Currently available blood and skin tests are of almost no diagnostic value. However, too much attention to the diet can sometimes be a mistake—food intolerance continues to be in fashion.

Another well-known textbook cause of persistent infantile vomiting without diarrhoea, especially in boys (4:1) is **pyloric stenosis**, but a GP should expect to see a case only once every several years; some may have a positive family history.

Vomiting usually starts in the second or third week, or very occasionally not until the child is six or eight weeks old. Initially the vomiting occurs infrequently and is non-projectile but after a few days it becomes more forceful and finally projectile, spurting out of the baby's mouth and covering a wide area of floor and mother's lap. Vomiting generally occurs during or shortly after a feed, but at times the infant may only be sick several hours later and some feeds may be retained altogether. The baby is usually not ill but remains hungry after vomiting and will quickly feed again. Constipation may be partial or complete, depending on how much milk reaches the intestine. In the undiagnosed baby there is steady loss of weight and eventual dehydration. A palpable, pyloric 'tumour' is felt in most proved cases, but repeated examination may be necessary until the diagnosis is confirmed. Diagnosis can also be reliably made by ultrasound. Clinical examination is easiest during a feed. The mass, which is like an olive, is best felt with the index finger on the right side of the abdomen at the level of the umbilicus. It is palpable intermittently and is sometimes easiest to feel after the infant has vomited. Visible peristalsis from left to right can often be seen if the baby is in an oblique light. It is most obvious immediately after feeding and just before the baby is sick. Urinary tract infection in babies may also lead to projectile vomiting and is commoner (p. 238). It is worse to miss a urinary tract infection than it is to delay for a day or two the referral for surgery of a well child with pyloric stenosis. Before deciding to refer such a baby for an opinion, or to a paediatrically competent ultrasound department, it may be very useful for the health visitor to visit the family at home to observe the feeding.

It is difficult to be dogmatic about when a recurrently vomiting baby requires more detailed investigation to exclude rare problems such as hypercalcaemia, uraemia, or raised intracranial pressure. A general rule would be to investigate those with associated poor weight gain or with definite abdominal distension, or where there are other hints of general disease, such as abnormal thirst, developmental delay, a rather large head, or just an appearance of ill-health.

Except for travel sickness, or as part of the 'periodic syndrome' (p. 268), recurrent vomiting is rather rare in children after babyhood. Amongst the rare causes in this group are intermittent hydrophrenosis, with loin pain and tenderness; recurrent urinary tract infection; intermittent intestinal obstruction with upper abdominal distension; cerebral tumour with morning headache and perhaps a squint of recent onset. In the teenage girl, early pregnancy or bulimia are possible causes. So is excess alcohol in teenagers of either sex. Constipation does not result in vomiting.

GASTRO-ENTERITIS

Gastro-enteritis in children can be caused by a number of different pathogens (Table 13.1), of which the commonest in Britain, especially in preschool children, are viral.

Table 13.1 Causes of acute gastro-enteritis

Type (Incubation period–days)	Comment	Diagnosis
Viruses		
Rotavirus (2–5)	Vomiting may be severe and diarrhoea watery; often fever; may be mild in neonates (maternal antibodies). Respiratory symptoms, including otitis media.	Electron-microscopy Stool immunoassay
Adenoviruses	Less vomiting and fever than rotavirus. Respiratory symptoms; severe with some subtypes.	Electron-microscopy Viral culture
Astrovirus	Similar to rotavirus. Less dehydration.	Electron-microscopy Immunoassay
Norwalk–like viruses (2)	Vomiting, mild diarrhoea, older children.	Electron-microscopy Immunoassay
Bacteria		
Salmonellae (1–2; usually 10–12 days for paratyphoid)	Contaminated food, especially meat Gram-negative motile bacillae; any age; fever; antibiotics indicated in young babies or patients with systemic disease; they may prolong carrier state.	Culture of faeces
Shigellae (1–3 may be longer)	Contaminated food or water Non-motile gram-negative remains in blood and stool; lasts 2–10 days; any age. May be associated with CNS symptoms. Usually self-limiting, but ampicillin or trimethoprim for toxic children.	Culture
Toxigenic *E. coli*	Gram-negative bacillus; certain toxigenic and invasive strains are important causes of diarrhoea especially in infants; cause of travellers' diarrhoea; any age; lasts from few days to 2 weeks; antibiotics may shorten the illness, e.g. trimethoprim.	Results of stool culture difficult to interpret. Lab. reports of 'Enteropathic' *E. coli* relate poorly to true pathogenicity.

Table 13.1 *continued*

Type (Incubation period–days)	Comment	Diagnosis
Campylobacter (1–3)	Gram-negative, thin motile curved rods. Infected meat especially poultry, or person-to-person. Usually excreted for up to 3 weeks; abdominal cramps and often bloody diarrhoea. Erythromycin may shorten duration of the illness.	Culture
Staph. aureus		
(a) toxic food (2–5 hours)	Forms toxin in custard, creams and cooked meats; multiple cases characteristic; acute symptoms last about a day	None routinely available.
(b) antibiotic enterocolitis	Rare; watery diarrhoea, high fever and sometimes shock; usually patient on a broad-spectrum antibiotic—stop it (same picture can also be caused by Clostridia).	Gram stain and culture of stool.
Protozoa		
Giardia lamblia	Important cause of persistent diarrhoea.	Microscopy of fresh stool.
Cryptosporidium		Microscopy of fresh stool.
Entamoeba histolytica	Foreign travel.	Microscopy of fresh stool.

Management

The main objective of the physical examination is to exclude other diagnoses, especially surgical emergencies, and to assess the state of hydration.

The potentially disastrous pitfall in the management of gastro-enteritis is failing to realize how dehydrating an attack in a small baby is going to be during the first few hours of the illness. The GP must be very ready to send a young baby with severe diarrhoea into hospital. Fortunately, the reduced mineral content of modern cows' milk preparations and the easy availability of oral rehydrating solutions has made severe dehydration less common. Nevertheless, it can still occur and be dangerous. The younger the child, the more easily will he become dehydrated. Sunken eyes, a dry tongue, inelastic skin, and a depressed anterior fontanelle are late signs, and any infant who is that dry needs urgent rehydration in hospital. Because urine output decreases when the child vomits or has diarrhoea, the frequency of micturition will provide an indication of the severity of dehydration. If the infant has a dry nappy, despite being changed several hours previously, he has probably lost a significant amount of fluid. In severe cases the faeces may be like water and be mistaken for urine, so that the doctor may be of the incorrect opinion that the child is not dehydrated because the nappies are very wet. If the infant's temperature is taken rectally it may be followed by a spurt of liquid faeces, a useful diagnostic point.

Loss of weight is another useful pointer to the severity of fluid loss if the infant's present weight can be compared with weight at a recent visit to the practice's child health clinic. In a young infant weight loss of up to five per cent (a significant amount) can occur before the signs of dehydration become obvious. By the time 10–15 per cent of body weight is lost there is a danger of peripheral circulatory failure, shown by an increasing tachypnoea, tachycardia, and a thready pulse. The signs of fluid loss are particularly difficult to assess in the fat baby or toddler who can have severe dehydration without apparent loss of tissue turgor (because fatty tissue is largely water-free). Infants who have lost five per cent or more of body weight will need closely supervised rehydration.

Apart from signs of fluid loss, general examination of children with uncomplicated gastro-enteritis is usually non-contributory. The abdomen may be a little distended with hyperactive bowel sounds. A rectal examination may be helpful in a difficult case by demonstrating local tenderness in pelvic appendicitis or precipitating a gush of watery stool in gastro-enteritis.

The mainstay of home treatment of gastro-enteritis is, during the acute phase, to give only fluids by mouth. Babies who are breast-fed should continue to take the breast during an attack of diarrhoea. In others milk and solids should be briefly stopped. Oral rehydration solution (ORS) should be used to supplement the breast if there is any possibility of dehydration and to replace the milk and solids briefly for the artificially fed. It is important to emphasize the correct dilution of ORS, as a solution which is inadvertently made up too concentrated may cause dangerous hypernatraemia in young babies. If the baby will only take a little at a time or is vomiting, the mixture can be given very frequently, even every 15–30 minutes. Provided the solution is accurately diluted and offered frequently enough the baby's thirst will govern how much needs to be taken. Usually about 1 litre per 24 hours at six months and 1–1.5 litres at one year, is required. The physiological reason for using ORS is that glucose and sodium when together, and only when together, are well absorbed by the small intestine and thus water is absorbed too, even when there is simultaneous diarrhoea. There is no convincing reason for using such solutions for other illnesses, or for vomiting alone.

The subsequent management of resolving gastro-enteritis is somewhat controversial. Most young babies respond satisfactorily to the return of full milk and normal diet, especially starchy foods, after 12–24 hours (Chew *et al.* 1993). Even though diarrhoea may continue to some extent, nutrition is better preserved.

There is no need to start with diluted milk, although a brisk relapse of diarrhoea is an indication for a more gradual introduction of normal feeds and is considered below under 'Chronic diarrhoea'. It is a common mistake to continue too long with clear fluids alone in babies, adding malnutrition to the primary problem. Some degree of loose stools for a week or two is acceptable (and quite common) provided the baby is having an adequate calorie intake and is well otherwise. If the infant continues to have bothersome diarrhoea beyond this time and especially if he fails to thrive, then lactose intolerance may be the cause.

Anti-diarrhoeal medicines have no place in the management of acute diarrhoea in the infant or toddler. In later childhood, kaolin or small doses of codeine phosphate may make life more comfortable for the patient and his family. Antibiotics are of no use in viral gastro-enteritis, and in some types of bacterial diarrhoea may prolong the carrier state. However, in campylobacter gastro-enteritis, erythromycin is probably helpful, and for the toxic child in shigellosis and with salmonellae, who may be septicaemic, trimethoprim or amoxycillin are indicated. For a mildly unwell child it is reasonable to await the stool results; for a very toxic older child, or a sick baby, referral will be needed, but for those in between, starting one of these drugs while awaiting the cultures may be reasonable. Finally, and not to be forgotten, it is essential to discuss with the family measures to minimize the chance of spread of infection.

Specimens of faeces (from which pathogens are more likely to be isolated than from rectal swabs) should be sent to the laboratory in the following circumstances:

1. The child has recently returned from abroad or has been in contact with somebody from abroad who has diarrhoea (several specimens may be necessary).
2. The child has diarrhoea and attends a nursery.
3. The child's parents handle food for the public.
4. Before starting antibiotics.
5. The child has persistent diarrhoea and giardia is suspected (see below).
6. Presence of blood.

Many laboratories only culture the stool and need to be asked specifically to look for virus (electron-microscopy) or protozoa (microscopy of fresh stool).

CHRONIC DIARRHOEA

It is not uncommon for a healthy toddler to toddle bouncily into the surgery with a mother who complains that the child has got persistent diarrhoea. Toddler diarrhoea—or, as it is appropriately named, 'the peas and carrots syndrome'—usually starts in children between the ages of six months and two years. There seems to be a decreased mouth-to-anus transit time so that the stools contain little bits of undigested food. If the child looks healthy, has normal weight gain, is without abdominal distension and does not have a history suggestive of the rarer conditions discussed below, no investigation is needed beyond a microscopic examination of fresh faeces for *Giardia lamblia*, perhaps on several occasions.

The most satisfactory management for these patients is to reassure the parents that the child is not ill and therefore does not need treatment, to commiserate with them, perhaps recommending a simple barrier cream to protect the child's bottom from getting too sore, and to encourage them to accept philosophically what is usually a temporary change in the child's bowel habits. The condition is less unpleasant for the parents once the child is out of nappies, and the stools usually revert to normal by about the end of the fourth year—admittedly a long time for the family to have to wait.

Lactose intolerance due to the absence of lactase may be the cause of sometimes rather frothy diarrhoea (perhaps with a sore bottom) because the unabsorbed lactose is degraded to lactic acid and CO_2 in those who are intolerant (usually older children and adults) who are given more than a small amount of cows' milk. It is a common recessively inherited condition in those ethnic groups whose ancestors were hunter-gatherers (e.g. many Africans and Asians) rather than cow-herders (Anglo-Saxons). The enzyme is present in their young children but 'switched-off' after the age of six (Platz 1989). This genetic variant needs no treatment, except to remember not to force milk on such children if they do not like it because it gives them mild abdominal pain or diarrhoea. Diagnosis can be made by measuring a raised hydrogen excretion in the breath (collected by the subject blowing up a balloon) following a standard lactose load, but is not routinely necessary. Temporary lactose intolerance is often seen following acute gastro-enteritis, as lactase is located on the tips of intestinal microvilli and is thus vulnerable to transient damage. A temporary intolerance to cows' milk protein may sometimes occur simultaneously. The simplest management for both is to try excluding milk for a few days, and in a baby, replacing it with a soya-based milk and lactose free product such as Wysoy. Butter and yoghurt are all right unless the intolerance is very marked. Unless there is a prompt improvement, it is not worth continuing the regime. After gastro-enteritis, the cows' milk and lactose avoidance, if effective, may need to be continued for a few weeks. If there is persistent intolerance with weight loss on reintroducing cows' milk, in a young infant referral is indicated.

Malabsorption from cystic fibrosis, coeliac disease or even rarer conditions is often thought of, but is seldom the cause of chronic diarrhoea in small children, and almost never if growth is good. The recessive inherited disease, **cystic fibrosis**, is the commonest genetic condition in Europeans, occurring in one in about 2500 births. The gene codes for a protein which regulates the normal transport of chloride ions through the epithelial cells lining sweat glands, and ducts and glands in the lung and the intestinal tract. If cystic fibrosis has not been diagnosed at birth (because of intestinal obstruction due to meconium ileus) the child will usually present in the first few years of life with recurrent chest infections and failure to thrive. Malabsorption occurs because thickened secretions reduce the outflow of pancreatic enzymes. Patients with cystic fibrosis have a high sweat sodium chloride concentration because of poor reabsorption by the sweat duct cells, and the 'sweat test' has been the mainstay of diagnosis. DNA examination of blood or buccal smears is becoming more important.

Coeliac disease causes persistent diarrhoea, sometimes becoming apparent fairly soon after the introduction of solid food which contains gluten. The child fails to thrive, may be anaemic, miserable, and have a poor appetite. On examination there is usually abdominal distension and evidence of wasting. Later presentation may be with poor growth, anaemia or amenorrhoea. The definitive diagnostic test is a peroral jejunal biopsy. It is essential that the child is not commenced on a gluten free diet until the biopsy has been performed.

Crohn's disease with insidious or acute abdominal pain and perhaps a mass, fever, anaemia, iritis, or arthropathy, and especially growth failure, may cause recurrent or persistent diarrhoea (sometimes bloody). It may be associated with mouth ulcers or perianal abscesses and skin tags. It is a good idea to look at the mouth and anus of a puny child presenting with recurrent diarrhoea. The diagnosis of Crohn's disease is often delayed, quite frequently the initial label being psychogenic abdominal pain. There may be a family history.

Ulcerative colitis is another rare cause of chronic diarrhoea which often contains mucus and blood. The child may have tenesmus and lower abdominal pain.

Giardiasis is due to an intestinal protozoan which is common in the UK and is also a common cause of diarrhoea in travellers returning from abroad. Outbreaks starting in camps may result from contaminated water. Some infections are asymptomatic; in others the child may have mild abdominal discomfort with chronic diarrhoea. Acute diarrhoea is also seen. By contrast with most intestinal pathogens, persistent symptomatic infection is sometimes seen and malabsorption may result with failure to thrive. It may be necessary to examine several stool specimens before the pear-shaped flagellate and its cysts are found. Giardiasis can be effectively treated with a three-day course of metronidazole. Tinidazole can also be given as a single treatment repeated after 7–10 days.

Amoebiasis is much rarer in the UK, being almost never seen except in returned travellers. It may lead to mild recurrent diarrhoea, perhaps with abdominal discomfort, tenesmus, and some blood and mucus in the stools, or to severe dysentery associated with large quantities of fluid and blood-stained faeces. Colonic ulcers may lead to perforation and peritonitis. There is sometimes serious systemic spread, for example to the liver. An ultrasound may show an hepatic abscess. Again, two or three fresh, warm, stools may need to be examined before the *E. histolytica* trophozoites are identified. Amoebic infection is one of the reasons for examining the faeces of newly arrived refugees from hot countries.

WORMS

Threadworms are often asymptomatic but may cause pruritis ani or, in a girl, vulvitis with dysuria, sometimes mistaken for urinary infection. The harmless infestation is diagnosed by parents when they notice the 1 cm long worms in the child's faeces or around the anus. Threadworms can be a source of great anxiety about horrible infestations and indeed the sight of several wriggly white worms around the anal margin can be quite frightening.

The doctor was called late one evening, despite his protestations, to see a nine-year-old girl with 'lots of worms coming out of her bottom'. She did, indeed, have a heavy infestation with threadworms.

More often they are seen in the faeces. It is sometimes recommended that all members of the family should be treated at the same time. Even if this is done, the infestation often returns. We usually only treat members of the family in whose stools the worms have been noticed. There seems to be a tendency in any case for excretion of threadworms to disappear with time. The patient can be treated with mebendazole (Vermox—one 100 mg tablet—or Pyrantel as a single dose), both repeated after two weeks. These drugs are also used for patients with the unpleasant-looking roundworms (*Ascaris lumbricoides*), which measure some 20 cm in length and somewhat resemble the earthworm. Very occasionally ascaris can cause either a pneumonic illness or a low-grade intestinal obstruction.

More serious is the Toxocara of dogs. If Toxocara eggs are eaten by toddlers the larvae may migrate to the eye and cause blindness; alternatively they may spread elsewhere in the body, causing failure to thrive. Fever, eosinophilia, hepatomegaly, and wheezing can occur. An antibody test confirms the diagnosis. Treatment is unsatisfactory but infection can be prevented if young pets, especially puppies, are regularly dewormed. Children returning from the tropics with persistent gastro-intestinal symptoms or with anaemia should have their stools examined for hookworms.

Bibiography

Chew, F., Penna, F. J., Peret Filho, L. A. *et al.* (1993). Is dilution of cows' milk formula necessary for dietary management of acute diarrhoea in infants aged less than 6 months? *Lancet*, **341**, 194–7.

Elliott, E. J. (1992). Viral diarrhoeas in childhood. *British Medical Journal*, **305**, 1111–12.

Farthing, M. J. G. (1993). Travellers' diarrhoea. *British Medical Journal*, **306**, 1425–6.

Faruque, A. S. G., Mahalanabis, D., Islam, A. *et al.* (1992). Breast feeding and oral rehydration at home during diarrhoea to prevent dehydration. *Archives of Disease in Childhood*, **67**, 1027–9.

Griffin, G. E. (1987). Travellers' diarrhoea syndrome. In *Advanced medicine*, Vol. 23, (ed. R. E. Pounder and P. L. Chiodini). Baillière Tindall, London.

Lewis, H. M., Parry, J. V., Davies, H. A., Parry, R. P., Mott, A., Dourmashkin, R. R. *et al.* (1979). A year's experience of the rotavirus syndrome and its association with respiratory illness. *Archives of Disease in Childhood*, **54**, 339–46.

Walker-Smith, J. A. (1980). Toddler's diarrhoea. *Archives of Disease in Childhood*, **55**, 329–30.

14 The skin

The epidermis, which is about 0.1 mm thick, is completely replaced every month through the mitotic division of cells in its basal layer. These cells gradually migrate towards the surface, become flattened, lose their nuclei and become filled with keratin. As well as the squamous cells or keratinocytes, which form the bulk of the final layer or stratum corneum, the epidermis contains other cell types including the pigment producing melanocytes. In diseases such as psoriasis, where there is an accelerated turnover of the epidermis, the more rapid movement of the keratinocytes to the surface prevents production of the usual well formed protective layer of dead cells. This surface layer is then an ineffective barrier and is more easily breached.

GENERAL PRINCIPLES OF MANAGEMENT

The skin is a single organ and when one section of it has been affected by a disease, it is likely that other areas will be affected as well. Although it is not always practical for a GP to see every child with a rash naked, diagnosis is sometimes difficult without doing so.

The following principles are important in treatment:

1. **Topical steroids**. If they are used, the weakest effective formula should be applied. The side-effects are proportional to the strength of the steroid and the duration of its use. A topical steroid should not be used purely for the lubricant properties of its base; it is better to use a plain preparation like emulsifying ointment or aqueous cream. The BNF divides topical steroids into groups according to potency; 'mild' (hydrocortisone 0.5–1%)–'very potent'(clobetasol 0.05%). It is useful to become familiar with one member of each group.

Prolonged use of topical steroids on the face may lead to persistent redness and telangiectasia, and thinning of the skin which may result in striae and purpura. Systemic side-effects such as suppression of the pituitary–adrenal axis are uncommon, unless strong preparations are used over wide areas of the skin.

2. If the skin is weeping, a lotion or cream should be used (a handkerchief moistened with tap water can be quite soothing). A localized area of weeping and crusting is usually a sign of bacterial infection, and addition of an oral anti-staphylococcal antibiotic, while continuing the steroid, is the best approach. A small patch of impetigo or infected eczema may be cleared with a topical antibacterial cream such as chlortetracycline. Creams, which are emulsions with a relatively high water to oil ratio, are better for most skin lesions than the more greasy ointments, which are usually reserved for areas of dry, corrugated 'lichenified' skin.

3. An unusual rash in a child may be an allergic reaction to a medicine. Some topical preparations are also potent skin sensitizers. They include antihistamine creams (which should not be used), local anaesthetic preparations, some antiseptics and antibiotics such as hydroxyquinolines (Vioform) and neomycin. Unusual rashes of recent onset are also often viral, especially if the child is unwell (p. 162).

4. In fungal infection, suppression of inflammation with local steroids gives a false impression of improvement. Relapse will occur when the steroid is stopped, the infection surging ahead with renewed vigour. If the doctor is uncertain whether the child's annular lesion is caused by a fungus, a topical antifungal preparation should be used first. Reserve topical steroids for those rashes which do not respond within two weeks.

Parents often have unvoiced fears that should be anticipated when they consult about a child with a rash. In eczema, the mother may blame herself wrongly that it is all due to her bottle-feeding and not breast-feeding. They wonder if the child is infectious to others, if the neighbours will think the child is dirty and neglected, or if the rash will persist into adulthood. Sometimes their fears of criticism are well justified.

Three-year-old Daniel had severe infantile eczema. His face was red and excoriated. Mrs K took him into the local grocer's shop where a fellow customer criticized her for bringing a dirty child into the shop.

THE INFANT

During the neonatal period a number of temporary skin blemishes may appear:

Sucking blisters. Oval blisters which occur on the peripheral parts of the lips of infants at birth. They resolve fairly quickly without treatment.

Milia. Multiple small pearly white papules over the face. These superficial epidermal inclusion cysts require no treatment.

Toxic erythema is a blotchy, erythematous, macular rash. Sometimes the lesions contain a central pustule or vesicle. They may be sparse or profuse, usually appearing on the face and trunk usually within 48 hours of birth, and fading away over a few weeks. A similar rash—neonatal acne—can be more persistent over the first two or three months; it is harmless and probably due to a stimulation of sebaceous glands by maternal androgens.

Neonatal staphylococcal skin infection. Staphylococcal pneumonia or osteomyelitis in neonates may be preceded by apparently minor skin infections. These should therefore be treated with a five day course of oral flucloxacillin (62.5 mg four times a day). Sometimes it is hard to be certain whether a minor lesion is definitely staphylococcal. However, clear cut paronychiae, especially more than one, convincing septic spots (very like toxic erythema but with slightly larger pustules at the centre of the redness), or erythema around the umbilical stump are all indications for treatment. If supra-umbilical erythema is flame shaped it may imply spread into the liver and is one indication for referral. Another is the occasional baby severely affected by staphylococcal skin sepsis, whose skin may peel off in sheets with slight trauma, such as rubbing with the finger—staphylococcal toxic epidermal necrolysis.

Birthmarks

Several types of birthmarks are common:

Stork marks (salmon patches) are pink areas over the nape of the neck, the upper eyelids, and the central forehead seen in about 50 per cent of infants. They are not of clinical importance as, with the occasional exception of those on the nape of the neck, they fade and disappear completely by the time the child is a year old. Their mythological pathogenesis is bruising from the beak of the bird bringing the child to the delivery.

Strawberry naevi (capillary haemangioma) are raised, red, compressible lesions that can be found anywhere on the body. They are not visible at birth but appear in the first four to six weeks. Most of them have a phase of rapid expansion lasting 6 to 10 months, with the majority reaching their maximal size by 12 to 18 months of age, followed by a stationary phase. Finally, spontaneous involution occurs, often preceded by patchy blanching of the lesion—an encouraging sign to parents. The majority are small. They do not require referral unless they are immense, or obstruct the eye or respiratory passages or ear. Parents will need careful explanation of the natural history of the lesion, especially during the phase of rapid growth. Most have regressed by the time the patient is five years old. Occasionally they leave a very mild puckering or scarring of the skin.

Port-wine stain. These permanent lesions are masses of dilated capillaries and are present at birth. They are well-defined, purply-red, and quite flat. They show little or no tendency towards involution and usually require covering with tinted, opaque, waterproof, cosmetic cream such as Covermark. Prescriptions should be endorsed 'ACBS'. Pulsed dye laser treatment, in expert hands, can be curative. It involves emission of short bursts of energy which specifically destroy the dilated blood vessels in the lesion but spare surrounding tissues. Between four and six treatment sessions over a couple of years are required.

Port-wine stains in the distribution of the ophthalmic division of the trigeminal nerve may be associated with underlying cerebrovascular malformations in the Sturge–Weber syndrome (fits, ipsilateral glaucoma, contralateral hemiparesis, and ipsilateral intracranial calcification).

MOLES (ACQUIRED PIGMENTED NAEVI)

The GP may be consulted about pigmented moles in children and adolescents, not only for cosmetic reasons, but also because of increasing public awareness of skin cancer. Moles arise from epidermal melanin-containing cells. Three types are described depending on the position of the naevus cells in the skin. Most moles seen in children are junctional; the cells lie in the lower epidermis in contact with the dermo-epidermal junction and are flat. In the raised ones the naevus cells have a compound position, including intradermally. Moles can appear anywhere on the body, are relatively small, varying in size and in shade of brown. They usually appear in early childhood or adolescence, may be flat or raised.

Malignant change in a mole is extremely rare. Rapid growth, irregular colour change, satellite lesions, repeated irritation, or bleeding are indications for excision. Even when one does refer a child whose mole meets these criteria it is extremely uncommon for it to be found to be malignant. Many benign moles do gradually grow in adolescence and may change colour.

Moles are occasionally present at birth. They are of varying size and grow with the patient. Very large black, congenital moles over 2 cm in diameter, and usually much larger, are an altogether more sinister category and up to 10 per cent may become malignant; they require a dermatological opinion. So do large lesions with hair on them—the giant hairy naevus—especially if they are over 1.5 cm in diameter.

Freckles develop in response to the sun with an increase in melanin pigment but no increase in the number of melanocytes. In many coloured infants large bluish-black areas are seen over the back, sacrum, or buttocks or occasionally more widely. These are Mongolian blue spots, a form of naevus which tends to fade with age.

ECZEMA AND SEBORRHOEIC DERMATITIS

These two may co-exist, and are sometimes difficult to differentiate. The skin of most infants with seborrhoea clears within a few months, a few are atopic and develop eczema. This is particularly likely if there is a family history of the latter.

Eczema

Severe atopic eczema is one of the most stressful medical conditions a family with a young child will have to cope with; endless broken nights, disfigurement, time-consuming treatment, behaviour disturbance and family demoralization are commonplace. Fortunately, most cases are milder. Atopic eczema is an inflammatory skin disease occurring in some degree in up to 10 per cent of all children. A family history of allergic disorder is frequent, and patients with eczema often develop subsequent asthma.

Atopic eczema usually begins in the first twelve months after birth, although in some children it only starts later in childhood. The earliest lesions are usually red, excoriated, occasionally weeping patches, often on the face; sometimes involvement is more widespread. Flexural lesions, so common in older children, are not dominant at this stage. As well as the flexures, the lower buttocks, wrists, and ankles are often also involved later. In the very severely affected toddler almost the whole surface of the skin is dry and covered with a mixture of scratch marks and weeping eczematous lesions. As the child gets older there is a tendency for the skin in affected areas to become thick and fissured. In African and African-Caribbean children the acute lesions are often hypopigmented and chronic eczema may be hyper- or hypo-pigmented.

Eczema is intensely itchy and the skin is torn by persistent scratching which can lead to weeping, crusting, and secondary infection. A careful history may reveal that the child's skin becomes worse after he has eaten a particular food, or worn a particular fabric, such as wool.

The patient and family who have to cope with this frustrating disease, are told that there is no simple cure, but that the eczema can be controlled by therapy. At times it will be quiescent, tending to improve, and often disappear, as the child gets older. Only a small proportion of all patients with infantile eczema will still be affected by adolescence.

Nails should be kept short and smooth with a nail file to minimize the damage done by scratching. Certain materials may make the child more itchy, and loose-fitting cotton washed in non-biological washing powders is better than nylon. Whilst children should not be overdressed, and therefore hot and sweaty, their skin is commonly too dry. Although dry skin alone is sometimes inherited as a familial trait, it is frequently present as an associated exacerbating factor in eczema. Frequent baths are soothing and beneficial for some children, others find they aggravate the eczema. Emollients such as Oilatum Emollient (Stiefel) added to the water may be helpful.

It is often recommended to avoid all soaps, as they tend to leach out the small amount of oil in the skin, making it even drier. Emulsifying ointment can be used as a substitute; 0.5–1 kg will need to be prescribed at a time. It is massaged into the skin before a bath, used as a soap in the bath, and applied afterwards if the skin is dry. Alternatively, after the child is washed and dried, aqueous cream can be used to prevent the skin from drying out, being used several times a day. It is uncertain how much impact these time-consuming procedures have on the course of the disease.

In addition to keeping the skin greasy, which is the key to successful control of dryness, local improvement will often be produced by one of the weak steroid preparations. Occasionally, stronger ones are necessary, but should not be used on the face. The strength and concentration of the steroid application can be reduced as the eczema improves and often the steroid can then be entirely replaced by enough use of emollient. A sedative antihistamine, such as trimeprazine, is moderately useful in helping the child to sleep at night. Whatever treatment is used, a relapsing course is the rule rather than the exception.

Two categories of infection are important in eczema. First, bacterial superinfection with staphylococci and often also with streptococci. It can be difficult to decide when colonization merges into bacterial infection, but the diagnosis should be suspected if there is weeping, crusting, and a purulent exudate, or an increase in severity of the eczema. David and Cambridge (1986) suggested that it might be worthwhile giving the child with a troublesome exacerbation of eczema a course of flucloxacillin rather than increasing the strength of steroid cream, even if the signs of infection are not obvious. However, the steroids should not be stopped. As with impetigo, small localized patches of infected eczema can be effectively treated by a topical antibiotic.

A second and potentially more serious infection is eczema herpeticum, infection with the herpes simplex virus (David and Longson 1985). The hallmark of primary infection is large vesicles or pustules with a central depression; the main feature of a recurrent infection is a crop of vesicles repeatedly appearing at the same location. They quickly rupture. A sudden worsening of eczema, especially if any vesicles can be seen, may mean eczema herpeticum. Secondary bacterial infection is almost invariable, and the vesicles soon become purulent. Occasionally, in a primary infection with HSV, there are severe systemic effects leading to admission and treatment with intravenous acyclovir and antibiotics. If a few vesicles are seen in a well child, no treatment other than close observation is reasonable.

It is uncertain how useful it is to attempt to avoid precipitating factors such as the house-dust mite, contact with pets and dietary allergens. Unfortunately skin tests and other antibody measurements are of no proven value. If a food appears to aggravate the eczema, or if the eczema is so bad it is causing a major degree of stress, the diet deserves more detailed consideration if, and only if, vigorously applied simple treatment has failed. Expectations should not be very high. Commoner dietary culprits are cows' milk, egg, soya, wheat, nuts, or citrus fruits. With obsessional attention to food labels, these can be omitted (including prepared foods containing them) in turn for a few weeks each. Partial exclusion of a possible culprit is likely to be useless. Longer term use of strict diets requires dietetic supervision as they may be deficient in calcium and other important components. Another danger is the occurrence of severe or even fatal anaphylaxis on reintroduction of an excluded item.

It is occasionally necessary to admit a child with widespread eczema to hospital to bring the eruption under control. Oral corticosteroids should be avoided as dramatic improvement is always followed by relapse when the drug is stopped. Their long-term use is only very rarely indicated. Most families will wish for an orthodox or unorthodox second opinion at some stage in the course of their child's disease. Unorthodox alternative treatments come and go. Some herbal preparations do have some non-placebo benefit, but preparations are poorly formulated, and some may lead to hepatotoxicity and cardiotoxicity. Furthermore, some have added steroids.

There has been controversy for many years over the role of different early feeding practices in the management of infants from families at risk. Does prolonging breast-feeding, with or without modifications in the mother's diet, soya milk preparations or goats' milk have any long-term benefit? There is no clear message, except to point out that special formulations may be nutritionally harmful (e.g. goats' milk has little folic acid and some soya preparations inadequate calcium; they may also be expensive).

Seborrhoeic dermatitis

Seborrhoeic dermatitis typically begins on the scalp as cradle cap during the first month or two of life. In many infants it does not extend any further, but in others an erythematous, slightly greasy, sharply demarcated, scaly rash may appear behind the ears, on the face and neck, and in the axillae and nappy areas. If large areas or the whole face are involved, the condition may be mistaken for severe infantile eczema, or for toxic epidermal necrolysis. In fact, seborrhoea can clear up quite quickly and the child is relatively undisturbed as the lesions are not itchy.

Cradle cap can be cleared by repeatedly washing the scalp with a mild detergent shampoo alone or following the application of olive oil. Lesions on the body and the face may be treated like atopic eczema, remembering the possibilities of superadded thrush (see below) and secondary bacterial infection.

Seborrhoeic dermatitis becomes common again in adolescents, who may suffer from dandruff, scaling of the eyebrows, dermatitis behind the ears, otitis externa, and inflammation of the nasolabial folds. The chest, axillae, groins, and perineal regions may also be involved with the development of red, somewhat greasy, areas. Topical therapy along the line of eczema management is the mainstay.

NAPPY RASH

In a non-seborrhoeic baby this is usually caused by prolonged contact of the skin with urine and faeces. It presents in many different forms ranging from a mild erythema to multiple flat topped ulcerated papules. Secondary infection with bacteria and candida is common. Widespread involvement of the skin in the absence of seborrhoea may be the sign of a neglected child. The following is one plan of management:

1. As the rash may clear when left in the open air, this should be encouraged when possible during the day. Disposable nappies need to be changed often to prevent wet, soggy skin.
2. When the nappy is changed, the perineum is carefully cleaned with warm water on cotton wool, and in mild cases a simple barrier cream is used (zinc and castor oil).
3. Candida may be a pathogenic factor, especially if the rash has satellite lesions, and sometimes if it does not. The application of nystatin cream three times a day, combined with the above measures, may be all that is needed, although it is often necessary to add 1% hydrocortisone after a few days if the rash is not obviously clearing. Canesten HC is a simpler alternative.

FUNGAL INFECTIONS

Candidiasis

Oral thrush is common in the newborn; the lesions are white, adherent, thready plaques occurring mainly on the inside of cheeks, but also on the tongue and fauces. The mouth should be examined for thrush if a baby has a nappy rash with outlying red spots. One ml of nystatin suspension (100 000 units/mL) delivered in the mouth four times a day is usually effective; it may also be necessary to remove the dummy. Alternatively, 2.5 ml of miconazole gel b.d. may be effective for intractable cases. Debilitated babies, or those given antibiotics, are often affected, but most infants with oral thrush are fit.

James, aged nine months, was brought to a doctor because he appeared to have a pain on swallowing. His mouth was covered in thrush and the doctor was not surprised to learn that James was on prophylactic antibiotics following a urinary tract infection.

Tineal infections

Dermatophytes are fungi which invade and proliferate in the outer layers of the epidermis. Some species also invade the nails and hair. In adolescents the feet and groin are the commonest sites. Pulled out hairs or diseased nail cuttings sent to the laboratory may sometimes lead to a positive identification.

Tinea pedis

The characteristic appearance of athlete's foot is of sodden white, peeling skin between the toes. Lesions may spread to the sole of the foot and are very irritating.

They may be sore or tender as well as itchy. Topical antifungal preparations such as tolnaftate (Tinaderm) or clotrimazole (Canestan) are effective against most dermatophyte species and should be applied twice daily for three or four weeks, the time, as mentioned earlier, that it takes for the epidermis to renew itself. A powder (for example, zinc undecenoate) may then be helpful in preventing recurrence.

Not all scaly, macerated skin around the toes is caused by fungi. Excess sweating or eczema can also mimic tinea pedis. Some children develop a dermatitis with burning, red, cracking skin on the plantar surface of the forefoot and toes, especially the first toe. This is probably due to synthetic footwear not allowing the sweat to evaporate.

The child should wash his feet and change his socks daily, using his own towel to dry between the toes. Sandals are better than shoes in allowing effective ventilation.

Tinea capitis

Ringworm of the scalp usually presents as a roughly oval patch with broken hairs of variable length affecting any part of the scalp. It may be secondarily infected. The important feature is a scaly base, in contrast to alopecia areata. Another occasional misdiagnosis is psoriasis, which may start with a fungal looking, scaly patch on the scalp. Suspicious hair can be sent for identification of the fungus. Griseofulvin (10 mg/kg per day) is given for six to eight weeks; it may interact with barbiturates or cause photosensitivity. Though topical treatment alone may reduce superficial inflammation, it is inadequate as a sole therapy.

Tinea cruris

This is an irritating red rash on the inner aspect of the thigh and perineum. The margins become well demarcated as the rash spreads; there may be superadded bacterial or candidal infection. Not all itchy rashes in the groin are fungal infections; intertrigo from moist areas of skin in contact with each other, or seborrhoea, are possibilities. The fungus usually clears with clotrimazole or miconazole, with or without hydrocortisone, followed by a bland dusting powder to absorb moisture. Loose cotton trunks are better than tight briefs.

Tinea versicolor

Tinea versicolor is an innocuous chronic fungal infection but one which is troublesome to treat because of the widespread lesions and the frequent recurrence of the infection. On white skins it has a slightly scaly, pigmented appearance, and on pigmented skins the lesions are often paler than the surrounding area. Clotrimazole applied twice a day for two to four weeks is likely to be effective, but is expensive if applied to a large area. Treated skin takes some time to regain the colouring of its surrounding.

ALOPECIA AREATA

This is a common condition usually affecting children and young adults. The patient presents with a well demarcated round or oval bald patch or patches. The involved scalp is hairless but appears normal and uninflamed. There are short broken hairs around the patches. The condition is often recurrent. The hair usually regrows within some months. Treatment is not usually helpful, though intradermal, and even systemic, steroids have been used for extensive alopecia. The prognosis is less good with very extensive baldness.

Alopecia areata needs to be distinguished from compulsive pulling out of hair which also leaves a normal scalp. In the latter, lesions are not so well defined and hairs remaining in the affected patches are of varying length.

WARTS

Warts are DNA virus-induced epidermal lesions. They are moderately contagious and usually regress within two or three years leaving no scar. There are several different types. The common wart is a raised brown lesion with a rough clefted hyperkeratotic surface, often found on the back of the hands and fingers. Other warty lesions include plane warts and thin filiform projections. Plantar warts (verrucae) are sometimes painful and, because of pressure on the sole of the foot, are not usually significantly raised above the surface of the skin. It is often difficult to distinguish verrucae from callouses. The former usually have an irregular surface. If the hyperkeratotic layer of a verruca is gently pared down with a razor blade or scalpel small black dots, thrombosed capillaries, and bleeding points appear. Condylomata acuminata are fleshy papillomatous lesions which occur around the genital and perineal areas. Both they and smaller perineal warts can be sexually transmitted and in childhood raise the possibility, though not the certainty, of sexual abuse. DNA analysis may be helpful if needed. A more common explanation is that the child has spread his warts from his finger to his perianal region as a result of scratching his bottom.

The general principle that the existence of multiple approaches to treatment implies that none are very effective is true for warts. Therapy, unpredictable and not very satisfactory, is often forced upon the reluctant GP by pressure from school or parents. Salactol which contains lactic and salicylic acids in a collodion base may be conveniently painted on the wart each day after paring it down and protecting the normal skin with a little Vaseline.

It seems very unlikely that excluding every verrucous child from swimming or PE will have any effect on the epidemiology of the condition. To save face, a reasonable compromise may be to allow the child to go swimming after a couple of weeks treatment, with the wart covered by a waterproof plaster.

Resistant lesions, or those on visible sites such as the hands, can be treated radically with carbon dioxide snow, liquid nitrogen, curettage, or cautery. All have their advocates and have become popular in practice minor surgery clinics.

A local anaesthetic cream (for example, Emla) should be used prior to such procedures. We prefer to wait for spontaneous regression, if such a course is socially acceptable to the child and parents.

Molluscum contagiosum

Molluscum contagiosum, caused by a large pox virus, is another common epidermal infection. The lesions are pearly, dome-shaped papules, sometimes with an umbilicated centre. They vary from 1–5 mm in size and occur in crops anywhere on the body. They can gradually spread locally and be transmitted to others. Widespread infections have been reported in immunosuppressed patients. The papules will eventually disappear if left alone—usually the best advice. Various methods of treatment have been devised on the principle that damaging the lesion causes involution. These include piercing the central core with a sterile needle after prior application of local anaesthetic cream.

IMPETIGO

Impetigo of the face or upper limbs, or elsewhere, is common in children. It is usually caused by a mixed infection involving *Staphylococcus aureus* and *Streptococcus pyogenes*. Each lesion starts as a purulent blister which soon ruptures to release an exudate. By the time the GP has been consulted, this has usually dried into a yellow or grey–black scab. Impetigo may sometimes be superimposed on other skin conditions such as eczema or scabies. Acute nephritis occasionally follows *Strep. pyogenes* impetigo occurring in hot countries but not in the UK.

After taking a swab from the crust, if there is diagnostic doubt, oral flucloxacillin is indicated for children who have extensive lesions. Those less severely affected will be cured by the topical antibiotic, mupirocin. Sometimes thick crusts need to be soaked off before treatment. As impetigo is highly contagious, care with personal hygiene is important. Some school authorities may prefer the child to stay at home until the lesions are obviously healing.

INFESTATIONS

Scabies

This common disorder is caused by the mite *Sarcoptes scabiei Var.hominis*. It is often difficult to diagnose but should be suspected in any child who has no history of atopy but who presents with an acute onset of itchy rash, often worse at night. Itchy papules may be seen between the fingers, on the wrists, genitalia, abdomen, and around the axillae. In infants, eczematous eruptions of the face and trunk may occur. The classical slightly curved burrow is rarely visible, being altered by excoriation and secondary infection.

If a well non-atopic child does not have obvious insect bites and presents with pruritis and a somewhat vague rash below the head, a trial of treatment seems reasonable. This is especially true if the rash is worse at night and if other members of the family are also affected. The treatment must be applied to all the skin surface area from the neck downwards. As the mite spreads from one person to another by close bodily contact the whole household and any other close contact must also be treated simultaneously. Various preparations are used such as 1% lindane (Quellada) or, for younger children, Malathion. Antibiotics may be necessary for secondary infection whilst residual irritation, which may remain for several weeks until the dead antigenic mite is shed from the skin, can be relieved by 0.5–1% hydrocortisone cream.

Pediculosis (lice)

Pediculosis is likely in any child who presents with an itchy scalp which looks reasonably healthy. There may, however, be a mild contact dermatitis on the neck or pinnae. The female louse lays numerous eggs which are cemented to the hair shaft (nits) close to the surface of the skull. Since hair grows 1 cm per month the duration of infestation may be dated by the distance of the nits from the scalp. Nits are pale, grey, ovoid bodies firmly attached to the hair shaft. Unlike dandruff, they cannot be easily brushed or blown off, and on inspection with a hand lens or an auroscope, have a uniform smooth surface. Secondary infection may lead to enlargement of occipital and posterior cervical glands.

Malathion (Prioderm) or permethrin (Lyclear) containing lotions/shampoos may be used for treatment and control of head lice. They should be rubbed well into the hair and left for at least eight hours before being washed out using a shampoo. The hair can then be combed out while wet, with a fine comb to remove unsightly nits. Treatment should be repeated a week later. Injured lice die and the regular use of a fine comb is therefore usually sufficient continuing prophylaxis after treatment. It is probably advisable to treat all members of the household (particularly children) at the same time, even if they have no symptoms. The school nurse should be told. Pediculosis pubis is usually sexually transmitted.

INSECT BITES AND PAPULAR URTICARIA

Biting insects can produce a variety of very irritating lesions in children, including papules with or without a central punctum and erythematous urticarial flares. Most lesions are grouped and are on the arms and legs, but occasionally they will be found on the trunk. There may also be acute urticarial eruptions with subsequent blister formations, sometimes quite large and frightening for the patient. As a result of scratching the lesions may become secondarily infected.

Insect bites have to be differentiated from simple urticaria, from mild chickenpox (lesions mainly on the trunk), and from scabies (usually causing a more generalized itching). It is often difficult to convince the parents of a child with persistent itchy papules that he indeed has insect bites, for often only one member of the family is affected. The problem is not the bite, but the ensuing allergic reaction in some people. Fortunately, with the passage of time, most affected children lose their tendency to over-react to bites. Symptomatic treatment includes cold water compresses or calamine lotion. For acute local lesions, hydrocortisone cream is useful to allay irritation, and oral antihistamines may be helpful. Better management is to avoid or kill off the offending insects. A family cat or dog is frequently the source, but biting insects may also come from other sites in the house or garden. Papular urticaria is a persistent eruption thought to be a hypersensitivity reaction to insect bites. Typically the spots are very irritating hyperpigmented papules.

URTICARIA

It is not uncommon for concerned parents to bring along a child with a florid, itchy, urticarial rash continually changing in shape and size. Often, there is no obvious provoking factor and the rash disappears after a few hours or days. Usually the cause is not established, though a viral infection, or, rarely, physical exercise or cold may be responsible. In a few, ingestion of certain drugs, such as aspirin or penicillin, reaction to food colourants or additives, or specific foods, such as fish, nuts, or eggs, may be the cause (David 1993). Antihistamines (for example, terfenadine or cetirizine) may be helpful. In a few children the urticaria comes and goes over several months, but usually dies out in the end.

PSORIASIS

This affects 1–2 per cent of the general population. There is usually a family history. An adolescent may consult with typical well-demarcated red lesions covered with silver scales. This often affects the extensor surfaces of the limbs; the scalp may also be involved. Guttate psoriasis with a widespread, slightly scaling, pink rash, which may be difficult to differentiate from pityriasis rosea, appears to be a more common presentation in younger children. Creams containing tar and hydrocortisone (Tarcortin) may help and are more acceptable for many than tar preparations. In older children with chronic plaque psoriasis, dithranol treatment (for example, starting with 0.1% dithrocream) may be needed.

ACNE

The peak age for acne is the second half of the teenage years but lesions can start in younger children and continue well into the third decade of life. The underlying cause is increased production of sebum under the influence of the burst of androgenic activity seen during adolescence. The openings of the pilo sebaceous ducts become obstructed with sebum and keratin, leading to the typical lesions, comedones, papules, pustules, and cysts. Pitted scars from previous assaults are often found. Besides the face, the forehead, the shoulders, back and chest may be affected. The role of infection is uncertain but the sebaceous follicles are colonized by various species of bacteria.

It is often stated that adolescents use their acne as the key to open doors for a discussion with the GP about their anxieties associated with various parts of their body. Although this is true in a proportion of cases, the majority of such consultations do not, in fact, extend significantly beyond the surface of the skin and its social implications.

The natural history should be explained to the adolescent, and also the fact that effective treatments are available to help him. There should be a discussion of any factors which appear to make the spots better or worse. There is no place for punishing diets, in which the young patient is asked to abstain from most foods he enjoys, although, if he feels that a particular food or item of clothing increases his acne, he may wish to avoid the provoking factor for a few months to see if there is an improvement. As for warts, so for acne; local preparations are legion. They are not very effective for anything but the mildest of cases, but have value in passing the time until natural remission occurs. The most fashionable preparations at the moment are topical keratolytics such as benzoyl peroxide (Panoxyl) in varying strength, or tretinoin (Retin A—expensive and teratogenic; it may also cause photosensitivity). The patient must be warned that, initially, the skin can become redder and more uncomfortable, which may be helped with 1% hydrocortisone, and also that the preparation may have to be applied to the skin for a few weeks before there is significant improvement. Even though told that the initial discomfort will be transient, many young patients find the treatment worse than the disease and return asking for a blander preparation. Salicylic acid and sulphur cream, or a skin cleansing agent, such as Betadine Skin Cleanser, solution can be used. Occasionally, topical antibiotics, such as clindomycin (Dalacin T), can be a helpful alternative.

More severe acne can often be effectively treated by antibiotics such as tetracycline. If the teenage patient is severely affected this can be started at 250 mg four times a day, the moderately affected patient begins with 250 mg thrice or twice a day given between meals (not with milk, as insoluble calcium salts are formed). Side-effects are rare although sometimes the patient can feel a bit sick. Absorption of the contraceptive pill may possibly be impaired. Again, patients must be warned that improvement will be slow. They will have to take the drugs for at least three months before deciding how effective the treatment is proving. If the starting dose is 1 g a day this can be reduced gradually after a few weeks to a maintenance dose of 250–500 mg daily, and, occasionally, some months later, to 250 mg every other day. If tetracycline does not work, an alternative is erythromycin 250 mg four times a day. We do not recommend treatment with minocycline because of adverse effects of drug induced hepatitis, SLE and eosinophilic pneumonitis (Ferner and Moss 1996). Systematic treatment is often given for a year or more.

Cyproterone acetate, an anti-androgen combined with oestrogen (Dianette) is occasionally recommended by dermatologists for post-pubertal young women. It may be used as an oral contraceptive. Another more toxic, but effective, new preparation for very severe acne is Isotretinoin (Roaccutane). It is extremely teratogenic and should therefore not be used by girls of childbearing age. Acne vulgaris can be a very distressing condition but the potential toxicity of some of the newer preparations is alarming.

Bibliography

David, T. J. (1993). *Food and food additive intolerance in childhood*. Blackwell, Oxford.

David, T. J. and Cambridge, G. C. (1986). Bacterial infection and atopic eczema. *Archives of Disease in Childhood*, **61**, 20–3.

David, T. J. and Longson, M. (1985). Herpes simplex infections in atopic eczema. *Archives of Disease in Childhood*, **60**, 338–43.

Ferner, R. E. and Moss, C. (1996). Minocycline for acne. *British Medical Journal*, **312**, 138.

Ridley, R. and Sarfanek, N. (1992). Common skin conditions. In *Clinical guidelines: report of a local initiative*, (ed. A. Haines and B. Hurwitz). Royal College of General Practitioners, London.

Rogers, M. and Barnetson, R. St. C. (1992). Diseases of the skin. In *Forfar and Arneil's textbook of paediatrics*, 4th edn, (ed. A. G. M. Cambell and N. McIntosh). Churchill Livingstone, London.

15 The eye

At birth the size of an infant's eye is about three-quarters that of an adult, full size being reached at puberty. In infants the sclera is relatively thin and translucent, giving the eye a bluish tinge. When this is very marked osteogenesis imperfecta is a possible diagnosis.

EXAMINING THE EYE

A clear red reflex, best demonstrated using a + lens on an ophthalmoscope, rules out a significant congenital cataract. A white reflex suggests a retinoblastoma. Screening for visual acuity is discussed on p. 29. Occasionally developmental abnormalities affecting the eyes and eyelids may occur. These include congenital ptosis and haemangioma (which may extend to the face, scalp or conjunctiva). Both will need treatment if there is a risk of vision being obscured. As limited acuity in one eye, and even blindness, may be overlooked by both a child and his parents, it is important to test visual acuity in each eye separately. Visual fields can be roughly and easily tested in babies by introducing an interesting toy into the field of vision, first on the left and then on the right. Field losses are seen in some children with cerebral palsy or with pituitary lesions. An acute deterioration of vision or of the visual field usually indicates serious disease, although it can be seen as a temporary phenomenon in some attacks of migraine. Fundoscopy is easier if the curtains are partially drawn; if necessary the GP should dilate the pupils with 0.5 or 1% tropicamide. The doctor kneels and looks at the child's right eye with his right eye. Meanwhile another adult crouches close behind the doctor and attracts the child's attention over the doctor's shoulder. A brief glimpse of the sharp disc edge (pinker in infants than adults) excludes chronically raised intracranial pressure. Red flares from retinal haemorrhage may confirm suspected violence to the head.

ERRORS OF REFRACTION

The GP's responsibility is to be able to diagnose that the child cannot see clearly, and then to ask the optician or ophthalmologist for advice.

Michael was eight when he was discovered to be short-sighted, although his father, a GP, had suspected myopia a year before. 'But Michael', his father said, 'I asked you whether you could see the black-board clearly at school!' 'I can see the black-board all right' said Michael, 'but I can't see what's written on it.'

Most infants are somewhat long-sighted (hypermetropic), but become less so as childhood proceeds. Important refractive errors may come to attention because the child is noticed to have a squint, or he sits too close to the television, or because he lacks interest or behaves badly at school, or because he screws up his eyes; as with the camera, so with the eye, reducing the aperture improves the depth of focus. Sore eyes, headaches, or clumsiness are less convincing presentations which often have non-ocular causes. It is particularly important to screen children with a family history of myopia regularly. It is reasonable to refer the myopic school-age child, whose eyes appear to be otherwise normal, direct to an optician. We usually refer younger children, with a suspected refractive error to an ophthalmologist or orthoptist.

The wearing of glasses neither speeds nor slows the progress of refractive errors. Failure of parents to realize this can make the life of a child who needs glasses and does not like wearing them unnecessarily difficult. Myopia may progress quite rapidly; a child with short sight should have his refraction rechecked annually.

Peckham *et al.* (1978) found that 9 per cent of 11 000 16-year-old children had mild myopia and in 16 per cent it was more severe.

SQUINTS

Children over six months old do not grow out of a squint spontaneously, and treatment is needed to prevent secondary loss of sight (amblyopia) in the squinting eye, as well as for cosmetic reasons. Even a very slight squint may be associated with marked amblyopia. Inspection of the corneal light reflex, and the cover test are useful in assessing the alignment of the eyes. The first is very simple, and involves comparing the position on the two eyes of the reflection on the cornea of a light. Unless there is a squint the reflection will be visible at the same point on both corneas, usually slightly nasal to the centre of the pupils, when the child looks at a pen-torch a few feet away. If the reflections are displaced significantly from the centre of the pupils, a squint is suspected. This test helps to distinguish a true squint from the apparent convergent squint of the child who has prominent epicanthic folds with perhaps a broad bridge of the nose. The cover test provides the definitive evidence for the presence of a manifest squint; however, it is difficult to perform on young children. The common squint of childhood is non-paralytic, the angle being relatively constant in all directions of gaze. Initially, the squint is often more obvious when the child is tired or unwell.

Young babies have to perfect the use of both eyes together, just as they have to perfect other motor skills, and various obstacles can cause a failure in this development. The most important common concomitant squint in childhood occurs during the preschool years in hypermetropic children. The increased accommodation required to produce clear vision in long-sighted patients leads to over-convergence of eyes and a squint. Conditions such as cataract, retinal scars, or retinoblastoma, which prevent normal formation of the retinal image may also present as a squint, as may neurological disease causing delay in psychomotor development, or leading to paralysis of one or more extraocular muscles. The most sinister cause of the latter is raised intracranial pressure leading to a sixth cranial nerve palsy and failure of lateral movement of one or both eyes. It is characteristic of paralytic squints that they are most obvious on looking in the direction of action of the paralysed muscle, when the older child may complain of double vision. The commonest presentation of paralytic squint in infants is an abnormal head posture.

Most squints are due to long-sightedness or non-refractive primary muscle imbalance. Squints are more common in children with physical and intellectual disabilities. However, most childhood squints are isolated disorders. Aims of treatment are to correct amblyopia and to align the visual axes, either to establish binocular vision, or for cosmetic reasons. The management of amblyopia usually includes occlusion of the non-squinting eye, normally the one with better acuity, in order to force the squinting eye into activity. Such a paradoxical treatment may take a lot of explaining to the family. It may help to know that untreated squints are responsible for over half the cases of monocular blindness found in military recruits. If the child has significant hypermetropia this will need to be corrected by lenses. A squint is a major social handicap and production of a satisfactory appearance is also an extremely important aim of treatment.

EYE INJURIES AND FOREIGN BODIES

An ordinary 'black eye' with swollen bruised eyelids resolves spontaneously in about a week. A quick check of visual acuity, ocular movements, pupil, clarity of the media, and integrity of the bones of the orbital margins is usually all that is necessary, unless there is anxiety about non-accidental injury. Most conjunctival foreign bodies will not become troublesome; they get washed away by the flow of tears. Many of those that remain can be located by careful examination using a good light. Sometimes a magnifying glass is helpful. Loose lashes and similar objects that have fallen into the conjunctival sac, or blown into the eye, will usually be found in the lower fornix. They can easily be removed from a co-operative child if he looks upwards. There is a risk that foreign bodies under the upper lid may scratch the cornea, and these can only be removed if the upper lid is everted. To do this the doctor stands behind the patient who is asked to look downwards. The doctor grasps the eyelashes of the upper lid between finger and thumb using one hand while applying the tip of a cotton-wool covered probe to the upper lid, just above the tarsal plate, with the other. He then pulls the lid away from the eyeball at the same time as applying slight downward pressure with the probe;

the lid everts to cover the tip of the probe. The exposed foreign body is most easily removed with the tip of a triangle of thin card.

Corneal foreign bodies are very uncomfortable. In a co-operative child the GP can attempt to brush it away with a cotton-wool bud or corner of a piece of paper. If that does not work it is essential to refer the child. One-third of all blind eyes in UK children result from trauma. Arrows, darts, sticks and stones, tools, and chemicals are the main culprits. If there has been any chemical injury, the eye should be washed copiously with tap water for about 15 minutes and the patient referred. Any child who may possibly have a perforating eye injury (for example from broken glass following a road traffic accident) needs to be sent to hospital, even if the signs are not obvious. It is reasonable to put a pad over the eye after first instilling a couple of drops of an antibiotic.

Other acutely painful corneal inflammations, which may also reduce visual acuity, include corneal ulcers and herpes simplex keratitis. There may be a localized or diffuse corneal haze, with the latter visible even before fluorescein has been used. This dye will stain the ulcer and may outline the branching tree-like herpetic lesions. Redness will be less peripheral than in conjunctivitis; referral is indicted for definite diagnosis and if ocular herpes simplex is confirmed, treatment with idoxuridine or acyclovir is advised. Whilst simple corneal abrasions can be managed by the GP, other diseases of the cornea or uveal tract require prompt referral. Local steroids will aggravate herpetic and other viral eye infections and the GP should not treat the acute red eye with eye drops containing antibiotics with steroids.

ACUTE RED EYE

Conjunctivitis is the commonest cause of a 'red eye'. Inflammation is usually most marked peripherally, on the inner aspects of the lids, in the fornices and towards the angles. It is usually bilateral, although one side is often affected first, or more severely than the other. The older child with conjunctivitis will complain of sore, gritty eyes, and initially may think he has a speck of something 'in the eye'. Vision may be distorted because of discharge, but blinking will usually clear the visual field. The pupil looks normal and reacts normally to light. The eyelids are stuck together on waking.

Mucopurulent conjunctivitis is usually caused by *Staphylococcus aureus*, pneumococci, *Haemophilus influenzae* or streptococci; adenovirus conjunctivitis is also common. Conjunctivitis may be part of a systemic viral infection, as in measles, in which case there is usually a non-purulent watery discharge. Measures to prevent spread of the infection are important, and the child should avoid sharing towels or flannels. Gentle washing of the eyes with cotton-wool dipped in warm water may give relief, while a bacterial infection usually responds to chloramphenicol eye drops instilled every two hours during the day for a couple of days at least, and then less frequently. Chloramphenicol eye ointment applied at night is helpful in preventing the lids sticking together.

Other causes of conjunctivitis include chemical irritation from eye drops of various sorts, including those prescribed by the doctor, from household sprays or from chlorine in swimming pools. Though allergic conjunctivitis presenting with itchy, watery eyes is most frequent during the hay fever season, it can occur at any time of the year caused by allergens other than pollen. The oedema of the conjunctiva can be quite frightening and is aggravated by the child rubbing his eyes. It usually subsides within 24 hours without treatment. Systemic antihistamines may be helpful. Sodium cromoglycate (Opticrom) eye drops can be used as a prophylactic measure in the chronic form, or for recurrent acute attacks.

If suspected bacterial conjunctivitis is not clearly improving after 48 hours of treatment with a broad spectrum antibiotic, the diagnosis should be reassessed lest the problem is in fact a missed foreign body, a keratitis, or uveitis. Referral is usually indicated. If it is decided that conjunctivitis is the correct diagnosis, a swab should be taken and the treatment changed, possibly to systemic antibiotics.

Corneal abrasions cause intense photophobia, blepharospasm, and a sensation of something being in the eye. A drop of fluorescein (Minims Fluorescein Sodium) will reveal the breach in the corneal epithelium as a bright green stained area. Treatment consists of the instillation of chloramphenicol eye drops and the application of a firm pad for about 24–48 hours. Many abrasions will have healed in this time, but the child needs to be referred if this has not happened. Although abrasions heal quickly, they may unfortunately recur.

The uveal tract consists of the iris, ciliary body, and choroid. In contrast to conjunctivitis, in the much rarer acute uveitis redness is greatest around the iris. There is lacrimation but no purulent discharge. There will also be pain, photophobia, usually impaired vision, and the pupil may be small and irregular. There may be no obvious cause, or the uveitis may be associated with juvenile chronic arthritis, sarcoidosis, and tuberculosis, or may be secondary to injury. In antinuclear antibody positive children with pauci-articular juvenile chronic arthritis, the uveitis may develop silently and therefore these children must have six-monthly slit lamp examination (p. 289). Children with an acute keratitis (inflammation of the cornea) and/or uveitis present in a similar fashion. While simple corneal abrasions can be managed by the GP, other diseases of the cornea or uveal tract require prompt referral.

ORBITAL CELLULITIS

This is usually secondary to an unnoticed ethmoid sinusitis, perhaps from a cold. A somewhat, or very toxic child presents with a painful red eye, with strikingly swollen, inflamed eyelids. It thus can be confused with severe conjunctivitis. It may be difficult to open the eyelids far enough apart to see the globe, but in contrast with conjunctivitis of this degree of severity, there is little or no discharge. The globe is often pushed forward by inflammation at the back of the orbit, ocular movements are restricted, and vision may be reduced. Treatment with systemic antibiotics is urgent, as there is a risk of spread of the infection to the cavernous sinuses or meninges. Staphylococci, streptococci, pneumococci, or, in younger children, *Haemophilus influenzae,* are the commonest causative bacteria. Admission will usually be needed.

BLEPHARITIS AND STYES

Some children with sticky eyes have no obvious reddening of the conjunctiva but rather a sticky discharge limited to the eye lashes, and sometimes responding to antibiotic (not needed in mild cases). The condition is often recurrent, as in seborrhoeic blepharitis, in which the scalp is also often involved, causing dandruff. Sore areas may be seen behind the ears.

Seborrhoeic blepharitis is a difficult condition to eradicate. Vaseline, to remove crusts on the margins of the eyelids, combined with anti-dandruff treatment may help. Repeated soaking of the margins of the eyelids with a weak solution of sodium bicarbonate or a mild baby shampoo may also remove the crust. A week or two of chloramphenicol eye ointment may help if there is evidence of infection, perhaps if the blepharitis is associated with conjunctivitis. Antibiotic ointment has some drawbacks, especially if used long-term, in that the child may develop a local allergy to neomycin or even to chloramphenicol. A few days of carefully applied 1% hydrocortisone ointment to the lid margins may be helpful in resistant cases, remembering that steroids may get into the eye and can cause a rise in intraocular pressure.

The common stye is an abscess occurring in the hair follicles on the eyelid. Frequently styes occur in crops, one following another. The offending organism is usually *Staphylococcus aureus.* Warm compresses may be soothing. Occasionally the infection can be aborted by pulling out the affected eye lash. Chloramphenicol ointment may help to prevent the spread of infection from producing other styes or, more rarely but more seriously, cellulitis of the eyelid. Neomycin and chlorhexidine cream (Naseptin) up the nostrils may help to reduce staphylococcal colonization of the anterior nares, and thus recurrent styes.

A stye presents as a tender localized swelling at the lid margin. Away from the lid margin a tender red swelling is an infected meibomian cyst. This should be treated as if it were a stye until the infection subsides. If it does not resolve spontaneously (most do) the child will need to be referred for its removal, usually under general anaesthesia in younger children. Uninflamed but generally puffy eyelids may be a presenting sign of oedematous states, notably the nephrotic syndrome, in which there will be a large amount of protein in the urine. Most puffy eyes, however, are a purely local phenomenon, especially when associated with local erythema or scaling.

STICKY EYES IN THE NEWBORN

Most mild sticky eyes do not matter. The mother need merely remove the discharge with cotton-wool moistened with water. There are, however, more severe cases. Some are from staphylococci. In others the eye has become infected during delivery, conjunctivitis developing a few days later. The most serious intrapartum eye infection is gonococcal ophthalmia which, if untreated, may lead to corneal damage and blindness. The gonococcus may be easily missed on routine culture. If it is seriously suspected, as in a baby under one-week-old with severe conjunctivitis, the child should be referred, for a culture and gram stains to be made under optimal conditions. If bacteria are grown, local treatment with eye drops of the appropriate antibiotic is adequate, unless inflammation is severe, or the baby has gonococcal ophthalmia.

A significant proportion of sticky eyes in the neonate are due to chlamydia acquired from the mother's genital tract. This small intracellular organism is also responsible for many cases of non-specific urethritis. When suspected, swabs should be put in special transport medium and quickly sent to the laboratory. Chlamydia does not grow on routine bacteriological media. Chlamydial conjunctivitis needs treatment with systemic erythromycin (50 mg/kg daily) and 1% tetracycline eye ointment. These should be continued for three weeks. Parents of a neonate with a gonococcal or chlamydia infection will also need to be referred to a genito-urinary clinic.

BLOCKED TEAR DUCT

The advice of the GP is frequently sought because a young infant has a constant or frequently recurring 'running eye'. Symptoms start soon after birth, when it is noticed that one eye is more sticky than the other and tends to water, the discharge being more obvious in the morning. In such cases the tear duct is usually blocked. If the mother is advised to express the contents of the lacrimal sac three or four times a day by firm finger pressure through the lower lid at the inner corner of the eye, any resulting discharge can be cleaned away with moist cotton-wool. This conservative treatment is all that is needed in most cases. Probing of the naso-lacrimal duct is not usually necessary in infants unless symptoms persist beyond the first birthday.

Bibliography

Jackson, C. R. S. and Finlay, R. D. (19). *The eye in general practice,* (10th edn). Churchill Livingstone, London. (A clear concise text.)

Peckham, C. S., Gardiner, P. A., and Tibbenham, A. D. (1978). Vision screening of adolescents and their use of glasses. *British Medical Journal*, **1**, 1111–13.

16 Urinary problems and diabetes mellitus

URINARY TRACT INFECTION

Approximately five per cent of girls and two per cent of boys will suffer from at least one symptomatic urinary tract infection (UTI). Thus, girls are more likely to develop UTI than boys, except in the neonatal period, when the reverse is true. The hall marks of childhood UTI are their, difficulty in diagnosis in infancy, recurrent nature, and association with renal tract malformation and with risk of renal damage.

Antibiotics for an imaginary UTI, and failure to diagnose a genuine one are common errors. The former results from treating all dysuria as urinary infections, or from taking the growth found in poorly collected or poorly stored specimens to be a positive culture; the latter because symptoms of UTI in childhood are commonly non-specific.

Dysuria and frequency are more commonly indicators of perineal soreness (perhaps associated with the use of bubble baths) or balanitis, than of a UTI. Similarly a complaint of a 'smelly' or 'strong' urine usually means that the nappy smells of ammonia from urea-splitting bacteria rather than infection.

Although an older child with a UTI may present with the classic symptoms of frequency, dysuria, fever, and suprapubic and loin pain, often only one or two of these are present, or the abdominal pain may be rather vague. A child with a urinary infection may also present with enuresis after a period of continence. A child with only low fever or listlessness may have a UTI which is scarring the kidney. The same may be true of an infant presenting with failure to thrive, diarrhoea, vomiting, a feeding problem, or prolonged neonatal jaundice. A urine culture is vital in an infant who has a rectal temperature of more than 38.5 °C for no obvious reason, and who does not recover within 24–48 hours (Guidelines for the management of acute urinary tract infection in childhood, 1991).

The only reliable way to diagnose a UTI is by culturing one or more satisfactorily collected urine specimens. Cloudiness of the urine and proteinuria should not be relied on as evidence of infection.

A positive albustix may be found with fever alone, after severe exercise, or with orthostatic proteinuria, in which protein is absent in the first urine passed after rising in the morning. It may also be a result of vaginal secretions. Conversely, non-infectious renal disorders, ranging from nephrotic syndrome to glomerulonephritis, can also give rise to proteinuria. Cloudiness may be due to the presence of phosphate and urate crystals as well as to pus cells. Pyuria, defined as greater than 10 pus cells per cubic millimetre of freshly collected, unspun urine, may indicate infection, especially in boys. It is, however, also found with balanitis, vulvitis, irritation from topical agents, trauma to the kidney, renal stones, and, occasionally, with inflammation in a neighbouring structure to the urinary tract, for example, acute appendicitis.

There is now a dipstick (Multistix GP, Bayer) which contains tests for two markers of urinary infections, leucocyte esterase and nitrites. The former will be present in urine if there is pyuria, the latter if nitrate is degraded to nitrite by pathogenic bacteria. These tests are not substitutes for a urinary culture when a UTI is seriously suspected, but, if both are negative, may be useful as a means of excluding UTI in a child with non-specific abdominal pain (Woodward and Griffiths 1993).

The chance of a false-positive culture can be minimized by attention to detail. The toilet-trained child can micturate directly into a sterile container, after washing the perineum or penis with water (not antiseptic) and drying it. In babies, a midstream specimen of urine (MSU) can also be collected by an alert and patient parent or carer. Failing this an adhesive bag needs to be stuck to the child's washed and dried perineum and the child given a drink and if possible kept in an upright position until the urine is passed. Urine left in the bag at room temperature soon develops an overgrowth of contaminants. For this reason the bag must be removed as soon as the specimen is passed and the urine put in a sterile pot. The urine specimen should be transported to the laboratory within two hours of collection or it can be refrigerated at 4 °C for up to 48 hours without substantial change in its bacterial count. The practice refrigerator needs checking regularly to make sure that a temperature of 4 °C is maintained. Alternatively the specimen can be transported in bottles containing 1.8% sodium borate (Jewkes *et al.* 1990) which preserves pus cells and bacteria. Problems of collection and storage may be reduced by using dip slides. The slide is momentarily held in the stream of urine as it is voided, or flowing out of a cut corner of the bag. The slide can then be kept in the practice at room temperature for 24 hours before reading (results are easier to read if the slide has been incubated overnight at 37 °C). Positive slides can be sent to the laboratory for further culture and sensitivities.

A negative culture before antibiotics excludes a UTI whereas a MSU in which more than 10^5 organisms/mm^3 are grown in pure culture is fairly reliable evidence of its presence. A lower count of a mixed growth is unlikely to be significant but a 10^4 pure growth means that another MSU should be collected. False-positive cultures are common from bag urine collections.

If a UTI is seriously suspected the GP should ideally obtain two urine specimens before antibiotics are started. The diagnosis is considered confirmed, and the child therefore in need of renal tract imaging only if they both show a significant growth of the same microorganism with the same sensitivities. This may be a counsel of perfection. Occasionally, in real life (perhaps during a weekend) if the alternative is a probably inappropriate admission, one may choose to give antibiotics to the febrile infant, without collecting a prior urine specimen. The child should be reassessed a couple of days later. If the child gets the same symptoms a second time, a urine specimen is mandatory. If it is impossible to collect a satisfactory specimen at home the infant should be referred to the local paediatric department for a supra-pubic aspiration of urine. However, if the GP is concerned enough to consider this course of action, the child probably needs to be admitted.

In the child with a urinary infection, questioning may reveal previous episodes of undiagnosed fever or malaise which may be retrospectively interpreted as previous infections. There may also be a family history of renal disease. Physical examination should include measurement of height, weight, and blood pressure and examination of genitalia. A minor degree of hypospadias or other malformation may be present. The abdomen is palpated for enlarged kidneys or a palpable bladder and the spine inspected for spinal lesions.

Most UTIs are caused by bowel flora which colonize the bladder, except in the neonate, when the infection is usually blood borne. Although the majority (80 per cent) of UTIs are caused by *Escherichia coli*, *Klebsiella aerogenes, Proteus mirabilis,* and *Enterococcus faecalis* may also be responsible. Provided there is no obstruction to the urinary tract, the infection will be rapidly eliminated by any antibacterial drug to which the pathogen is sensitive; usually trimethoprim is the first choice as many urinary pathogens are resistant to amoxycillin. If an infant appears to be acutely unwell (Chapter 2) hospital admission is indicated for treatment with intravenous antibiotics. Neonates are particularly vulnerable because of their increased risk of an accompanying septicaemia. Most children and infants with a UTI can be managed at home, provided they tolerate their antibiotics and are able to drink enough fluid. The urine culture should be repeated 48 hours after starting treatment and after completing a seven to ten day course of antibiotics. If there is no clinical improvement within 48 hours the antibiotic sensitivity should be reviewed and an urgent ultrasound scan of the kidneys and urinary tract requested to exclude obstruction. An ultrasound is also indicated for any child whose urine continues to show significant infection or pyuria two to four days after starting appropriate antibiotics. A high fluid intake may ease dysuria and reduce bacterial colonization by stimulating frequent emptying of the bladder. In children under five years, prophylaxis with a low-dose of an antibiotic such as trimethoprim (2 mg/kg per day) given at bed-time, is indicated, once the initial course is completed, until investigations have shown there is no abnormality of the renal tract that is likely to predispose to infection.

Imaging investigations after a proven UTI reveal obstructive malformations in up to 2 per cent of girls and 10 per cent of boys, and vesicoureteric reflux in 30–40 per cent of both sexes. About 10–15 per cent will develop scarring of the kidney, especially after repeated infections associated with vesicoureteric reflux (VUR) (Jodal 1994). Normally the vesicoureteric junction does not allow reflux of urine from the bladder into the ureter. When reflux is present the abnormal back flow of infected urine from the bladder into the renal pelvis may result in scarring and poor growth of the kidney. Extensive, bilateral scarring is an important cause of hypertension and chronic renal failure in children and young adults (Smellie 1991). Most scars have started to develop by the time the child is five years old; infants are particularly vulnerable. Kidney damage is more likely if there has been a history of more than one urinary infection. Imaging of some type following a UTI is essential if this important minority is to be identified soon enough to prevent further renal damage.

Thus, all children with proven UTIs require investigations at a centre experienced in paediatric imaging. A plain abdominal X-ray will rule out renal stones and spinal defects, and an ultrasound will detect abnormalities, such as a hydronephrotic, or polycystic kidney, or a ureterocele, or the thickened bladder wall seen in a boy with posterior urethral valves causing outflow obstruction. Ultrasound is not good at detecting renal scars. These are best seen on intravenous urography (IVU) or through radionuclide imaging after intravenous injection of ^{88}Tc dimercaptosuccinic acid (DMSA). This has the advantage of a considerably lower radiation dose than an IVU.

Most paediatricians will recommend that, following a definite UTI, children under the age of one year should have a micturating cystourethrogram to exclude VUR, though this is an unpleasant test that involves catheterizing the urethra. An ultrasound and a DMSA scan three months later to look for renal scars are also necessary. In an older child, following a first infection, an ultrasound and either an IVU or a DMSA scan should be sufficient. Continual low-dose antibiotic prophylaxis with sugar-free preparations (trimethoprim, 2 mg/kg or nitrofurantoin 1 mg/kg) should be given as a single evening dose to those children who have an abnormality of the renal tract, and to those who have reflux. Both these groups should have their urine cultured every three months or so. In all but severe cases, VUR can be treated conservatively as, in about 80 per cent of cases, it ceases spontaneously after some years. When it is confirmed that this has occurred, the antibiotics can be stopped. Surgical correction of VUR is indicated if it is gross, and thus less likely to resolve spontaneously, or when there are repeated break-through infections, perhaps associated with poor compliance. Practices should keep a register of children on antibiotic prophylaxis. Their notes can be checked twice a year and the child recalled for a urine culture and measurement of the blood pressure, unless there is evidence of assiduous attendance at paediatric out-patients. A urine culture should also be routine if these patients present with an unexplained fever.

Urinary infection is a long-term problem; recurrences are common. The risk of further infections in those with an underlying renal abnormality may be reduced by encouraging a high fluid intake and regular voiding. In that way any bacteria that find their way up the urethra can be expelled before multiplication can get under way. This is particularly important in children who have VUR, in whom micturition twice in quick succession, 'double micturition', helps to empty the bladder of the urine that has refluxed during the first micturition. Other measures include avoiding bubble baths and scented soaps, prevention and treatment of constipation if present, wiping the bottom clean from front to back and easy access to toilets at school.

VAGINAL DISCHARGE AND VULVITIS

A sore red vulva with dysuria is common and, even though the urine should be tested for glucose and sent for culture (it may have pus cells in it from the vulva), a urinary tract infection or diabetes are unlikely. Most can be managed by discouragement of excessive cleanliness, especially with perfumed soaps and bubble baths, together with a bland preparation such as aqueous cream. However, a sore vulva may be one presentation of sexual abuse and the perineum should be inspected for bruising and laceration. If sexual abuse is suspected, the child should be referred, ideally to a paediatrician with special interest in child protection.

Slight vaginal discharges are common and, if pale and non-offensive, usually require no intervention, especially in the older pre-pubertal girl. They are also normal in neonates. In the older child, if profuse, a swab should be taken and, if they are offensive or blood-stained, referral to a paediatrician, or to a gynaecologist known to have a particular interest in children, is indicated, for bacteriological studies for sexually transmitted diseases (for example, gonorrhoea) and for exclusion of foreign bodies in the vagina (for example, a teddy bear's eye or a piece of toilet paper).

NEPHRITIS, HAEMATURIA, AND NEPHROTIC SYNDROME

Acute glomerulonephritis after a streptococcal infection, with facial oedema, hypertension, oliguria, and smoky urine, is now rare. Slightly more common is the nephrotic syndrome which presents with more marked oedema and a heavy proteinuria. It has a relapsing course, each relapse responding to steroids, which should be prescribed under hospital supervision. Various rare nephritides may present with haematuria, proteinuria, hypertension, and renal failure.

Red urine, if shown to be from blood and not beetroot or red crayons, always requires investigation in a child. It can be the first sign of urinary tract infection, calculi, renal tract malformation, tumour, nephritis, or a bleeding tendency.

ENURESIS

Bed-wetting usually ceases with the passage of time. The classical study of Rutter *et al.* (1973) showed that five per cent of seven-year-olds wet their bed at least once a week; half of those will be dry by the age of 10, and less than one in six of these will be still wetting at age 14. It is by no means always a symptom of psychological disturbance, although stress, such as the loss of a mother, family break-up, admission to hospital, or the birth of a new sibling, may precipitate its onset. It is common to find that more than one member of the family has had the problem.

A urine culture is essential, though a UTI is an uncommon cause of primary enuresis. However, it may be secondary to the persistently sore perineum; curing the infection often does not help the enuresis. Other organic causes, such as diabetes mellitus, renal failure, or a bladder abnormality, are very rare; their hallmark is excessive thirst or a poor urinary stream. Where there is day- as well as night-wetting, psychiatric disturbance or a UTI is more likely to be found, although minor degrees of wet pants are common in the first year or two of primary school and should not be cause for serious concern. In general it seems that in children who are enuretic between the age of five and seven, delay in development plays a major role, while in children who are still wetting at 11 years, behavioural difficulties and lower educational attainments are more likely to be present.

In assessing the situation, symptoms of urinary infection or of diabetes mellitus and evidence of recent family stress may be sought. Is the enuresis a relatively recent problem or has the child never had a prolonged dry period? Secondary enuresis is more likely to be associated with a precipitating event, such as the birth of a sibling. Slow development may occasionally present as enuresis. A discussion about the family's housing and sleeping arrangements may help. It is important to ask whether, apart from the wetting, there are any other symptoms worrying the parents which might indicate emotional disturbance. The family may have already tried to cope with the situation in various ways; how well these have worked will be important in deciding what action to take. It may be reassuring for the child to discover that one of his parents was not dry at night until late in childhood.

Abnormal physical findings are almost never noted, but the conscientious GP will examine the abdomen for a palpable bladder or renal masses and look for abnormal genitalia. Also important is examining the back for signs of a spinal lesion; checking perineal sensation and tendon reflexes in the lower limbs. The blood pressure should be recorded, the urine cultured and tested for sugar and protein. If the teenage girl is still wetting by day, the vulva should be looked at to see if there is a continual trickle of urine which may come from an ectopic ureter. Renal imaging is practically never fruitful, but occasionally it is worthwhile if there are any hints to suggest renal tract abnormality, such as loin pain, any trivial malformations of the genitalia, or un-improving enuresis in a teenager. Although enuretic children appear to pass urine more frequently, their bladders are not smaller than those of other children.

Most patients can be managed in the practice provided wetting is not a symptom of organic disease or of serious emotional disturbance. We do not advocate giving drugs or introducing an enuretic alarm until the child is six or seven, unless he is very keen and unusually mature. Simple measures are helpful while waiting for the spontaneous improvement which occurs in most children. These include protecting the mattress with a plastic sheet. More optimistically, a pot should be put underneath the bed or the route to the lavatory well lit. A chart with each 'dry night' marked with a star, along with positive reinforcement from parents for dry nights are useful incentives. It is worthwhile for a trial period to try restraining night time fluids, and 'lifting' the child when the parents go to bed. Many children feel guilty about their bed-wetting and the family should be involved in an attempt to reduce criticism; a small daily reward after a dry night is more helpful than a rebuke after a wet one. The mother is bound to feel fed up because of the extra washing the problem creates and may want to discuss her feelings privately with the doctor.

The only treatment of long-term value is the enuresis alarm, but attention to detail is crucial. It is a waste of time for uninterested doctors to treat unwilling children whose parents have not got the stamina to help them. Success is likely when both parent and child wish to work for a cure and are treated by a practice nurse, partner, or clinical medical officer who is prepared to take a special interest in the problem. The device consists of an auditory alarm linked to two electrodes in the form of perforated metal or foil pads placed underneath the lower sheet of the child's bed. The electrodes themselves are separated by a further cotton sheet and when the child wets the bed the urine completes an electrical circuit and the buzzer goes off. It is better for the child not to wear pyjama trousers so that the sheet wets quickly.

Ideally, the child is woken by the alarm when he wets. Waking up does not prevent wetting on that occasion. However, over ensuing nights the child gradually associates wetting with waking up, and this leads to dry nights in order to avoid being woken. When the alarm goes off because the child is wet, he should get out of bed, turn it off, and, with the parents' help, put clean sheets on the bed before switching it on again. The treatment is rigorous and may lead to being woken two or three times a night initially. When applied with persistence it works in 50 per cent within six weeks and 85 per cent within four months. Failures occur when the above criteria are not met, or if the alarm fails to wake the sleeping child because he switches it off in his sleep (put the switch further away from the bed), or if it not loud enough (a parent should sleep in the room to do the waking). The first sign that an alarm is working is when the patch of urine in the bed begins to diminish in size. Gradually the wetting ceases altogether, usually over two to three weeks, although it is wise to keep the alarm available for a further couple of months because relapses are common. They appear to respond well to the re-use of the alarm if this is done promptly. Newer body-worn 'mini-alarms' are more compact, easier to use and tend to arouse the child as the first few drops of urine make contact with the detector worn in the pants.

Housing circumstances (including sleeping arrangements of siblings) permitting, an alarm is a treatment of choice in the co-operative child whose enuresis is not part of a more serious emotional or family problem. Tricyclic antidepressants, such as imipramine, can suppress wetting completely in 30 per cent and reduce it in 85 per cent of children. Improvement occurs within a week or two of starting the drug. We do not, however, recommend treatment of a benign and a self-limiting condition like enuresis with a potentially lethal drug like imipramine.

Nasal desmopressin, 20–40 µg, or desmopressin acetate tablets, 0.2–0.4 mg nightly, reduces urine volume and is effective in up to two-thirds of patients during treatment, though less than a third remain dry, even after three months of continuous treatment (Stenberg and Lackgern 1993). It can be used as a temporary expedient; for example, during 'sleep over parties' and school trips.

The Enuresis Resource and Information Centre (65 St Michael's Hill, Bristol, BS8 8DZ, tel.: 01272 264 920) provides helpful advice and information for children, parents, and professionals.

DIABETES MELLITUS

Insulin dependent (type 1) diabetes mellitus is the most common endocrine problem of childhood. A practice of 10 000 may have two or three affected children. Type 1 diabetes is associated with a variety of genetic markers in the HLA system, in the DR and DQ loci. It is possible that an environmental factor, such as a virus, can cause irreversible autoimmune damage to pancreatic islet cells in susceptible children.

Onset is usually fairly acute with symptoms of thirst, polyuria (including secondary enuresis), lethargy, and weight loss developing over days or a few weeks. If untreated the child will go on to develop keto-acidosis (sweet-smelling ketotic breath, nausea, vomiting, abdominal pain, dehydration, deep and heavy breathing), then coma, and, eventually, death. It is not uncommon for vomiting and abdominal pain to be mistaken for gastro-enteritis, appendicitis, or urinary tract infection, or breathlessness for asthma or pneumonia. GPs and practice nurses should have a low threshold for testing urine for glucose in a thirsty child presenting with these symptoms. The diagnosis is easily confirmed by a random blood glucose of >10 mmol/L. A glucose tolerance test is rarely necessary in childhood.

Once the diagnosis has been made, the child must be referred to the local paediatric diabetic team so that the treatment can be started promptly. For example, the fully active child with some weight loss can wait a day or two. Any child who is poorly must be seen on the day of diagnosis. In most centres, a child with mild symptoms will be treated as an out-patient and monitored by home visits from a diabetic specialist nurse. The family will need to learn about the disease and its dietary management, how to give insulin injections, monitor blood glucose, test urine for ketones, and recognize and manage the hypoglycaemic symptoms. The aim is to give parents and older children control over day-to-day management of diabetes. There are many useful commercially sponsored handbooks for the patient and family, such as *Diabetes, a book for children and their families*, which is available from Boehringer Mannheim House, Bell Lane, Lewes, East Sussex BN7 1LG. The diagnosis of diabetes may profoundly affect the family, who may experience a mixture of shock, sadness, anger, fear, and guilt. Parents should be encouraged to talk about their feelings and may require counselling. Sometimes meeting with another family with a diabetic child is helpful, but the family need to be aware that approaches to detailed management of the disease may differ between experts.

INSULIN AND MONITORING

Availability of a range of pre-mixed insulin mixtures and easy to use pen injection devices with ultrafine needles have greatly simplified the administration, and reduced the discomfort associated with subcutaneous insulin injection—the preferred route; intramuscular injection leads to too rapid absorption. Rotation of injection sites is important to prevent fat hypertrophy which may lead to erratic blood levels and is unsightly. Most children will manage with two injections per day, each consisting of a mixture of short-acting neutral insulin (30 per cent) and intermediate-acting insulin (70 per cent). Two-thirds of the dose is given 30 minutes before breakfast and one-third 30 minutes before the evening meal. Alternatively, an intermediate-acting or long-acting insulin in the evening can be given to provide continuous basal activity, supplemented by short-acting, neutral insulin injections prior to meals. This mimics physiological insulin secretion and may produce even better glycaemic control. Adolescents often prefer this regime because it allows a more flexible lifestyle. The actual dose of insulin is adjusted according to blood glucose measurements. In most children the total daily dose required ranges from 0.5 to 1.5 units/kg a day, but after the diagnosis there is usually a 'honeymoon' period, lasting a month or longer, during which less insulin is required. The child and parents need to learn to make adjustments to the dose based on home blood glucose testing. Most children measure their blood glucose two or three times a day, and more frequently when unwell, using a glucose oxidase reagent strip (for example, Glucostix) and a reflectance meter (for example, Ames glucometer). Blood glucose measurements at different times on different days help to build up a profile of blood glucose concentrations over the week. The aim is to maintain the value between 4 and 10 mmol/L pre- and post-prandially. Measurement of glycosylated haemoglobin (HbA_{1c}) is useful periodically as it indicates how well the diabetes has been controlled over the preceding three months.

Diet and exercise

Rigid diets are out. The child's should be based on the family's previous eating habits, with emphasis on foods with plenty of fibre (wholemeal bread, jacket potatoes, etc.), low in refined sugars and low in fats. The diet should be sufficient for normal growth. Judicious use of treats such as ice-cream and 'fast food' once or twice a week helps to prevent the child feeling too different from his peers. So does exercise which fosters a sense of well-being, as well as lowering insulin requirement and helping to maintain fitness and avoid obesity.

Acute complications

Hypoglycaemic episodes which result from too much insulin, vigorous exercise, or too little food, are common in patients on the more intensive insulin regimens (Diabetes Control and Complication Trial Research Group 1993). Symptoms include hunger, irritability, bad temper, sweating, shakiness, blurring of vision, headache, confusion, or convulsions. It may be difficult for parent, patient, or doctor to decide whether irritable behaviour is metabolic or psychological until a blood glucose measurement clarifies the situation. If not treated immediately with glucose tablets (which the child should carry at all times) or a sugary drink, the hypoglycaemia may result in convulsions and loss of consciousness. If confused or unconscious the patient should be given glucose gel (Hypostop) which is absorbed through the buccal mucosa, or intramuscular glucagon (0.5 mg for children under five years and 1 mg for older children). Parents should keep glucagon at home and should be taught how to administer it.

Illnesses. Infections lead to an increase in insulin requirement, blood glucose levels rise and ketosis may develop, even if the child is not eating. If untreated, diabetic keto-acidosis may develop. It is essential during any illness that the blood glucose is checked more frequently, urine tested for ketones (with reagent strips), and additional insulin given (usually an increase by 10–20 per cent in the total daily dose) as short-acting neutral insulin (for example, Actrapid) every four hours until ketonuria disappears.

Long-term complications

Microangiopathy is a serious complication resulting in nephropathy which may lead to renal failure, retinopathy which may lead to blindness, and neuropathy 10–15 years from the time of diagnosis. Large blood vessel disease contributes to coronary heart disease, stroke and peripheral vascular disease. Results of the recent Diabetes Control and Complication Research Group Trial (1993) suggest that development and progression of microvascular complications are less common in patients with near normal metabolic control achieved by an intensified insulin regimen. Children who have been diabetic for more than five years should have an annual retinal examination and measurement of urine microalbumin excretion, the earliest laboratory evidence of nephropathy. If present, treatment with ACE inhibitors may slow the progression of renal deterioration and efforts at improving diabetic control need to be increased. However, it is better if excellent control is instituted from diagnosis.

Bibliography

Urinary tract infections

Guidelines for the management of acute urinary tract infection in childhood. (1991). Report of the Working Party of the Research Unit of the Royal College of Physicians. *Journal of the Royal College of Physicians of London*, **25**, 36–42.

Jewkes, F. E. M., McMaster, D. J., Napier, W. A., Houston, I. B., and Postlethwaite, R. J. (1990). Home collection of urine samples—boric acid bottles or dipslides? *Archives of Disease in Childhood*, **65**, 286–9.

Jodal, U. (1994). Urinary tract infections: significance, pathogenesis, clinical features and diagnosis. In *Clinical Paediatric Nephrology*, (ed. R. J. Postlethwaite, 2nd edn), 151–9.

Smellie, J. M. (1991). AUA Lecture: reflections on 30 years of treating children with urinary tract infections, *Journal of Urology*, **146**, 665–8.

Woodward, M. N. and Griffiths, D. M. (1993). Use of dipsticks for routine analysis of urine from children with acute abdominal pain. *British Medical Journal*, **306**, 1512–3.

Enuresis

Rutter, M., Yule, W., and Graham, P. (1973). Enuresis and behavioral deviance: some epidemiological considerations. In *Bladder control and enuresis*, (ed. I. Kolvin, R. MacKeith, and R. Meadow). Clinics in Developmental Medicine, Nos. 48/49. Heinemann, London.

Stenberg, A. and Lacgern, G. (1993). Treatment with oral desmopressin in adolescents with primary nocturnal enuresis; efficacy and long-term effects. *Clinical Pediatrics*, Special Edition, 25–7.

Diabetes

Diabetes Control and Complication Trial Research Group. (1993). The effect of intensive treatment of diabetes on the development and progression of long-term complications in insulin-dependent diabetes mellitus. *New England Journal of Medicine*, **329**, 977–85.

Johnston, D. I. (1989). Management of diabetes mellitus. *Archives of Disease in Childhood*, **64**, 622–6.

17 Anaemia and bruising

PHYSIOLOGICAL CHANGES

A constant supply of oxygen is needed by the tissues and it is the function of haemoglobin to combine reversibly with oxygen, allowing the red blood cells to pick up the gas from the lungs and release it in the capillary bed. Interestingly, a litre of blood after leaving the lungs contains the same volume of oxygen as a litre of air—200 mL. Because of the different haemoglobin values at different ages (Table 17.1), it is important for the GP to know the normal range, making it less likely that he will treat a child for a non-existent anaemia. Haemoglobin concentration at birth is high by adult standards (16–18 g/dL). It initially falls rapidly and then more gradually to a low at two months of age, when the normal range is about 10.5–14.5 g/dL. After that there is a gradual rise throughout childhood but the haemoglobin concentration remains below adult values until adolescence.

Children's white blood cell counts are rather higher than adults'. Normal counts may be as high as 21×10^9/litre during the first few days of life, with a mean of 12×10^9/litre up to the age of six months and $8–10 \times 10^9$/litre throughout childhood. There are usually more lymphocytes than polymorphs present until the second year of life, then roughly equal numbers until the age of seven.

All normal haemoglobin molecules produced after the first eight weeks of gestation are composed of four protein subunits, two α-chains and two non-α-chains.

Table 17.1 Haemoglobin concentrations (in g/dL) according to age

Age (years)	Median value	Lower limit[1]
0.5–5	12.5	11.0
5–9	13.0	11.5
9–12	13.5	12.0
14–18	F: 14	12.0
	M: 15	13.0

[1] 97 per cent of children have values above this.
Adapted from Dallman and Siimes (1979).

Each subunit carries one haem group and can carry one molecule of oxygen. The clinically important haemoglobins are HbA($\alpha_2\beta_2$), HbA$_2$($\alpha_2\delta_2$), and fetal haemoglobin, HbF($\alpha_2\gamma_2$). HbF resists denaturation by strong alkali, a property which underlies the Kleihauer test for fetal haemoglobin. Gene mapping and antenatal diagnostic techniques have proceeded apace in recent years. The β, γ, and δ genes are closely linked on chromosome 11, whilst there are two sets of genes for α-polypeptide chains on chromosome 16.

In late fetal life most haemoglobin is of the F variety but the proportion of HbA gradually increases. By term, HbA provides 30 per cent of the total, HbF 70 per cent, and HbA$_2$ less than 1 per cent. By six months of age most haemoglobin is HbA, 3 per cent or less is HbA$_2$, and only up to 1 per cent is HbF. These proportions are altered in the haemoglobinopathies.

THE PALE CHILD

Parents often suspect that their pale offspring is anaemic but this is usually not the case. His features may be constitutionally sallow, or he may be unwell for some other reason, or he may be temporarily pale because he is tense, frightened, or just cold. It is not unusual to have a rosy-faced child brought for a 'blood test' because he is easily tired, not eating as the parents wish he should, or just 'playing them up'. Conversely, genuine anaemia may not be very obvious and an anaemic child can have fairly rosy cheeks. The presence of a low haemoglobin can to some extent be confirmed by comparing the appearance of the palms, or the colour of the nail beds, or the finger tips, to that of the doctor, as well as by looking at the mucosae and the conjunctivae. But a blood test is the only foundation for a secure diagnosis.

If a genuine anaemia is present or suspected, enquiry should include the following areas—depending on the age of the child and whether he appears well or sick:

1. General symptoms of ill-health, such as breathlessness, tiredness, anorexia, fever, and poor growth.
2. Nutritional history. Is there a history of delayed weaning, or weaning on iron-poor foods? The volume of cows' milk drunk is an important question. Many parents do not recognize that it is nutritionally inadequate. It has a low iron content, its iron is poorly absorbed, and intolerance to it is common causing minor degrees of blood loss and an increased iron requirement. Furthermore, if most of the calories are coming from milk, there is little pressure from the baby for solids. The pale toddler who drinks two to three pints a day is probably iron-deficient.
3. Evidence of chronic disease, such as pyelonephritis, or of malabsorption (appearance of the faeces).
4. Evidence of blood loss, including unexplained bruising.

5. Any family history of anaemia?
6. Has the child had access to drugs, such as aspirin, or toxins, such as lead, that could cause anaemia?
7. Travel abroad with possible exposure to parasites.

During the examination of the child note his ethnic origin. Thalassaemia occurs particularly in people from the Mediterranean and the Middle and Far East, and sickle cell anaemia in African and African-Caribbean children. The child with a haemolytic anaemia may be obviously jaundiced. The patient (usually of non-Caucasian origin) who has glucose-6-phosphate dehydrogenase deficiency may have eaten one of the foods or medicines that cause haemolysis of their enzyme deficient red cells.

A tachycardia and cardiomegaly, with a systolic murmur, may occur in severely anaemic children, especially if the anaemia is of rapid onset. Investigation beyond a full blood count and differential white count depends on the history and examination. The doctor should look for petechiae and other signs of abnormal bruising, lymphadenopathy and an enlarged liver or spleen.

IRON-DEFICIENCY ANAEMIA

Iron-deficiency anaemia is the commonest haematological disorder in toddlers and young children in the UK. Several studies suggest that, contrary to earlier belief, even mild degrees of iron-deficiency may be associated with poorer developmental progress in toddlers and that iron supplementation can cause measurable improvement in performance (Aukett *et al.* 1986). Iron-deficiency anaemia has an incidence of between 4 per cent and 30 per cent in different populations (Stevens 1991). The incidence is particularly high amongst children of Asian immigrants living in inner city areas, who tend to rely heavily on cows' milk and be weaned onto non-meat-based foods. Their families may be vegetarians, or wish to feed their children a vegetarian diet because of a lack of ready-prepared Halal baby foods.

In order to maintain a positive iron balance children need to consume a diet containing about 10 mg of iron daily; about 10 per cent of this will be absorbed. Breast-milk is, like cows' milk, low in iron, but what it contains is better absorbed. Most formula milks and infant cereals are fortified but the amount of iron in the food is not a good guide to absorption. Relatively little iron is absorbed, for example, from food of vegetable origin (including spinach—2 per cent absorbed!), while that from animal sources is better utilized (about 15 per cent; Nathan and Oski 1981). Absorption from vegetables is increased by ascorbic acid (for example, fruit juice with meals) and may be reduced by tannin in tea and phytate in cereals, including the flour used for making chapatis. If body stores are low, more iron will be retained. This is also true when there is increased haemopoiesis, a benefit after haemorrhage, but a drawback in chronic haemolytic anaemias, such as thalassaemia, in which iron overload may reach toxic levels.

Iron-deficiency is uncommon in full-term infants under six months of age. Most iron in the newborn is contained in circulating haemoglobin, which is initially at high concentration, and declines after birth. In preterm infants iron-deficiency is more common. Unless extra iron is given from the first few weeks these children will consume their body stores prematurely. Such low-birth-weight babies, including twins, should receive iron supplements (2 mg elemental iron/kg per day) from soon after birth until mixed feeding is established.

Other causes of iron-deficiency are rare in this country. Malabsorption may present as anaemia. Recurrent nose bleeds, perhaps unnoticed because the blood has been swallowed, occasionally lead to iron-deficiency. Other occult gastro-intestinal blood losses are very uncommon but should be considered as a possibility in patients whose anaemia persists, despite adequate dosage of iron (if it is certain that the child has taken the medicine). Chronic, heavy, hookworm infestation may result in anaemia in children from the tropics.

Mild iron-deficiency is usually picked up as a result of a blood count when perhaps the child has been seen for an intercurrent infection. More severely affected children may easily become tired and flop around. Many children with severe chronic iron deficiency are reasonably fit, but sometimes the child will be fat or underweight and may show other evidence of inappropriate nutrition. However, this may not always be the whole story.

James was the 18-month-old fourth child of English parents. He presented with a complexion as white as a newly laundered sheet. His mother said that he had been fed on a diet of cows' milk with a small amount of mashed potatoes and butter, `because it slips down so easily'. He was fairly well but he had to be carried everywhere. He responded quickly to treatment: 12 June. Hb concentrations 5.7 g/dL, white blood cell count (WBC), 14.6 × 10^9/litre; packed cell volume (PCV), 20.1 per cent; mean corpuscular volume (MCV), 50 fl; mean corpuscular haemoglobin (MCH), 14.9 pg; mean corpuscular haemoglobin concentration (MCHC), 29 per cent. 22 October. Hb concentration 12.0 g/dl; PVC, 36.5 per cent; MCV, 72 fl; MCH, 23.5 pg; MCHC, 32.9 per cent.

Ten years later James was admitted to hospital with melaena following six weeks of recurrent abdominal pains. A Meckel's diverticulum containing a peptic ulcer was removed at laparotomy!

As with small stature, or failure to thrive, the further a Hb value is below the normal, the more likely is an organic disease, rather than the psychosocial environment, to be the cause. A Hb of 5 g/dL requires much more careful evaluation and follow-up than one of 9 g/dL.

The development of progressive iron-deficiency proceeds, before frank anaemia, through depletion of body stores of iron and a subsequent fall in the level of the iron-binding protein ferritin in serum and tissues. Serum ferritin is the single most sensitive indicator of iron-deficiency. Later, the serum iron decreases and the total iron-binding capacity (TIBC) of the serum rises. As the process continues typical changes in the red blood cells ensue. They become smaller (remembering that toddlers have a lower mean MCV than do adults), with a decreased haemoglobin content. The blood smear eventually shows the classic picture of microcytosis and hypochromia with some irregularly shaped red cells.

It is important to distinguish iron-deficiency anaemia from other causes of a hypochromic microcytic blood picture if the child is not of northern European origin. The heterozygous form of β-thalassaemia (thalassaemia trait) gives the same picture but long-term extra iron is contra-indicated. Haemoglobin electrophoresis shows a raised HbA_2 concentration and is diagnostic. The picture may be confusing if there is co-existing iron-deficiency because this may diminish HbA_2 production. In children with a chronic infection the result-ant anaemia, although usually normocytic, may occasionally be microcytic, but in these cases TIBC is reduced instead of increased. Chronic lead poisoning with pica and a raised blood lead concentration also causes a microcytic, hypochromic anaemia.

Dietary iron-deficiency is by far the commonest cause of a mild or moderate anaemia during childhood and the majority of these children will respond satisfactorily to oral iron. A therapeutic trial without further investigation of children with a moderate microcytic anaemia is usually justified, if β-thalassaemia trait has been excluded. Children whose Hb and red cell indices do not return to normal after a course of iron require investigations. Oral iron is well tolerated by children. It may stain the teeth temporarily (regular brushing is recommended) and cause the motions to turn black, a good indication that the medication is being taken, but one which may frighten the unwary into believing that the child has developed a gastro-intestinal bleed. The GP should familiarize himself with one of the less exotic preparations. Sytron with 27.5 mg iron in 5 mL has the benefit of being sugar-free. It should be given before meals. A daily dose of 6 mg elemental iron/kg is adequate to achieve a rise in haemoglobin concentration of some 0.25 g/dL of blood per day, but a patient with intercurrent infection may not respond until the infection has resolved. A significant reticulocytosis is found four to seven days after treatment is started, at which time the child with severe anaemia should have his reticulocyte count measured. The iron should be given for a couple of months after the anaemia has been corrected to rebuild iron stores, and the haemoglobin concentration checked again three months later, to make sure that anaemia has not recurred—an indication for more detailed investigation.

Dietary advice is necessary for all families whose child's anaemia is nutritional. It may be wise to reduce the amount of milk the child drinks, and to increase the proportion of iron-rich food in the diet, particularly meat.

A GP programme of screening young children for iron-deficiency anaemia may be justified particularly in areas of marked socio-economic deprivation. Intervention consisting of dietary advice and education can markedly reduce iron-deficiency amongst toddlers in a practice (James *et al.* 1989). Mothers should be advised to include meat in their infant's diet during the second half of the first year unless it is against their beliefs.

FAMILIAL HAEMOLYTIC ANAEMIAS

A child with haemolytic anaemia usually has, in addition to a low haemoglobin, a raised bilirubin and reticulocyte count, frequently with abnormal red blood cells; he may have a large spleen. Some episodes of haemolysis are immunologically induced during an intercurrent infection, but most arise from production, through genetic mechanisms, of functionally abnormal red blood cells. We here consider only the three commonest: sickle cell anaemia, thalassaemia, and glucose-6-phosphate dehydrogenase deficiency. Carrying the gene for sickle cell anaemia or thalassaemia as a heterozygote 'having the trait' gives some protection against malaria. Haemoglobinopathies are thus seen in children originating from Africa, the Mediterranean basin, and the Middle and Far East. Parents who learn that their children have the trait need to be reassured that they will not develop a blood disease. The haemoglobin concentration may be a little low, but extra iron is contra-indicated except in pregnancy, unless the serum iron or ferritin is low. It is possible to make a prenatal diagnosis in the first trimester for most mothers at risk of a fetus with a haemoglobinopathy; that is, when the father is also a carrier (p. 297).

In the thalassaemias, the production rate of one of the haemoglobin chains is impaired; in sickle cell anaemia, the amino acid sequence of the haemoglobin molecule itself is abnormal. They are diagnosed by haemoglobin electrophoresis. In glucose-6-phosphate dehydrogenase deficiency, an enzyme which plays a part in maintaining red-cell integrity is absent, or reduced in amount.

Sickle cell disease

Sickle cell disease (SCD), an autosomal recessive disorder, affects approximately 5000 people of African-Caribbean and occasional Asian origin in the UK. Sickle cell haemoglobin (HbSS) results from a substitution in the β chain, of the amino acid valine for glutamine. In the deoxygenated state, HbSS undergoes polymerization causing red blood cells to become crescent-shaped (sickle cell). These can cause occlusion of small blood vessels in various tissues including bone and spleen. The deformed red blood cells are rapidly destroyed and removed from the circulation by the spleen, leading to chronic haemolytic anaemia. The children are normal at birth and the symptoms of sickle cell disease usually appear after six months of age as the concentration of HbF falls and is replaced by HbSS rather than HbA. Affected children have a baseline haemoglobin concentration of between 7 and 10 g/dL. Folic acid requirements are increased due to chronic haemolysis and supplements should be given. Acute worsening of anaemia, which can sometimes be fatal, may occur with parvovirus B19 infection, which, in a pale-skinned child, causes a characteristic 'slapped-cheek appearance' (the "fifth disease"). This virus causes transient destruction of red cell precursors. The acute manifestations of sickle cell disease are traditionally called 'crises', and during childhood they include painful vaso-occlusive crises, splenic and hepatic sequestration crises and aplastic crises. Congestion of the spleen with sickled red cells leads to impaired function. Initially this spleen is palpable but by school age repeated infarction in fact renders it fibrotic and impalpable. An unwell young child with SCD will usually need to be admitted.

Infections

Children with sickle cell disease are susceptible to serious infections caused by *Streptococcus pneumoniae, Haemophilus influenzae* and Salmonella species, due to a mixture of hyposplenism (either functional or atrophic) and defects in immunity. This susceptibility is an important cause of the raised mortality of children with this disease, particularly in the first three years of life, and is an important reason for neonatal screening for HbSS disease. Risk of pneumococcal infections can be minimized by indefinite prophylactic penicillin-V therapy (62.5 mg twice a day <1 year, 125 mg twice a day between 1–3 years and 250 mg twice a day if >3 years) and by administration of pneumococcal vaccine (Pneumovax). The age for giving Pneumovax is debatable. The 1992 immunization guidelines recommend Pneumovax at the age of two years; however, some paediatricians give it at the age of six months, with boosters given every five years. All standard childhood immunizations should be given at normal times. Parents should be taught how to check their child's temperature (see Chapter 10) and to seek an urgent consultation with their GP if his temperature is >38 °C, as fever may be the only early sign of pneumococcal septicaemia. The GP must ensure that the child has quick and easy access to the practice.

Painful vaso-occlusive crisis

These are the most frequent clinical symptoms and may be precipitated by infection, dehydration, or exposure to cold. Infants may develop painful swelling of their hands and feet (hand–foot syndrome) caused by infarction of metacarpals and metatarsals. Recurrent episodes of ischaemic pain involving the bones, muscles, and abdomen occur throughout childhood. Strokes may occur in adolescents with severe disease. Pain due to vaso-occlusive crisis may be severe and demoralizing; it is frequently underestimated and undertreated by doctors. Oral analgesics, such as paracetamol (12 mg/kg every six hours), ibuprofen (5 mg/kg every six hours), or codeine phosphate (1 mg/kg every four to six hours) will suffice for milder cases (Grundy *et al.* 1993). Most children with severe pain, or those who fail to respond to oral analgesics within one hour of administration, will need hospital admission for treatment with parenteral opiates. A few older adolescents may be managed at home if the GP and or the district nurse are prepared to administer IM morphine at four to six hourly intervals. Patients should be encouraged to drink copious amounts of fluid to avoid dehydration and given a full dose of penicillin.

Sequestration crisis

Sudden enlargement of the spleen (or the liver) may be due to rapid pooling of large amounts of blood, leading to severe anaemia, shock, and death. These sequestration crises are usually precipitated by infections. Parents should be taught how to feel the lower edge of their child's spleen, so that they may recognize this problem by checking its position when he appears unwell.

Banke, a three-year-old girl with sickle cell disease who had recently arrived in the country from Ghana with her mother, was taken to casualty department complaining of abdominal pain. She was noted to be very pale (Hb 1.8 g/dL) and shocked. Her spleen was grossly enlarged and tender on palpation. She died four hours later despite emergency transfusion with O-negative blood. Autopsy revealed severe splenic sequestration.

Early identification of infants with sickle cell disease following ante-natal or post-natal screening, together with comprehensive care, has led to a decrease in mortality during childhood. The survivors, in addition to repeated crisis, may go on to develop complications such as leg ulcers, gall stones, priapism (painful, persistent penile erection), femoral head necrosis, retinopathy, nephropathy, and stroke during adult life. However, there is a wide range of severity; many individuals survive to middle age with rather little disability.

Thalassaemia

The important form, homozygous β-thalassaemia (thalassaemia major) presents as gross anaemia (Hb concentration 4–7 g/dL) usually before the first birthday. There is hepatosplenomegaly and compensatory bone-marrow expansion throughout the skeleton: which leads to an abnormal appearance. The symptoms, and the skeletal deformity can be completely suppressed by regular transfusions of enough blood to maintain a nearly normal concentration of Hb. Once regular transfusions are started the major therapeutic problem is multi-organ toxicity from iron overload. This can be reduced, and perhaps prevented, by regular treatment with the iron-chelating agent desferrioxamine. Chelation therapy currently involves subcutaneous infusion of desferrioxamine over 10 to 12 hours, three to seven times a week, although oral agents are under development. Parents and children are taught how to administer desferrioxamine at home using a portable infusion pump. The grossly enlarged spleen, by leading to excess red-cell destruction, may itself increase the frequency of transfusion necessary to maintain an acceptable Hb concentration. Many thalassaemic children sooner or later need a splenectomy. Any child who has had a splenectomy, particularly in early childhood, is at slight but real risk of sudden death from overwhelming septicaemia, usually pneumococcal, and such children should be given Pneumovax, preferably before splenectomy, and maintained on lifelong prophylactic penicillin subsequently. The GP should be aware that after splenectomy a febrile illness with malaise may be the first sign of fulminating septicaemia; he should be liberal with antibiotics for minor febrile illnesses in these children. Bone-marrow transplantation is now an important therapeutic option for children who have an HLA identical sibling donor, with a >90 per cent cure rate in some centres. As mentioned, heterozygotes have a mild hypochromic anaemia, which may be mistaken for iron-deficiency anaemia. These subjects require genetic advice.

Glucose-6-phosphate dehydrogenase (G6PD) deficiency

G6PD deficiency is a sex-linked disorder occurring in areas where malaria is or was endemic. In such areas about 7 per cent of the male population carry the gene. The red blood cells break down *in vivo* when exposed to oxidizing agents such as fava beans, sulphonamides, or some other drugs and chemicals. Very alarming haemolytic episodes can occur with jaundice, gross pallor, and even heart failure. It is an important cause of prolonged neonatal jaundice. Such a child keeps well if the list of dangerous substances is avoided. These include antimalarials (primaquine, pamaquine, and possibly chloroquine), sulphonamides, and certain antibiotics (nalidixic acid, possibly chloramphenicol).

Congenital spherocytosis

There are also a number of inherited haemolytic anaemias seen in white children, spherocytosis, which is dominantly inherited, being the best known. In it the red cells become spheres and are removed from the circulation by the spleen. Splenectomy is very effective as it increases the red cell survival. Pneumovax vaccine and lifelong penicillin prophylaxis are important to reduce the risk of post-splenectomy sepsis.

RHESUS INCOMPATIBILITY

Blood-group incompatibility between mother and fetus may lead to intrauterine or neonatal haemolytic anaemia. The most serious example is rhesus incompatibility, in which red cells of a rhesus-positive fetus are damaged by antibodies produced by a sensitized rhesus-negative mother. This has become less common since maternal sensitization has been prevented by the administration of rhesus anti-D antibody in the post-partum period.

Anaemia may damage the baby *in utero* and lead to hydrops. After birth, haemolytic jaundice develops rapidly, unlike the development of neonatal physiological jaundice which takes two or three days. Jaundice on the first day needs immediate investigation, as brain damage from hyperbilirubinaemia may supervene unless adequate treatment, by exchange transfusion or other means, is undertaken, sometimes within a few hours. Mild cases may present later with anaemia in the early weeks of life. Babies who have had exchange transfusions in the neonatal period occasionally develop dangerous degrees of anaemia after discharge from hospital. Non-rhesus incompatibility between a group O mother and a group A baby can also lead to a similar but milder clinical picture.

BONE-MARROW DEPRESSION

The commonest cause of more than transient depression is leukaemia, but drugs such as chloramphenicol or sulphonamides, or poisons such as benzene can be responsible. Frequently no cause is apparent. A moderately unwell child presents with intercurrent infection precipitated by granulocytopenia, or with unexplained bruising, a persistent nose bleed or anaemia. In the case of leukaemia there is frequently splenomegaly or lymphadenopathy. Blast cells are not always seen on the blood film in leukaemia, but anaemia or thrombocytopenia are usually found (see Chapter 23).

Isolated red blood cell aplasia is rarer and may be congenital. An otherwise well baby or child presents with gradually increasing pallor over two or three months as the circulating red blood cells come to the end of their lifespan and are not replaced. By the time of diagnosis the haemoglobin will usually be below 7 g/dL.

ABNORMAL BRUISING

Once they start walking, all children get bruises, particularly on the lower limbs. The commonest pathological cause is child abuse, with bruising especially of the face, arms, and bottom (see Chapter 5).

Sudden onset of a bleeding tendency is rare. Commoner than leukaemia is idiopathic thrombocytopenic purpura. A well child, sometimes after a viral infection, develops multiple bruises and petechiae. The platelet count is very low, often less than 20×10^9/litre. Most children with idiopathic thrombocytopenic purpura get better spontaneously after a few weeks. The only significant risk is that of cerebral haemorrhage, which occurs in less than one per cent of affected children. If the platelet count is exceptionally low, treatment with intravenous immunoglobulin infusions or oral steroids is indicated.

Henoch–Schönlein purpura, despite its name, does not really resemble a bleeding disorder. It is a vasculitis in which the child develops erythema, papules, and purpura, characteristically distributed over the extensor surfaces of the buttocks and the lower limbs. Intestinal, joint, or renal involvement may occur. Heavy proteinuria, with or without haematuria, is a serious sign prognostic of possible long-term renal impairment.

Congenital disorders of the clotting proteins, such as haemophilia, are usually found in boys. Extensive and indurated bruises due to bleeding into muscle, or painful joints from haemarthrosis, may not be noted until the toddler becomes mobile or until a severe haemorrhage occurs after dental extraction or surgery. In the case of haemophilia, regular self-injection of factor VIII has transformed the haematological prognosis and more or less abolished chronic joint problems. Tragically, many children treated this way have been inadvertedly infected with HIV. There can also be problems with antibody formation to factor VIII and with iatrogenic hepatitis. Some children with mild clotting-factor deficiencies need treatment only in the event of a joint bleed (which must be treated to avoid arthropathy), or after head injury, following cuts around the mouth and airway, or to cover surgery. Contact sports should often be avoided. Most children are now managed by regional haemophilia centres.

HAEMORRHAGIC DISEASE OF THE NEWBORN AND VITAMIN K PROPHYLAXIS

Newborn infants have marginal stores of vitamin K, while those born prematurely or to mothers receiving anticonvulsants during pregnancy may be vitamin K deficient. Thus haemorrhagic disease of the newborn (HDN), due to lack of vitamin K-dependent clotting factors may develop at any time during the first few weeks of life, resulting in spontaneous bleeding from the gastro-intestinal tract, the umbilicus, or, rarely, intracranially bleed. The HDN is completely prevented by a single dose of intramuscular vitamin K administered to all newborn infants, shortly after birth. Breast-milk is a poor source of this vitamin but infant formulae are supplemented. Thus HDN may occur in exclusively breast-fed infants who have not received vitamin K because of parental concerns about an unproven report linking an increased risk of childhood malignancies with intramuscular vitamin K administration in the neonatal period (Golding *et al.* 1992). Oral vitamin K is an alternative preparation.

Bibliography

Aukett, A., Parks, Y. A., Scott, P. H., and Wharton, B. A. (1986). Treatment with iron increases weight gain and psychomotor development. *Archives of Disease in Childhood*, **61**, 849–57.

Dallman, P. R. and Siimes, M. A. (1979). Percentile curves for haemoglobin and red cell volume in infancy and childhood. *Journal of Paediatrics*, **94**, 26–31.

Golding, J., Greenwood, R., Birmingham, K., and Mott, M. (1992). Childhood cancer, intramuscular vitamin K, and pethidine given during labour. *British Medical Journal*, **305**, 341–6.

Grundy, R., Howard, R., and Evans, J. (1993). Practical management of pain in sickling disorders. *Archives of Disease in Childhood*, **69**, 256–9.

James, J., Lawson, P., Male, P., and Oakhill, A. (1989). Preventing iron deficiency in preschool children by implementing an educational and screening programme in an inner city practice. *British Medical Journal*, **299**, 838–40.

Nathan, D. G. and Oski, F. A. (ed) (1981). *Hematology of infancy and childhood*, (2nd edn), Saunders, Philadelphia.

Stevens, D. (1991). Epidemiology of hypochromic anaemia in young child. *Archives of Disease in Childhood*, **66**, 886–9.

18 Fits and faints

One of the most frightening experiences for any parent, is to witness their child having a convulsion, particularly its first. They have visions of a dead or brain-damaged child, and it is common for him to be rushed directly to the Accident and Emergency department of the nearest hospital, bypassing the GP. A fit is usually unpredictable, and the child may have appeared reasonably well a few minutes before:

Jimmy was the 14-month-old baby of French parents. He was brought to the surgery with a fever and an upper respiratory tract infection. The GP told the mother that the child was not seriously unwell, had a self-limiting illness, and only needed paracetamol. A few hours later a very angry mother rang from the hospital. Jimmy had a convulsion five minutes after she had left the surgery. The parents had taken him directly to the hospital, where he was now better. However, she never wanted to see the doctor again, who was obviously quite unable to realize how sick her child had been.

FEBRILE CONVULSIONS

At least one *grand mal* or generalized convulsion may be expected in 2.5 per cent of children during their first five years (Ross *et al.* 1980). Apart from the fits seen in children with cerebral palsy or severe learning difficulties, the vast majority are relatively benign febrile convulsions, easily triggered off in certain preschool children by any fever, regardless of its cause. Most such fits occur between six months and five years of age in neurologically normal children. Based on a survey of 14 676 British children, Verity and Golding (1991) found that 398 (2.7 per cent) had at least one febrile fit and 17 of these had subsequent afebrile fits. The risk of developing subsequent epilepsy was higher if the child had had a 'complex' febrile fit—lasting more than 15 minutes—or focal or repeated fits in the same illness.

Febrile fits usually occur soon after the initial rise in temperature. Typically, the child who has been generally off colour due to a cold or mild gastro-enteritis, suddenly goes limp, his eyes roll up and he loses consciousness. His body then stiffens, followed by shaking movements of his limbs which usually go on for much less than five minutes, but sometimes for a little longer. He then drifts into a post-ictal sleepy period. A parent who telephones about a convulsing child should be instructed to keep him in a position where inhalation of vomit is unlikely—namely, lying on his side, slightly face down. There does not seem to be any point in sticking a gag into his mouth.

Prolonged febrile fits are rare but any *grand mal* convulsion that continues more than 10 minutes is potentially dangerous. A child may sustain brain damage and even die during a very prolonged seizure. In the rare cases in which the GP needs to give an anti-convulsant to a fitting child, the drug of choice is usually rectal diazepam (Stesolid: dose 5 mg for the child under 3; 10 mg for an older child) which is surprisingly rapidly absorbed. Diazepam may rarely cause respiratory arrest, dealt with by the GP giving mouth-to-mouth respiration until spontaneous breathing returns, usually very quickly. Usually, by the time the child is seen, the fit is over and the important decision is whether he requires admission.

First, could it be meningitis? Some paediatricians recommend a lumbar puncture after every first febrile convulsion. This seems an unnecessarily extreme position, but a careful search should be made for a purpuric skin rash, a full fontanelle, or neck stiffness. If there is any doubt about the exclusion of meningitis because of difficulty in the evaluation of irritability and drowsiness in the immediate post-ictal period, the doctor must arrange to see the child again a few hours later, or refer anyway. Most doctors will also remain uneasy if they cannot find a cause for the fever, particularly as an early sign of meningitis in a baby may be a fit, and it is wise to admit any child under one year.

Secondly, could the fit be symptomatic of some other problem requiring urgent treatment? Brain tumour, hypoglycaemia, drug overdosage, lead poisoning, reported or unreported head injury, encephalitis, Reye's syndrome, and hypertension are all uncommon or very uncommon possibilities. Thorough examination and a careful history with particular attention to developments over the few hours and days before the fit, will usually give the necessary clue.

Thirdly, is the child neurologically handicapped or, more rarely, suffering from a neuro-degenerative condition with gradual regression of development? Sometimes neurological handicap is not spotted until epilepsy starts. Again the history gives the clue. Has the child been delayed in development? Was there a difficult perinatal period?

Finally, if this is a simple febrile fit does the febrile illness require treatment in its own right?

In general, a child with sensible parents does not have to be admitted to hospital for a febrile convulsion unless the fit continued for more than 10 minutes, recurred during the same attack of fever, left residual neurological signs, or there is any question of meningitis.

Parents of any child who has had a febrile fit should know how to treat the child when he develops a fever. Tepid sponging has not been shown to be effective in controlling fever in children. Therefore, parents should be advised to give paracetamol (120 mg up to 1 year, 240 mg from 1 to 3 years and 360 mg for 4 years and over, at 6 hourly intervals), to cool the child by undressing him, and to encourage him to drink plenty of fluids. He should never be cooled in a bath lest he have a fit and inhales water while the mother's attention is distracted. Fever lasting for two to three days may occur about a week after an MMR immunization, with a small risk of febrile convulsions (Immunisation against infectious diseases 1992). The child with a previous history of febrile fits should be given the MMR vaccine, but parents should be vigilant for febrile episodes from day 5 to 8 after the MMR jab and treat as described above.

A Joint Working Group of the Royal College of Physicians of London and the British Paediatric Association (1991) felt that prophylactic anticonvulsants were rarely indicated in children with recurrent febrile fits as there is no evidence that they lessen the risk of subsequent epilepsy. It is helpful to have rectal diazepam available at home for use by competent parents of recurrent fitters, though the Working Group did not decide whether this should be given as soon as the fit begins or only after five minutes. A fact sheet giving explanation about the nature of febrile convulsions, advice about management of fever and any future fits may be helpful for the family to keep at home.

GENERALIZED TONIC–CLONIC SEIZURES

Fits definitely unaccompanied by fever are altogether more serious. The infrequent child who, despite normal development, continues to have fits without a fever after febrile convulsions, will require continuous anticonvulsant medication and a specialist assessment, at some stage, including an EEG, biochemical investigation, and perhaps a cranial CT scan. This is also true of children who develop *grand mal* attacks without preceding febrile convulsions. However, provided a single fit was short, and the child is free of neurological handicap or of intellectual deterioration, it is reasonable to await events and investigate and treat only in the event of a second afebrile seizure. Sodium valproate or carbamazepine are the drugs of choice.

Parents are naturally concerned to know what activities should be barred to a child who has fits. Whilst there are few hard and fast rules and the answer depends on how well the epilepsy is controlled, O'Donohoe (1983) gives useful guidelines emphasizing that normal life, both at home and at school should be encouraged:

1. Children with well controlled epilepsy, including an occasional fit, may swim if accompanied by an informed adult who is a qualified life saver.
2. Drowning in the bath is a recognized hazard and younger children need surveillance. Even older children should shower rather than bath with the plughole open and the bathroom door unlocked.
3. Sports are important to most children and, whilst climbing activities and body contact sports such as boxing have to be discouraged, many epileptic children partake successfully in athletics, tennis, or golf.
4. Bicycling in traffic is not advisable unless the epilepsy is under excellent control.

5. Most children are not particularly vulnerable in discotheques, but children who are aware that their fits may be triggered by stimuli, such as hyperventilation, music, or the flicker of a TV or a computer monitor, should be wary.

OTHER FITS

Brief lapses of attention at home or in the classroom can occasionally mean *petit mal* epilepsy. Interruptions of concentration that result may lead to the child being labelled as slow at school or as very unco-operative. Characteristically, there is a moment's vacancy and sometimes eye blinking that cannot be interrupted by the observer. The attacks can usually be brought on by hyperventilation. A good quality EEG showing regular 3 cycle per second spike and wave activity confirms the diagnosis, and drug treatment sometimes makes a big difference to progress in school. Sodium valproate or ethosuximide are the drugs of choice.

Complex partial epilepsy (temporal lobe epilepsy) may present with:

(1) perceptual disturbances, such as 'déjà vu' or feeling of familiarity, auditory or olfactory hallucinations, distortion of visual images, or emotional reactions such as feelings of intense fear;

(2) purposeless movements, such as repeated buttoning and unbuttoning, fidgeting, swallowing, or lip smacking movements;

(3) autonomic disturbance, such as facial flushing.

It is not surprising that temporal lobe epilepsy is often mistaken for a behavioural problem; misuse of hallucinogenic drugs is sometimes suspected. Occasionally a prolonged "absence" or staring may be the only feature, but attacks may also progress to a tonic–clonic phase with post-ictal drowsiness or sleepiness. The EEG usually shows discharges emanating from the temporal region of the brain. A CT scan may reveal an underlying cause, such as a vascular malformation or an abscess in one of the temporal lobes. Carbamazepine is the drug of choice but if an underlying cause, is present, it may be amenable to surgical treatment.

Nocturnal epilepsy is another occasional missed diagnosis which may lead to a bitten lip, a wet bed, or blood on the pillow. For infantile spasms or Salaam attacks see p. 128 and below.

THE DIFFERENTIAL DIAGNOSIS OF FITS—IS IT EPILEPSY?

Not all losses of consciousness in children are brought about by epilepsy and a careful description of the circumstances of the attack will usually be very helpful in clarifying the diagnosis. Robinson (1984) found that 75 out of 201 patients referred to him with the possible diagnosis of epilepsy proved to have other diagnoses, such as fainting or breath-holding attacks.

It is vital that the GP makes every effort to contact a person who has witnessed the fit (for example, a school teacher) to obtain a detailed history. The following questions may help to distinguish fits from other causes of loss of consciousness:

1. Did the child become extremely pale all over or blue around his lips before he fell? Did he bite his lips or become incontinent of urine or faeces?
2 Did the child lose consciousness, or was he able to respond to questions during the episode?
3. Was there any stiffening, and if so did it affect the whole body or just his hand?
4. Were there jerking movements of his limbs? Did the jerking occur on one side of his body; how long did it last for?
5. Was he sleepy or did he appear confused afterwards?

The following conditions may sometimes be misdiagnosed as fits:

Paroxysmal screaming associated with drawing up of the legs may be confused with infantile spasms or 'Salaam attacks' but the reverse can also occur:

Samantha, a two-month-old infant, was admitted via the casualty department because of a two-week history of episodic crying associated with drawing up of her legs. Her mother had put her on a soya formula and had been giving her 'colic drops' on advice of a health visitor. EEG showed 'hypsarrhythmia' characteristic of infantile spasms and this was treated with ACTH injections.

A **faint** occurs in an older child particularly when he, or more often she, is standing in a stuffy atmosphere; classically the child who has had no breakfast falling to the ground during school assembly. The patient often feels faint or giddy before she falls and a loss of consciousness is usually short-lived, without, or with only faint, twitching. If a teacher takes the pulse it will be very slow. **Syncope due to hyperventilation** may be triggered off in a young teenager who, when very upset, overwrought, or hurt by a fall in the playground begins to over breathe, presumably becomes hypocapnic, and then lapses into semi-unconsciousness. The description by bystanders is of her being unable to catch her breath, and adults may worry that she is having a heart attack. The diagnostic clue is the way the hands stiffen up in carpopedal spasm during the episode. The child remembers this when asked. Once the doctor has diagnosed the situation and given reassurance to the child, parents, and teacher the problem appears to resolve. We personally, have never had to resort to the textbook manoeuvre of rebreathing into a paper bag to raise the CO_2, though it is said to be highly effective if simple reassurance does not work.

Breath-holding attacks occur when the toddler who has been hurt or thwarted screams and then holds his breath in inspiration. He quickly goes blue around his face, and if he continues to hold his breath for many more seconds he will become limp, keel over, and lose consciousness, occasionally even twitching. They are almost all totally benign.

James, aged two, had numerous breath-holding attacks. He was brought to the GP to have some stitches removed from his head. When approached he started screaming and the doctor patiently waited for him to inevitably lose consciousness before removing the stitching without further fuss.

A substantial minority of generalized seizures in preschool children are not primarily neurological but follow a brief period of asystole. Such **reflex anoxic seizures** are often misdiagnosed as, for example, febrile fits. The attacks are usually precipitated by fright or by painful stimuli, and the hallmark is the child becoming deathly pale, 'as white as a sheet', falling down limp and unconscious, and, more rarely, having a few clonic movements. Recovery is usually rapid and the prognosis is excellent, with most attacks ceasing by the fourth year of life. It is obviously an error to treat these children with anticonvulsants. For the occasional child with frequent attacks, atropine is sometimes helpful. Such children have increased vagal tone and easily develop bradycardia at any time, for example, if the doctor presses gently on the eyeball—a useful diagnostic test, but not recommended in primary care because of the risk of asystole or of damaging the eyeball. Very much more rarely, other cardiac arrhythmias, particularly those occurring during exercise, can underlie fits and may be recorded on a portable 24-hour ECG tape. If there is a family history of sudden death, this is sinister, as arrhythmias can run in families. Occasionally an ordinary ECG will show abnormalities of the P-waves between attacks.

Other conditions which may be confused with fits include startle responses and shuddering movements of the jaw in infancy, tics and day dreaming, or night terrors in toddlers and older children. A number of children with florid behaviour disorders or temper tantrums masquerading as fits are reinforced in their behaviour by the use of regular medication and are sometimes inappropriately maintained on anticonvulsants for many years; a serious iatrogenic error. This is one reason why a too-ready trial of anticonvulsants in a dubious case is unwise. Such problems overlap with Munchausen syndrome by proxy, when a disturbed parent, who may have paramedical or nursing experience (usually the mother), may fabricate a convincing history of fits in her child or, more dangerously, induce them by suffocation or administration of drugs (Meadows 1984).

Bibliography

Immunisations against infectious diseases. (1992). HMSO, London.

Joint Working Group of the Research Units of the Royal College of Physicians of London and the British Paediatric Association. (1991). Guidelines for the management of convulsions with fever. *British Medical Journal*, **303**, 634–6.

Meadows, R. (1984). Fictitious epilepsy. *Lancet*, **2**, 25–8.

O'Donohoe, N. Y. (1983). What should the child with epilepsy be allowed to do? *Archives of Disease in Childhood*, **58**, 934–7.

Robinson, R. (1984). When to start and stop anticonvulsants. In *Recent advances in paediatrics*, (ed. R. Meadow), pp. 155–74. Churchill Livingstone, Edinburgh.

Ross, E. M., Peckham, C. S., West, P. B., and Butler N. R. (1980). Epilepsy in childhood: findings from the National Child Development Study. *British Medical Journal*, **280**, 207–10.

Verity, C. M. and Golding, J. (1991). Risk of epilepsy after febrile convulsions: a national cohort study. *British Medical Journal*, **303**, 1373–6.

19 Recurrent pains

Complaints of aches and pains at one site or another, recurring over several months or years, are common in childhood. Often they seem to peter out or, at least, the family becomes able to cope with the symptom at a domestic level, once the doctor has guessed or established the family's specific fear, and has been able to reassure them that the pains are not, for example, appendicitis, leukaemia or a brain tumour. Other family members may have dysmenorrhoea, indigestion, or migraine.

The abdomen and head and limbs seem to be the most common sites for recurrent pains in children; chest pains or chronic backache are rarer. Although, in most patients, there is no physical cause to account for the pain, careful assessment is necessary. Chronic backache, unlike the others, is more usually a symptom of some underlying organic pathology in a child. It, and limb pains are discussed in Chapter 21.

Children with a recurrent pain, predominantly in one site, not infrequently have one elsewhere during a subsequent period. Conversely, when a GP looks back through the records of a child or adolescent presenting with a somewhat vague health problem, he will sometimes note past attendances for recurrent pain. In any case, it may be worthwhile sitting back and occasionally reassessing the diagnosis (with the family) in a child who presents repeatedly over the years with persistent, apparently unrelated symptoms. Could there be a specific psychosocial problem such as parental alcoholism or sexual abuse? Have pointers towards an obscure physical cause so far been missed: night thirst (renal failure), loose stools or poor growth (Crohn's disease); has the GP considered measuring the blood pressure, the serum calcium (hyperparathyroidism) or the creatinine? Is there a family history suggestive of porphyria?

ABDOMINAL PAIN

Recurrent episodes of abdominal pain occur in about one out of every nine children; girls more than boys. The child complains of episodes of pain, more usually colicky than constant. The site and character of the pain is variable, though often around or near the umbilicus. Most attacks have a similar individual pattern. Children who have rather stereotyped attacks, lasting a few hours, of not very severe bellyache, recurrent vomiting, pallor, and headache are often described as having the periodic syndrome, or abdominal migraine, and some such children certainly develop classical migraine subsequently. A rare child who has neurological symptoms such as ataxia or marked lethargy during the attacks may be worth referring for exclusion of an inborn error of amino-acid metabolism; normal children develop ketosis if they vomit or do not eat. New physical causes for some cases of recurrent abdominal pain are frequently postulated. Current favourites include gastro-oesophageal reflux, even without acid regurgitation; abnormal patterns of bowel mobility; and malabsorption of lactose—all somewhat vague; gastritis due to *Helicobacter pylori* is not thought to be a cause.

The traditional view is that only about one in ten children with recurrent bellyache turn out to have an organic cause (Murphy 1993). The further from the umbilicus the pain occurs, the more likely is the cause to be organic. If the pain occurs in the loin an ultrasound examination is certainly wise in order to exclude a renal abnormality, even if microscopy and culture of the urine is clear.

Associated symptoms, such as weight loss, dysuria, or frequency, make a physical illness more likely. A regular periodicity may suggest dysmenorrhoea in the post-pubertal girl. The severity of the pain is not a good guide to diagnosis. Even severe discomfort can occur without any diagnosable organic disease.

The doctor's knowledge of the family may be helpful, although in many cases, even if the pain is the expression of an emotional disorder, the cause will not be obvious to the GP or to the family. There seems to be an increase in emotional disturbance in families with affected children, and this may lead them to have a lower threshold for reporting problems to the doctor, other families putting up with their children's recurrent bellyache. School refusal or neurotic symptoms such as irrational fears, can indicate that the recurrent pain is one manifestation of wider emotional disturbance.

The child should be weighed and his abdomen examined between attacks and, if possible, during one. If, for example, his abdomen is distended when he is in pain, an abdominal X-ray at this time, and perhaps a barium meal, are indicated; remember that if a lateral pain is due to an intermittent hydronephrosis, the ultrasound may only be abnormal during the attack. Assuming no significant pointer is noted in the history or on examination, investigation should be kept to a minimum. Microscopy and culture of urine are obligatory; a full blood count and ESR may be helpful especially if the history is not very prolonged.

Jane was an 11-year-old girl who came from an unhappy family background and had just started at her secondary school. She presented on three occasions in three weeks with vague upper abdominal pain and malaise. It was thought that her symptoms were due to stress but on the third occasion her temperature was mildly elevated and her spleen was palpable. A blood film showed a typical picture of infectious mononucleosis.

Only if the history of the complaint, the family history, or examination point to possible organic disease, will further investigation be necessary, for example, endoscopy if the pain persistently occurs in relation to meals and is epigastric. Only rarely will one want to go further to exclude, for example, pancreatitis, cholecystitis, lead poisoning, or spinal tumour.

If the doctor decides that there is no organic disease, this should be frankly discussed. The parent may have been worried about the possibility of appendicitis—not the cause of recurrent abdominal pain. It is often helpful to give the parent an explanation of the symptoms, perhaps merely the label 'recurrent non-organic abdominal pain'. It seems wise to avoid the almost always unjustified labels of constipation, allergy, or food intolerance, which often become the focus for an increasingly physical approach to personal health. They become used as an excuse to avoid considering emotional factors and the child's life is medicalized. 'It's when he has the allergy that he can't concentrate on his homework', rather than 'since my ex-husband forgot his birthday last week he has been down in the dumps'.

The absence of serious organic cause does not mean the cause has to be emotional; rather that the focus should be on getting on with life rather than pursuing rare or marginal causes. Usually it is useful to work out with the mother, and perhaps with the school, what line to take when the child gets the pain again. In the absence of evidence that the problem is symptomatic of serious psychosocial problems, a sympathetic acceptance that the pain is genuine, coupled with advice to avoid making too much fuss about it, will often allow people to cope with the situation. Paracetamol can be reserved for more than usually severe attacks. In any case, the GP should arrange to reassess the situation a few weeks later. It is reasonable to point out at some stage that, while this particular abdominal pain has been judged to be non-organic, if a totally different pain crops up they should consult the doctor as usual.

Follow-up of these patients shows that, though most of them recover, a higher proportion than in the rest of the population continue to have chronic abdominal symptoms as an adult and that some develop different recurrent pains.

HEADACHE

Recurrent headache with no obvious cause is common. The child is brought partly because of the symptom but also because the parents may be afraid that he has a brain tumour, or something wrong with his eyes or his sinuses. The doctor will deal with such patients with more confidence if he has developed a simple routine of assessment. The history includes a careful discussion of any significant event that may have occurred before the pain started, as well as questioning about school attendance and any obvious family stresses. Apart from the headache, is the child well or has he got an unnoticed intercurrent infection? Are there any other symptoms at all? Nausea is not uncommon and vomiting may also occur. Does the child have a recurrent pain elsewhere?

Some families express their tensions and stresses as headache. The examination should begin with an assessment of the child's demeanour. Does he look well? Has he been smiling and lively during the interview or withdrawn and depressed? It is important to check the optic discs, to take the blood pressure, and to note the visual acuity in each eye separately (a small child may become blind in one eye without apparently noticing it). Neck movements should be tested, and occipital muscles palpated for areas of spasm or local tenderness. Discomfort in the face or above the eyes may be due to an occult dental abscess or sinusitis, though these are unusual causes of recurrent childhood headache. If a child complains of aching eyes, headache after reading, or is seen to prefer to be close to the blackboard and to screw his eyes up to see properly, it is sensible to get his eyes tested, although wearing spectacles may not stop the headaches.

In most cases, an open discussion with the child present is helpful if it is felt that stress is precipitating the pain. However, if progress is difficult, it may be useful and a more satisfactory approach to see the parents alone and to ask them the question, 'What do you think the cause may be?' A report from the school obtained with parental agreement is sometimes useful. Nevertheless, we are often left with a somewhat sensitive child who has recurrent headaches for no very obvious reason. A simple explanation of how pain in the head can arise from stress and tension may help. There is no reason why the child should not take an occasional paracetamol tablet, if the headache becomes troublesome.

Some children have more classic migraine, although the diagnosis is often not clinched until months or years later when an attack with fortification spectra occurs. There is often a family history. Provoking features are legion and include emotional distress, dietary indiscretion, and travel, particularly long car journeys. Classically the aura consists of visual disturbances, but may include a variety of neurological phenomena, including vertigo and ataxia. In the full migraine syndrome, the aura will be followed by a severe, throbbing, unilateral headache associated with nausea and vomiting. The child may be in great discomfort, preferring to lie in a dark room, trying to get to sleep. At first he may manage to do this for a very short while, only to awaken again to be sick, still complaining of the pain which may take several hours to abate. Partial forms of migraine occur in which there is only an aura, or no aura at all, and the child just suffers from a unilateral headache. Accurate diagnosis with an explanation of the symptoms and an attempt to avoid provoking factors is usually more effective than drugs. These should usually be limited to paracetamol or possible ibuprofen taken at the time of the onset of symptoms, perhaps with an anti-emetic if vomiting is a prominent problem. There is rarely need for regular prophylaxis with, for example, a small dose of propranolol (for the non-asthmatic). Sumatriptan has not yet been evaluated in childhood migraine. The parents or the child may have learnt to avoid certain trigger factors, such as cheese or excessive tiredness. Reassuringly, in a study of 73 children diagnosed as migrainous, none were found to have a cerebral tumour or vascular malformation during a mean 5.4 years follow-up (Tal *et al.* 1984).

The headache of raised intracranial pressure, like that of hypertension, will usually remit and recur, gradually becoming more severe and prolonged as the pressure rises. It is almost always more prominent in the morning and may wake the child. The pain is often aggravated by coughing and straining at stool although this is also true of more benign headaches. Projectile vomiting is common. If the child with a headache has signs of neurological disease such as diplopia, or ataxia causing a staggering gait, a neurological opinion is essential. Of 60 children with brain tumours who had headache at the time of diagnosis, half had diffuse, and a quarter each, lateral or occipital headaches; 51 showed neurological or eye abnormalities within two months of the onset of the headache; two-thirds had papilloedema (Honig and Charney 1982). A CT or MRI scan will almost always confirm or refute the diagnosis.

CHEST PAIN

It is the adolescent, rather than the younger child, who appears to present most commonly with recurrent pain in the chest, and of 100 young people with chronic chest pain, over half were worried that there was something wrong with their hearts and 12 per cent feared cancer (Pantell and Goodman 1983).

Before reassurance that all is well, obvious disease of the heart, lungs, oesophagus, and spine needs to be excluded. Does the pain have the features of angina? is it accentuated consistently by exercise? are there shortness of breath, cough, or sputum? does eating or drinking bring on the discomfort? is the child well in himself? On examination is there a heaving displaced apex beat or a significant cardiac murmur or hypertension? are there added sounds in the lungs or a reduced peak flow? is the pain provoked by pressing the chest wall or spine or getting the young person to touch his toes? Organic causes are rare but surprises occur:

James, aged 15, who hadn't attended the surgery for 3 years, and whose father was on anticoagulants following a previous heart-attack, came to see his GP on a couple of occasions with pain over the sternum. Nothing was found on examination except for unconvincing tenderness and appropriate reassurance was given. A few days later his mother saw the GP to have her blood pressure checked 'Has James told you about the large bruise that appeared two weeks ago?' she asked. His full blood count disclosed leukaemia from which he subsequently died.

Bibliography

Apley, J., MacKeith, R., and Meadow, R. (1978). *The child and his symptoms: a comprehensive approach*, (3rd edn). Blackwell Scientific Publications, Oxford. (Useful and enjoyable classic.)

Christensen, M. F. and Mortensen, O. (1978). Long-term prognosis in children with recurrent and abdominal pain. *Archives of Disease in Childhood*, **50**, 110–4.

Honig, P. J. and Charney, E. B. (1982). Children with brain tumour headaches. *American Journal of Diseases of Children*, **136**, 121–4.

Lance, J. W. (1992). Treatment of migraine. *Lancet*, **339**, 1027–9.

Murphy, M. S. (1993). Management of recurrent abdominal pain. *Archives of Disease in Childhood*, **69**, 409–11.

Pantell, R. H. and Goodman, B. W. (1983). Adolescent chest pain: a prospective study. *Pediatrics*, **71**, 881–7.

Tal, Y., Dunn, H. G., and Chrichton, J. V. (1984). Childhood migraine—a dangerous diagnosis? *Acta Paediactrica Scandinavica*, **73**, 55–9.

Turner, R. M. (1978). Recurrent abdominal pain in childhood. *Journal of the Royal College of General Practitioners*, **28**, 729–9.

20 Surgical problems

ACUTE ABDOMINAL PAIN

An organic cause for recurrent abdominal pain is only found in under 10 per cent of affected children, a problem discussed in Chapter 19. Here we consider quite another issue, acute abdominal pain occurring without a previous history. Most affected children will have unimportant illness; a few will be starting the weary round of recurrent abdominal pain; an important small minority will have a serious organic cause. In these, other symptoms are almost always present and give a clue to the diagnosis.

After babyhood, the common causes are gastro-enteritis, with colicky pain, vomiting, and watery diarrhoea (p. 207); perhaps dietary indiscretion; and pain associated with upper respiratory tract infection. This latter in its severe form, 'mesenteric adenitis', may cause moderately severe abdominal tenderness which tends to have moved on re-examination. At operation enlarged mesenteric lymph nodes are found.

The catalogue of the rarer causes is long. It includes appendicitis, with anorexia, vomiting, and persistent and sometimes severe pain and local tenderness; and, especially in younger patients, intussusception, in which screaming attacks are associated with pallor and, later, bloody stools. Both are discussed later in this chapter. Hepatitis, especially in the pre-icteric phase, is a cause of upper abdominal discomfort; there is bile in the urine. Urinary infection surprisingly infrequently presents with acute abdominal pain as the most prominent feature, though loin tenderness may be found in older children. Renal stones or intermittent hydronephrosis may give rise to severe flank pain, often radiating towards the genitalia.

Disorders outside the abdomen are often forgotten. Pneumonia may start with abdominal pain and rigidity, together with a reversed respiratory rhythm and flaring of the alae nasi. Testicular torsion will be overlooked if the genitalia are not examined; the hernial orifices can be inspected and palpated at the same time. Rarer causes include pancreatitis, especially in mumps; septicaemia with rapidly progressive prostration; Henoch–Schönlein purpura with rash and joint pains; the ketoacidosis of diabetes; and, in African-Caribbean children, sickle cell crises. There are many other rarities.

THE BABY

In a baby, the big problem is to decide whether the abdomen is indeed the seat of a painful disorder or not. Quite apart from evening 'colic' in the first few months of life, painful screaming may be a symptom of conditions as diverse as otitis media, gastro-enteritis, a fractured limb from child abuse, or osteomyelitis. The more severely ill baby may be suffering from meningitis or septicaemia. In general, if the doctor notes that the belly is not abnormally distended (remembering that all babies' abdomens are rather full); if he finds no tenderness on gentle palpitation; and if he does a rectal examination without finding a gush of watery stool, blood on the finger, or an unexpected mass, the abdomen is unlikely to be the culprit although the urinary tract may be. Amongst abdominal causes, intestinal obstruction is more common in infants than in older children. If vomit is bile stained, an obstructive cause is more likely. Obstructed hernias, congenital bands and other malformations are the leading causes. Intussusception is also a baby and toddler complaint. Appendicitis at this age is often diagnosed late, for abdominal tenderness is very easy to miss in the early stages. Of course, gastro-enteritis and otitis media are much commoner than any of these in babies who seem to be in pain.

ACUTE APPENDICITIS

On average the GP will only see one child a year with acute appendicitis, but the incidence of perforation rises with delay in diagnosis. Although parents sometimes wait too long before calling the doctor, they more commonly call too early. If the child is seen less than six hours after the pain has started, it is often impossible to reach a diagnosis; reassessment is needed four hours or so later. There are several reasons why the diagnosis is often delayed:

1. The pain is often intermittent or relatively mild, or the child is keeping a stiff upper lip and not complaining, sometimes because he is afraid he will be sent to hospital. Truly continuous abdominal pain, even if mild, is rare in childhood and should suggest appendicitis, as should abdominal pain aggravated by coughing or by movement of the anterior abdominal wall.

2. The tenderness is at an unusual site, such as the right flank, or the pain began in the right iliac fossa rather than centrally, or it remained central.

3. The patient is very young. Appendicitis can occur at any age but is particularly difficult to diagnose in children under three who do not complain of localized pain. Fortunately, the GP need only expect one such case every 20 years. The high proportion of such patients with perforation—90 per cent in the preschool child (Rappaport *et al.* 1989)—is probably due to delay in diagnosis.

4. The GP forgets that it is diagnostically helpful to do a rectal examination in the doubtful case:

A doctor was called during the night to see Jimmy, a 5-year-old. He had just developed severe central abdominal pain and diarrhoea. No abdominal signs were discovered and he was re-examined 6 hours later. By that time the pulse was 104 and the temperature 38 °C. There was some suprapubic tenderness but no dysuria; he did have definite tenderness on the right on rectal examination. After admission to hospital Jimmy was observed for a further 24 hours, by which time he had developed an abscess from his acute pelvic appendicitis.

5. The occasional presentation without typical features is overlooked:

Richard, age 2½ years, was taken to casualty at a weekend because of apparent pain on micturition. Antibiotics were started after a urine culture, but the urine subsequently only grew a mixed growth of organisms. There was a mild improvement. Three days later the parents returned because Richard refused to stand on his right leg. An early out-patient appointment was made, but they returned the next day. It was then obvious the child was seriously ill. Despite the absence of clear abdominal pain at any stage, a retrocaecal appendix abscess was drained.

The trite truth is that a diagnosis of appendicitis is reached on the basis of history, examination and, often, re-examination. Diagnosis gets easier as time passes; the last doctor is the lucky one.

The child will usually have been sick within a few hours of the pain starting, but even if not, will be anorectic. The pulse rate and temperature (unless the child has recently had an antipyretic) are likely to be somewhat raised, but are not always. A few points of paediatric technique sometimes help with further assessment. Young children of three years or so may be willing to select from a choice of leading questions when they will not formulate an answer for themselves: 'Is it a coming-and-going pain, or is it a there-all-the-time pain?' 'Did the pain start where it is now, or did it start somewhere else in your tummy?' Observe the patient carefully, leaving abdominal palpation to the end. Typically he will lie relatively still, as movement or coughing aggravate the pain. In the early stages he may roll around to get relief. Young children usually breathe abdominally but, when they have acute appendicitis, they hold their abdominal wall rigid and take shorter quicker breaths using their rib cage. If the respiratory rate is markedly raised the child may have pneumonia or, rarely, diabetic ketoacidosis rather than appendicitis. The breath may smell and the tongue is usually furred. The presence of tonsillitis is a pointer to acute mesenteric adenitis but, unfortunately, can also occur in appendicitis.

It is often best to start the examination by focusing on a less uncomfortable area, usually the chest. In a small child the abdomen is most easily examined while he is sitting on the mother's lap, or while he is holding her hand if he is already in bed. First, ask him to point out the most tender spot, though, if the child is asleep when first seen, it is worthwhile trying to palpate the abdomen before he wakes up. Start palpation on the side away from the pain, moving gradually round towards it. All the while talk to the child and ask him questions, in an attempt to distract him from the examination. The maximum tenderness and guarding are usually on the right but sometimes are, unfortunately, in an atypical place. As in the above case history, an inflamed appendix lying on the psoas muscle may cause pain on extension of the hip. Localized tenderness is not easy to demonstrate in a child under three years, but if convincingly present is an important sign. Generalized rigidity may well mean peritonitis. A tender, ill-demarcated mass (an appendix abscess secondary to a missed appendicitis) may present late. Usually there will have been a preceding history of pain, vomiting, and malaise, and perhaps diarrhoea.

The child with mesenteric adenitis usually has a higher temperature, cervical lymphadenitis, and vaguer abdominal tenderness, which, as mentioned earlier, seems to move from place to place on repeated examination.

INTUSSUSCEPTION

There are 700 admissions a year for intussusception; one for every 40 GPs (Stringer *et al.* 1992). Classically, the infant is aged between 3–18 months with a peak between five and nine months. About a fifth are over two. It is often triggered by an intercurrent respiratory or gastro-enteric viral infection. A swollen Peyer's patch gets sucked down the gut by peristalsis, which then starts to pull the following segment of intestine inside out. The diagnosis may easily be missed against a background of non-specific malaise induced by the infection. Intermittent screaming attacks are characteristic; each bout associated with marked pallor and a drawing up of the legs. Early diagnosis is important, for the chance of avoiding bowel resection diminishes with each hour that passes. Also, in the early stages, treatment can be non-surgical by techniques such as a controlled barium enema.

Although initially the toddler may be surprisingly well between bouts of pain, later he becomes obviously languid and stops feeding. He soon becomes constipated and eventually bloody mucus is passed; the "redcurrant-jelly" stool. Passage of blood is a late sign and is present in less than 50 per cent. Vomiting may be a feature, initially of gastric contents, but later containing bile.

Attention to the intermittency of the symptoms and to the striking pallor when the baby screams should give the necessary clues at an early stage. If blood is being passed per rectum or there are any signs of persistent shock, treatment is even more urgent. On examination a mass may be palpable, but only if the patient is able to relax; rectal examination is vital in all infants in whom intussusception is suspected. If there is blood, with, perhaps, mucus on the examining finger, the child must be referred to hospital. In the first few hours of the disease normal stools may be passed and the GP may need to reassess the child a short while after the original consultation.

Crying babies and toddlers with vague tummy upsets causing anorexia and a few vomits may worry the doctor. They do not develop the striking pallor of a child whose intestine is being pulled inside out during each episode of peristalsis; neither does the infant with frank gastro-enteritis in whom watery diarrhoea (not a common feature of intussusception) is usually found. Gastro-enteritis with bloody diarrhoea, often from campylobacter infection, or possibly from shigella, poses more of a problem because these children have both abdominal pain and bloody diarrhoea. The belly of any child with gastro-enteritis and blood in the stool must thus be carefully examined for a mass. Re-examination after a few hours is often wise for, despite the usual prominence of pain and pallor in a typical case, one in seven children with intussusception have no obvious discomfort. About 10 per cent have recurrent intussusception, sometimes because of an underlying cause such as an intestinal polyp or a Meckel's diverticulum.

ACUTE INTESTINAL OBSTRUCTION

Obstruction is rare but important. As in adults, the hallmarks are severe colic, persistent vomiting, distention with visible peristalsis, and constipation. The main diagnostic error is to mistake intestinal obstruction for gastro-enteritis. There may be some loose stools passed in the former but only a small amount. A substantial gush of a watery stool is always a reassuring bit of evidence in favour of the much commoner gastro-enteritis. In doubtful cases a squirt can usually be elicited by a gentle rectal examination; one of the reasons we find this a useful procedure.

RECTAL BLEEDING

In a well child by far the commonest cause of specks of bright red blood in the faeces is hard stools. Presumably they cause minor abrasions and tears around the anal margin, although often no definite lesion can be seen. An attempt to soften the stool is a good initial move, being both diagnostic and therapeutic in many cases. Rectal bleeding is also seen with bacterial gastro-enteritis and, as mentioned, intussusception.

Much rarer are polyps which can be treated endoscopically but are hard to visualize. If bleeding without constipation (even in a well child) is really recurrent, referral is necessary, if possible to a centre at which paediatric endoscopy is available. Recurrent blood in loose stools may be a sign of cows' milk allergy, or of Crohn's disease, or ulcerative colitis. A substantial haemorrhage of fresh blood, although rare, may come from a Meckel's diverticulum, as may melaena.

Rectal bleeding due to haemorrhagic disease of the newborn is a possibility in the breast-fed newborn who may have not have received intramuscular vitamin K (p. 259).

RECTAL PROLAPSE

A rectal prolapse is an alarming event for both parent and doctor, but it is not of itself a dangerous symptom. Usually a swab or handkerchief placed over the offending mass will lead to reduction. A common cause appears to be a toddler sitting on a potty on the floor for long periods of time. Stopping the training for a few weeks helps. The symptom usually settles with time, especially if any associated constipation is relieved. Prolapse may occur in malnourished babies and toddlers, especially those with cystic fibrosis. For this reason, a sweat test (or DNA test) should be arranged.

HYDROCELES AND INGUINAL HERNIAS

Both result from a patent processus vaginalis (PPV) and can co-exist. In the hydrocele the opening is small, in the hernia large enough to admit contents from the peritoneal cavity. They are particularly common in premature infants with an incidence as high as 30 per cent in infants weighing <1000 g (Harper *et al.* 1975). A hernia may be noticed from birth onwards and usually presents during the first year of life. Often the mother brings the child to the GP because she has noticed a lump in the groin which may extend into the scrotum and is particularly prominent when the child cries. If the parent thinks the child has an intermittent swelling, but the doctor cannot detect it, the patient will usually turn out to have a hernia. Most inguinal lumps are hernias. Occasionally a lymph node or an undescended testis is responsible. If the swelling extends into the scrotum it may be confused with a hydrocele. It is not possible to get above the swelling if it is a hernia, whereas one can if it is a hydrocele.

If a hernia is present it can usually be reduced by gentle pressure. In babies this is often easily achieved after soothing them with a feed. If the hernia cannot be reduced after a good try the child should be admitted to hospital where sedation and elevation of the legs will usually be successful. After such incarceration the surgeon will want to wait a day or two before repair, as local oedema around the hernia makes the procedure more difficult.

Most surgeons operate as soon as a diagnosis is made, especially in children under one year. Prompt referral limits the small but real risk of strangulation following incarceration. In one series of children with inguinal hernias, 27/37 hernias in male neonates and 72/1994 in older children were irreducible on presentation (Wilson-Story 1987). Most of the latter reduced with conservative treatment, but strangulation of the bowel, especially in neonates, was an important complication. At surgery, a prophylactic repair on the unaffected side may prevent a contra-lateral hernia developing later. Inguinal hernias in girls are rather unusual. One per cent of girls with inguinal hernias turn out to be genetic males.

An infantile hydrocele is, in effect, a hernial sac without a hernia. Most resolve spontaneously. The swelling, often bilateral, is not usually tense, being in communication with the peritoneal cavity. If the swelling has not gone by the age of two to three years operative intervention should be considered, as after this age the PPV is unlikely to close spontaneously and may evolve into a later hernia.

It is important to be aware that hydroceles may be associated with hernias. Though hydroceles transilluminate, hernias in infancy may also do so. A hernia indicates a large PPV and the chances of spontaneous closure appear to be small. The 'cured' inguinal hernia often reappears later.

THE TESTES

Undescended testes

One or both testes are undescended in about 3.8 per cent of full-term and in almost half of infant boys weighing less than 2000 g at birth. This percentage falls to 1.6 overall by three months of age, after which age later descent is unlikely (John Radcliffe Hospital Cryptorchidism Study Group 1992). The cremaster muscle is relaxed in the first weeks of life and it is easy to assess whether the testes are fully descended or not. If a note is made at this stage that two testes are present, it can prevent bother later when the boy is brought to the GP because the parents cannot find them.

The doctor's most usual role in this area is to try and distinguish between normal retractile testes and those which are incompletely descended. Sometimes the problem can be solved by asking the parents to note if two testes are present when the child is in a warm bath.

The retractile testis is a normal testis from a normal scrotum drawn up into the superficial inguinal pouch by contraction of the cremasteric muscle. The boy should first be examined standing, when the presence of any inguinal bulge can be noticed as well as the normality, or otherwise of the external genitalia. If the scrotum is undergrown on one side, genuinely incomplete descent is likely.

If the doctor's warm finger is run gently down the line of the inguinal canal towards the scrotum a retractile testis will be felt in the superficial pouch (the subcutaneous tissue immediately superficial to the external ring). In this way most testes can be coaxed gently into the scrotum. If they can be made to enter the scrotum the parent can be reassured that there is no problem. Another sometimes successful manoeuvre in stubborn cases is to ask the boy to squat, which may relax the cremaster enough for the testes to descend. If the parents or older child are shown the descended testes, reassurance is more effective.

An undescended testis is one stuck in its normal course of descent. It may be in the abdomen, inside the inguinal canal, or at the inguinal ring. An ectopic testis may be easily palpable in the inguinal pouch superficial to the canal, but cannot be eased into the scrotum. Undescended and ectopic testes are an embarrassment to the teenage child. They are also more exposed to trauma than normal testes and may be associated with indirect inguinal hernias. They are at least 10 times more likely to undergo malignant change, and spermatogenesis is diminished in testes which are not in the scrotum. For all these reasons operative intervention to bring the testes down is recommended. To achieve optimal spermatogenesis later, it is thought that surgery should be done by the age of two (Spitz 1983). However, even with late operation between the ages of 7 and 14 years of age, 75 per cent of those with unilateral and 33 per cent of those with bilateral surgery achieved normal sperm counts after puberty (Puri and O'Donnell 1988). Early orchidopexy reduces the risk of cancer (Woodhouse 1992).

Torsion

Twisting of the spermatic cord is an important emergency in both neonates and pre- and post-pubertal teenage boys. It presents with abdominal or groin pain, vomiting, and a swollen tender testis and scrotum. Unless the torsion unwinds spontaneously, or is relieved surgically within six hours, the testis will be lost. The common error is to mistake a torsion for epididymitis, the latter condition being very rarely seen in children. Antibiotic treatment for an acutely inflamed testis in a teenager usually implies a bad diagnostic error. The tendency to develop a torsion depends on an underlying anatomical variant, usually bilateral. After one testis has developed torsion the other testis remains at risk and should be stitched down.

If the child presents with a history of severe self-limiting testicular pain and swelling, he may have had a torsion which unwound spontaneously. Because of the risk of recurrence it is worth considering referral for a bilateral anchoring of the testes. In some children with the clinical picture of torsion only the appendix testis has twisted; an unimportant event usually only diagnosed at surgery.

UMBILICAL PROBLEMS

The umbilical cord usually contains two arteries and one vein. Up to a third of all neonates with only a single artery in their cord have malformations, some of which may not be evident externally.

Umbilical hernias are particularly common in African children. The majority cure themselves by the age of three. Strapping is not advisable as it makes the skin sore. Hypothyroid babies have a very high incidence of umbilical hernias, which may be a diagnostic pointer in white babies, who may have escaped neonatal hypothyroid screening.

Umbilical granulomas are small tags of granulation tissue seen sticking out of the umbilical stump of young babies. They can be shrivelled by touching with a small stick of silver nitrate, protecting the surrounding skin with Vaseline. The treatment may have to be repeated. Those with a narrow base can be treated by tying a suture tightly around the base of the granuloma, which subsequently drops off. The rare umbilical fistulous polyp is a firmer brighter pink with perhaps leakage of urine or faeces.

LYMPH-NODE ABSCESS

Occasionally, a feverish child will present with a large tender lump below the jaw or high in the neck. Such inflamed lymph nodes are usually infected with staphylococci and will respond to a course of oral flucloxacillin. It is wise to continue the drug until the mass has almost completely resolved, otherwise the infection may flare up again. Sometimes the overlying skin becomes red, and the GP detects an area of softening over the gland. Such children will almost always have to have the abscess drained.

Other long-standing, mid line or lateral lumps in the neck may be ectopic thyroid tissue or congenital cysts, such as branchial cysts, which should be referred for diagnosis before superadded infection occurs.

Abscesses in the groin are seen in infants who may be so well in themselves, that the fluctuant lump is mistaken for a hernia. It is in a more lateral position. If an infected groin gland is not fluctuant it will again usually resolve with oral flucloxacillin.

THE PENIS

Circumcision

Apart from religious reasons, it seems odd that some parents should consider it necessary to arrange for a portion, however small, of their child's penis to be removed so soon after birth. There are few medical indications for circumcision. The operation probably does not significantly reduce the chance of the child's future partner developing carcinoma of the cervix, although it may protect the child himself from penile carcinoma, which is very rare in circumcised Jews. As this carcinoma accounts for only 0.1 per cent of deaths from malignant disease in men, any benefit is marginal. Most penile carcinomas develop in men whose tightly non-retractile foreskin has prevented cleaning of the glans for many years.

The foreskin is almost always unretractable at birth. However, by the age of four years, 90 per cent of boys have a retractile foreskin which means that very few need to be referred to a surgeon (Davenport 1996). The size of the hole in the foreskin, seen when it is pulled downwards over the glans, is misleadingly small. To get a true idea, the two opposite sides of the hole in the foreskin should be held with the finger and thumb of either hand and pulled upwards and apart. A large passage all the way down to the glans will usually be reassuringly revealed.

Balanitis is common in young children and is not an indication for circumcision unless it is recurrent and occurs in the older child. It may be a part of nappy rash. More likely it is a local infection, with sub-prepucial pus. Mild cases resolve with washing. More severely affected children will need systemic antibiotics. The child may find it so uncomfortable to micturate he is only willing to do so in the bath. It is worth noting that most cases of dysuria in boys are caused by balanitis.

Ballooning of the foreskin during micturition is an indication to check the patency of the orifice in the manner just described; it will usually be normal. However, bacteriologically confirmed recurrent urinary tract infections, if associated with a convincingly tight foreskin, may be an occasional indication for circumcision, or, preferably, for a stretch under anaesthesia.

Hypospadias

Hypospadias is the result of failure or delay of fusion of the urethral folds and occurs in 1:400 male births. The urethral meatus opens on the ventral aspect of the penis and there may be a ventral curving of the penis (chordee), more apparent when the boy has an erection. Operative reconstruction may be done early, so referral at the time of diagnosis is indicated. Repair may involve using the prepuce; thus, before full assessment, circumcision is strictly contra-indicated. An abdominal ultrasound examination is needed because of the possible association between renal tract malformation and hypospadias.

Bibliography

Davenport, M. (1996). Problems with penis and prepuce. *British Medical Journal*, **312**, 299–301,

Harper, R. G., Garcia, A., and Sia, C. (1975). Inguinal hernia: A common problem of premature infants weighing 1,000 grams or less at birth. *Pediatrics*, **56**, 112.

John Radcliffe Hospital Cryptorchidism Study Group. (1992). Cryptorchidism: a prospective study of 7,500 consecutive male births, 1984–8. *Archives of Disease in Childhood*, **67**, 892–9.

Puri, P. and O'Donnell, B. (1988). Semen analysis in patients who had orchidopexy at or after 7 years of age. *Lancet*, **ii**, 1051.

Rappaport, W. D., Peterson, M., and Stanton, C. (1989). Factors responsible for the high perforation rate seen in early childhood appendicitis. *American Journal of Surgery*, **55**, 602–5.

Spitz, L. (1983). Maldescent of the testis. *Archives of Disease in Childhood*, **58**, 847.

Stringer, M. D., Pledger, G., and Drake, D. P. (1992). Childhood deaths from intussusception in England and Wales 1984–9. *British Medical Journal*, **304**, 737–9.

Wilson-Story, D. (1987). Scrotal swellings in the under 5. *Archives of Disease in Childhood*, **62**, 50–2.

Woodhouse, C. R. J. (1992). Late malignancy risk in urology. *British Journal of Urology*, **70**, 345–51.

21 Bones, joints, and limbs

POSTURAL DEFORMITIES OF THE FEET AND LEGS

Parents frequently consult about their toddlers' posture or gait. Fortunately most children's legs and feet are normal, even if they point in slightly unusual directions. The best advice is, with few exceptions, to do nothing. Important but rarer deformities, such as congenital dislocation of the hip, which do require prompt attention, or club feet, may result from exposure to an abnormal pressure *in utero*. For example, they are slightly more common after amniocentesis, presumably from oligohydramnios associated with continued loss of amniotic fluid. Abnormal intrauterine moulding also underlies some of the milder abnormalities of posture.

The foot of an infant is very mobile; it can be plantarflexed, so that the forefoot becomes a continuation of the tibia, or dorsiflexed so that the dorsum of the foot touches the front of the leg, and abducted or adducted to about 45 degrees. If an infant's foot can be put through this full range of movements there is usually no need for great concern, although, if the foot is kept in a very abnormal position at rest, strapping under the direction of an orthopaedic surgeon may be necessary, especially if the foot cannot be easily restored to the neutral position and slightly beyond. Usual mobility is not present in the foot of a child with talipes equinovarus, the commonest form of club foot. The foot is so twisted that the sole faces medially, and, if neglected, the child will end up bearing his weight on the outer border of his foot or even on its dorsum.

The normal foot of a toddler is somewhat chubby, and the fat pad on the medial aspect makes it look flat. When he starts to walk it is on a flat base, sometimes with everted feet, giving the impression, for a while, of flat-footed gait. By the time the child is 2½ years, the heel of the shoe will show maximum wear on the outer aspect of the mid line, a useful way of reassuring the mother that 'flat feet' are not present. Over- and underlapping toes are also relatively common. They will often concern parents, but will need surgical correction only if it becomes a problem to find comfortable shoes. Usually a child's foot and leg can be rotated equally, both externally and internally, most of the movement taking place at the hip joint. In children with 'in' or 'out toeing', rotation is restricted in the opposite direction to that in which the feet point. No treatment is needed provided that there is no associated neurological abnormality and the hips are not dislocated.

Metatarsus varus is an uncommon condition in which only the front part of the foot turns inwards. In the normal foot a straight line extended distally from the middle of the heel should run between the second and third toes; the line lies further lateral in metatarsus varus. The condition causes little disability but leads to problems in finding shoes that fit properly. Treatment by splinting appears to be rather effective in early infancy but gets more difficult later on, so it is probably worth referring these children early, especially if the adduction cannot be easily corrected. We have never referred a child with flat feet or 'in' or 'out toeing' to an orthopaedic surgeon—so far this has not rebounded on us.

A few serious rarities may be mistaken for postural deformities of the foot. Congenital dislocation of the hip will cause shortening and is discussed below. Cerebral palsy (the motor defect from a non-progressive damage to the developing brain), or a spinal cord tumour or malformation will usually lead to an odd gait, asymmetrical posture, reduced muscle bulk, and brisk tendon reflexes, as well as, perhaps, to developmental delay, and urinary infections or dribbling in the case of a spinal lesion. A generalized muscle disorder such as muscular dystrophy will be associated with general hypotonia and hypermobility of the joints at first, followed by deformity, and contractures later in childhood.

The appearance of bow legs is common in infants. If, when the child is lying down with his legs extended and his medial malleoli in contact, a gap of more than 5 cm (2 in) is seen between the femoral condyles, an X-ray of the knees and the wrists may be wise to exclude rickets and rare epiphyseal disorders. Unilateral bowing should also always be investigated. Knock-knees as a normal variant are common and usually disappear by the time the child is about seven years old. If the gap between the medial malleoli of a 3- to 4-year-old is 10 cm or more, referral is indicated. For children with a gap of 5–10 cm, review after six months to assess whether the gap is narrowing seems sufficient action.

Vitamin D deficiency rickets is seen in non-white, especially Asian, toddlers and teenagers. As well as knock-knees or bow legs, the child will have wide wrists and may be hypotonic. The well known rickety rosary is not very easy to demonstrate; it is best seen as a row of bumps coursing downwards and outwards on either side of the sternum. It is surprisingly far lateral. An X-ray of the wrist or knee will confirm the diagnosis. In all ethnic groups, rickets is occasionally seen in children with renal failure, with malabsorption, or with one of a number of genetic defects of vitamin D metabolism, perhaps with a family history.

CONGENITAL DISLOCATION OF THE HIP (CDH)

The incidence of this condition in the UK is about 2 per 1000 live births but up to ten times this number of hips may show instability in the early weeks of life. About 40–50 newborn babies will be added to the average GP's list each year. This means he will examine an infant with unstable hip every one to two years, hardly enough to maintain his skill in examination. But it is still worth doing, for the paediatric senior house officer (SHO) is equally likely to find it a difficult test to perform. As with other screening procedures, children at higher risk deserve particular attention. These risk factors include a positive family history, breech delivery, Caesarean section, foot deformities, oliogohydramnios and fetal growth retardation. CDH is also commoner in girls than boys. Treatment in early infancy by splinting may allow normal development of initially dislocated hips which otherwise require surgery; not always successful. Early diagnosis depends on screening and techniques are clearly explained in a working party report (Special report 1986).

Neonatal diagnosis is achieved by testing for hip dislocatability using the Barlow test. The infant is laid on his back on a firm surface. The knee and hip on one side are flexed and the hip to be tested adducted. The pelvis is held still with one hand, while the other grasps the flexed adducted leg with the middle fingers placed over the greater trochanter and the thumb pressing on the inner aspect of the thigh. Joint stability is then tested by attempting to push the femur vertically downwards to dislocate the femoral head posteriorly out of the acetabulum. After this, the flexed leg is then abducted which will return a dislocated femoral head to the acetabulum with a palpable clunk. This rather uncomfortable procedure, which should be gently performed lest it damage a normal hip, is more easily demonstrated than described. 'Ligamentous clicks *without* movement of the head of the femur in or out of the acetabulum may be elicited in 5–10 per cent of hips and should be disregarded' (Special report 1986). If the hip is dislocatable or there is any limitation of abduction the child must be promptly referred to prevent permanent dislocation. Dislocatability is most easily picked up in the first two or three days of life and the test is only useful until about three months of age. 'Classical' signs are more useful from about six weeks of age onwards. Of these, limitation of abduction is the most important—with the infant supine and the hip flexed to about 90 degrees the thigh normally can be abducted to 75 degrees. Other signs include above knee shortening of the limb, detected by measuring the distance between the anterior superior spine and the medium malleolus, a flat buttock, asymmetry of the skin creases, persistent external rotation of the leg, and, in the second year, a limp or waddling gait.

Bilateral dislocation is always more difficult to spot than unilateral. Hip X-ray is little use until three or four months of age, when the femoral head becomes calcified, but ultrasound is helpful (Berman and Klenerman 1986).

Dislocation of the hip may present after the newborn period, either in a child in whom it was missed at birth, or in whom it has developed later, perhaps because of a poorly formed acetabulum, as in acetabular dysplasia. This is why examination of the hips is recommended on a number of occasions in the first few years of life. If a mother is worried because of her toddler's 'funny walk', she should not be dismissed out of hand.

Margaret aged nine, was brought to the GP with a 'rolling' gait. The mother said that she had first mentioned it to a doctor when Margaret was 2 or 3. On examination the left femur was 2 cm shorter than the right and there was wasting of the thigh muscles. An X-ray showed a poorly developed acetabulum, and a partially dislocated hip.

Late dislocation may also occur in neurological disorders in which muscular action around the joints is unbalanced, as in the spastic diplegic form of cerebral palsy.

THORAX

A prominent sternum (pigeon chest) or a concave sternum (funnel chest) occur in older children. When severe, they look quite disfiguring, causing psychological distress rather than impaired respiratory function. The former is very unusual. Occasionally these deformities are seen in certain syndromes, such as Marfan's syndrome. Harrison's sulcus, a circumferential indrawing about the rib margins, is usually due to undercontrolled asthma.

SPINE

Backache

Unlike the common spinal aches and pains after gymnastics and playing games, persistent central backache in children is uncommon and may be the sign of an underlying disorder. This is particularly true if there is associated limitation of movement. In these cases a neurological examination is important, as extradural tumours can present with backache, stiffness, and an abnormal gait. An X-ray, including a lateral view, is indicated to identify such entities as spondylolisthesis, in which one vertebral body slips forward on the one below, or Scheuermann's disease, a form of osteochondritis. It may also be abnormal with a spinal tumour. Prolapsed discs occur in teenagers, and ankylosing spondylitis, an uncommon disorder, may be found in an older boy who has pain and stiffness in the back and whose X-ray sometimes discloses involvement of the sacro-iliac joint. Over 90 per cent of patients with ankylosing spondylitis possess the tissue type HLA B27 and the clinical diagnosis of this disease is unlikely to be correct unless the patient carries this antigen on his white blood cells. An unwell child with persistent backache, limitation of movements, and, perhaps, a raised sedimentation rate (ESR), may be suffering from spinal tuberculosis or a low-grade osteomyelitis. Isotope bone scans are helpful in the diagnosis.

Scoliosis

In idiopathic scoliosis a side to side curve and spinal rotation develop in the presence of apparently normally formed vertebrae and in the absence of muscular weakness. It is most easily recognized when the patient, usually a girl, is asked to bend forward with her arms hanging freely. The doctor looks along the now horizontal thoracic spine from behind. In this position a gross prominence of one side of the rib cage (usually the right) indicates scoliosis. Most cases of scoliosis occur in adolescent girls, but can also occur in infants and young children, usually involving mid- or lower thoracic region with curve to the left in almost all cases. Infantile scoliosis tends to resolve spontaneously, but the adolescent form may progress rapidly, ending up as a grossly 'hunched back' which may compress the lungs and lead to serious pulmonary disease in adult life. The problem is to identify which mildly scoliotic teenager is at risk of this. Treatment by bracing is only required if serial X-rays show the curve to be becoming progressively marked (about one in seven affected children). It is then urgent if very major surgery is to be avoided. The GP could thus test for scoliosis when he happens to be examining the torso of his early teenage patients. However, routine clinical screening is not at present recommended, as the test identifies many children with mild spinal curves, best left alone rather than referred (Hall 1991).

CONGENITAL TORTICOLLIS (STERNO-MASTOID TUMOUR)

In this condition, a young infant presents with his head tilted slightly to one side. On examination there is often a firm swelling in the mid portion of the shortened sterno-mastoid muscle—the 'tumour'. It is probably a haematoma arising as a result of tearing of muscle fibres, perhaps during a difficult delivery. Repeated gentle rotation of the head to stretch the shortened muscle (perhaps under the direction of the physiotherapist) is usually associated with gradual resolution over the first few weeks of life, though the face may remain slightly asymmetrical. In a gross case, a neck X-ray is useful to exclude an underlying vertebral anomaly.

PAINFUL JOINTS

A detailed history (most are due to trauma) and a thorough and unhurried examination are vital in clarifying the wide range of differential diagnosis of a child with a painful joint or joints. Partial or complete loss of function rather than pain *per se* is the most obvious feature of acute joint disorders in very young children. Although the leg is more commonly involved than the arm, the same diagnostic approach applies to either. A checklist of questions is useful.

1. *Is the joint swollen?*

It is also important to distinguish between arthritis, which is usually characterized by inflammation causing swollen, red, hot, painful, and stiff joints, and arthralgia, where there is only joint pain. On the whole, arthralgia is less likely to have a serious underlying cause.

2. *Is the child of African-Caribbean origin?*
Sickle cell disease may cause joint or bone pain in an older child, and painful, swollen fingers and toes—the hand–foot syndrome—in toddlers (p. 254).

3. *Is the child unwell?*
An ill, febrile child with a single, painful, swollen joint has septic arthritis until proven otherwise. There is usually a striking limitation of joint movement, but in babies this feature is not quite so reliable as it is in older children. If the diagnosis is suspected, the child should be referred for an urgent needle aspiration or exploration of the affected joint, perhaps preceded by an ultrasound examination. Even with early diagnosis, surgical lavage of the joint, and intravenous antibiotics, the child may be left with a handicap. The risk of a fixed joint or a poor limb growth or necrosis of the femoral head in the hip joint, increases with delay in treatment. Thinking of septic arthritis in a child with fever and a stiff joint is as important as thinking of meningitis in a child with a cold and a severe headache. In either, antibiotics may mask the clinical picture. Septic arthritis of the hip is particularly easy to miss because the joint is difficult to inspect; always check hip movements with special care.

4. *How many joints are affected? How long have the symptoms been present for?*
Juvenile chronic arthritis (JCA) is a rare condition of which there are three main clinical sub-types. For formal diagnosis, symptoms must last for more than three months and other causes, such as post-viral arthritis, be excluded. A positive test for rheumatoid factor is very rare. Pauciarticular JCA affects up to four joints, usually knee, ankle, or elbow. Anti-nuclear antibodies may be found. The affected child should have slit lamp examination of the eyes every six months. Fifty per cent of these children develop asymptomatic uveitis and may go blind if untreated. Older boys with pauciarticular JCA sometimes develop juvenile ankylosing spondylitis. They will be HLA-B27 positive. In polyarticular JCA there is involvement of five or more joints. The third commonest subgroup present with systematic features: swinging pyrexia, lymphadenopathy, hepatosplenomegaly, anaemia, and a pink macular rash (typically during spikes of fever). Polyarthritis affecting small and medium-sized joints may occur weeks after the systemic symptoms. Glandular fever, endocarditis, tropical infections, and leukaemia must be considered in the differential diagnosis of systemic onset JCA.

Sally, aged 9, was seen with vague malaise and aches and pains. She was brought back 10 days later, by which time she had developed a limp and pain in the groin. She was somewhat pale with a moderate degree of lymphadenopathy. A blood count unfortunately disclosed the typical picture of acute lymphoblastic leukaemia.

5. *Does the child have a family history or symptoms of an inflammatory bowel disease?*
Of children with Crohn's disease or ulcerative colitis 10–15 per cent develop arthritis, which sometimes precedes bowel symptoms.

6. *Was there a preceding history of an illness?*
Joint symptoms starting one to three weeks after a streptococcal sore throat and associated with fever, carditis, erythema marginatum (erythematous macular rash with circinate borders), and subcutaneous nodules are diagnostic of rheumatic fever. The pain moves from one joint to another every two or three days. This disease has almost totally disappeared in the United Kingdom, except in recently arrived immigrants, although there have been recent outbreaks in the USA. After one attack, long-term penicillin prophylaxis is indicated to prevent progressive cardiac damage.

Viral infections, such as rubella, may also be followed by transient polyarthritis, as may parvovirus B19 infection (p. 162). Reiter's syndrome (non-bacterial urethritis, conjunctivitis, and arthritis) may follow gastro-intestinal infection with, for example, *Shigella flexneri.*

7. *Does the child have a rash?*
Children with Henoch-Schönlein (anaphylactoid) purpura have a rash which is often initially urticarial and, later, maculo-papular with purpuric elements. It is characteristically found on the extensor surfaces of the lower limbs and buttocks. Other features include a migratory polyarthralgia or polyarthritis affecting mainly knees, ankles, and elbows, swelling of the dorsum of hands and feet, colicky abdominal pain, and sometimes melaena or haematuria, with or without proteinuria. A small proportion of children with haematuria/proteinuria may progress to renal failure. Rash may also occur in children with Lyme disease (p. 169) and, as mentioned before, with systemic onset JCA and rheumatic fever.

8. *Is there a family or past history of bleeding disorders?*
If so, in boys a painful swollen joint may be due to haemarthrosis from haemophilia (p. 258).

9. *Is there a history of foreign travel?*
Brucellosis caused by *Brucella abortus* contracted from infected milk products may cause arthralgia along with low grade fever, rigors, malaise, and depression.

THE CHILD WITH A LIMP

Limp is more commonly a complaint in an older child. A toddler may present with refusal to get to his feet, usually on waking. In the infant the leg or arm is merely moved less than its fellow—pseudoparalysis. Examination of a limping toddler, in particular, is difficult. This group of patients always merits the five minutes necessary to gain their co-operation. Often they will have to be examined on their mother's lap before or after watching them walk along a corridor. Septic arthritis, appendicitis, and unexpected fractures may all be missed if the examination is not reasonably thorough, and it is almost impossible to be thorough if the child is screaming his head off. Do not accept too readily a history of minor trauma as the cause of the limp. A full range of knee movements should lead to the examination of the hip, as the diseased hip may cause pain around the knee. The differential diagnosis of a limp will vary according to the age of the child, whether the child is unwell, and whether the limp is a chronic one or of recent onset:

1. *Is the child well?*

In a toddler a short-lived limp may be the result of an injury sustained during an unobserved fall, while gait returning to normal when walking barefooted should make one think of ill-fitting shoes.

Transient synovitis of the hip or an 'observation hip' (as observation is the only intervention required of the GP) occurs in children (usually boys) around the age of five. There is a history of discomfort, pain perhaps in the knee, and of refusal to bear weight on the affected leg. There is modest limitation of abduction and internal hip rotation. If limitation is marked, if there is local tenderness and heat, or if the child is systematically ill, other more serious diagnoses are likely. With an obviously mild case in an older child, it is reasonable to try rest at home for a few days before proceeding, if the symptoms are not resolving, to an X-ray or an ultrasound scan (to look for fluid in the hip joint), full blood count and ESR. The symptoms can last up to two or three weeks and sometimes recur.

Perthes' disease results from avascular necrosis of the femoral head, in which the classical X-ray changes may be delayed for several weeks. It presents as a 'persistent observation hip' in a 4 to 11 year old boy, often small for his age. It is a condition which may cause rather little disability in childhood but which is believed to predispose to serious osteo-arthritis in early adult life. It may be bilateral in 15 per cent.

In the adolescent, slipped capital femoral epiphysis or problems in or about the knee (e.g. Osgood–Schlatter disease) are more common causes of a limp. X-ray will diagnose either.

2. *Is the child unwell?*

In the sick child osteomyelitis, septic arthritis, muscle spasm around the hip joint from a retrocaecal appendicitis, or, with a more indolent picture and anaemia, leukaemia or neuroblastoma are more likely.

In osteomyelitis the critical diagnostic point is to look for sharply localized bony tenderness. If osteomyelitis is suspected the doctor can, while chatting with the patient, feel gently over the entire surface of his limb. If the child has osteomyelitis, touching the site of the infection will lead to severe pain; the child gasps and spasms away from the examiner. This is characteristic and will be repeated whenever the doctor's finger, feeling gently over the bone, arrives at the same crucial exquisitely tender spot. This physical sign is only hard to elicit if the deeply placed bones, such as the pelvis or the upper femur, are affected. Pain and diffuse tenderness in this region in a febrile child may mean osteomyelitis.

X-ray changes in osteomyelitis take 10 days or longer to develop, an important cause of diagnostic error. Treatment must be started early, so that osteomyelitis has to be a clinical diagnosis unless radionuclide scans are available. These are positive earlier. Incidentally, a patient with cellulitis may be difficult to differentiate from one with osteomyelitis in whom there are overlying skin changes. An area of simple cellulitis is uncomfortable if prodded, but there is no single, acutely tender spot.

3. *How long has the child been limping?*
With a more long-standing picture, cerebral palsy, juvenile chronic arthritis, a missed congenital dislocation of the hip, or perhaps even late onset muscular dystrophy are all uncommon diagnoses. Limp as a behavioural disorder also occurs, but it is unlikely if there are reliable signs of limited hip mobility.

LIMB TRAUMA

It may be difficult to decide whether a child with a history of straightforward trauma to a limb requires an X-ray, usually following a visit to casualty. The answer is probably yes if there is any obvious deformity, marked swelling, or local tenderness, or if pain and lack of movement in a limb continues beyond a day or two. It is also often unwise to decline to X-ray a child whose parents are pressing for it, as fractures can occasionally occur without obvious signs. Bruising and skin discolouration following an injury may take a day or two to develop.

Infants and babies are difficult to assess. Refusal to use a limb or bear weight may result from a fracture. If this occurs immediately after the fall or knock and there are no other signs of a fracture, re-examination some hours later may save an unnecessary X-ray.

LIMB ACHES

1. *Is there really anything wrong with the joints at all?*
A recurrent complaint of arthralgia with unconfirmed reports of fever and no physical signs are more likely to indicate parental anxiety or school refusal than any of the many serious rarities mentioned. More common than any of these diagnoses is the clinical picture, seen in children of school age, of persistent mild to moderate aches and pains in the limb. So called 'growing pains' are nearly always completely harmless but may wake the child at night.

2. *Non-traumatic pain in and around the knee*
Occasionally it is referred pain from the hip or a sign of juvenile chronic arthritis. Osgood–Schlatter disease, due to osteochondrosis, is a relatively common cause of pain, associated with a tender prominent tibial tuberosity. An X-ray will usually confirm the diagnosis. There is no active treatment, and the usual orthopaedic advice appears to be to let the patient do as much physical exercise as he or she wishes, until the symptoms eventually settle down, often only after months or years.

Chondromalacia patellae leads to discomfort, most marked when walking up or down stairs. The patella is tender and it hurts when it is pushed back against the femur. Again, treatment is symptomatic, except in the most severe cases, when surgery can be considered. Low grade tenderness of the heel can also be due to osteochondrosis.

ISOLATED BONY SWELLING

A growing rather painless swelling identified for the first time in a teenager and initially thought to be an unexplained 'bony bruise' may be the first sign of an osteosarcoma. They often occur round the knee but may be seen anywhere on the skeleton. Initial diagnosis depends on X-ray. Prognosis after excision and chemotherapy is poor but improving.

Bibliography

Berman, L. and Klernerman, L. (1986). Ultrasound screening for hip abnormalities: preliminary findings in 1001 neonates. *British Medical Journal*, **293**, 719–22.

Hall, D. M. B. (ed.) (1991). *Health for all children,* (2nd edn). The report of the Joint Working Party on Child Health Surveillance. Oxford University Press.

Special report. (1986). Screening for detection of congenital dislocation of the hip. *Archives of Disease in Childhood*, **61**, 921–6.

22 Congenital disorders and genetic disease

Genetics is becoming more and more relevant to primary care. The aim of this chapter is to put this major development which affects existing and future babies and children, into context. Practice staff have an important role in educating and counselling carriers of common recessively inherited conditions (haemoglobin disorders, cystic fibrosis), in providing information to those offered testing elsewhere, and in referring carrier couples for genetic counselling. Many women attending for family planning advice intend to have a baby in the near future. This may be an ideal opportunity for preconception counselling. Antenatal care often includes several screening tests often inadequately explained. Being alert to the genetic components of handicap or chronic disease is important, so that the need to refer parents of children affected by these conditions for genetic advice is not overlooked. All members of a primary health care team who come into contact with parents or potential parents must be able to give basic genetic information. However, it may be advisable for larger practice teams to arrange for one member, perhaps a health visitor or practice nurse, to receive additional training in this area.

PRECONCEPTION ADVICE

It is helpful for the doctor and the health visitor to have a check list of topics to discuss with couples who intend to start a family (Table 22.1).

THE FAMILY TREE IN PRIMARY CARE

A basic family tree is a useful shorthand method of highlighting important family events (for example, separation or divorce, or premature death or severe illness of a parent or sibling) which the doctor needs to know to understand the family and its members' worries. In addition, issues of genetic significance may become

Table 22.1 Topics to cover in preconception advice

Previous obstetric history
Maternal (and paternal) smoking and drinking habits
Vitamin (especially folic acid) supplementation
Consequences of maternal disease (e.g. diabetes)
Effects of drugs at the time of conception (e.g. anti-epileptics)
Rubella/HIV status
Family history to identify genetic risk, unexplained stillbirth, or neonatal death
Ethnic group (haemoglobin disorders, Tay–Sachs disease)
Implications of advancing maternal/paternal age
Are the couple related?
(consanguineous marriage may increase the risk of a recessively inherited disorder)
Need for referral to clinical geneticist because of:

- family history
- previous stillbirth or child with congenital abnormality
- carrier couple at risk for an autosomal recessive condition

Symbols

Male, female (unaffected)	Deceased (and affected)	Twins
Sex unknown	Individual without offspring	Monozygotic twins
Affected male and female	Consanguineous marriage	Heterozygote (autosomal recessive)
Three unaffected males	Illegitimate offspring	Heterozygote (X-linked)
Examined personally	Abortion or stillbirth	Propositus

Figure 22.1. Symbols for use in a family tree.

apparent when information to draw a tree is obtained (the full range of symbols is in Fig. 22.1). These include:

1. Families which have more than their fair share of cancer, or cardiovascular or autoimmune disease. For example, a lipoprotein profile may be suggested for children one of whose parents has died prematurely from ischaemic heart disease.
2. The presence of clear cut inherited disease. With the exception of late onset dominant conditions such as Huntington's or polycystic kidney disease, these tend to reveal themselves in childhood. A family history of these conditions is an indication for referral to a clinical geneticist. Some intrauterine deaths, stillbirths, or neonatal deaths may also be due to a chromosomal abnormality or an inherited metabolic disease.
3. The report that a close relative is carrying a recessive trait—the rest of the family should be offered testing.

Table 22.2 Prevention of congenital abnormalities (or their effects)

Preventive measure	Examples
Avoiding abnormalities by preconception care	Malformations in diabetes Fetal alcohol syndrome Congenital rubella Spina bifida (folic acid)
Early detection by screening in pregnancy including ultrasound, followed by prenatal diagnosis and selective abortion	Haemoglobin disorders Cystic fibrosis Down syndrome Many structural abnormalities (for example, heart)
Medical treatment following neonatal screening	Phenylketonuria Congenital hypothyroidism
Early paediatric surgery following ultrasound in pregnancy or clinical examination of the newborn	Some heart or renal abnormalities Undescended testes; hypospadias Inguinal hernia

CONGENITAL DISORDERS

About two per cent of newborn infants have a major malformation obvious in the neonatal period. Many more have minor or moderate abnormalities, such as birthmarks or digital anomalies. Further undiagnosed defects, particularly of the heart and renal tract, gradually become apparent in later childhood, as when a congenital renal abnormality is discovered following a urinary tract infection. While only 15 per cent of congenital malformations are due to identified environmental factors such as infections, maternal diseases, drugs, or radiation, Czeizel and colleagues (1993) calculate that about half of current congenital abnormalities could in principle be either prevented or effectively treated (Table 22.2).

Even when treatment is not practicable, it is important to try and make a precise diagnosis when a child has a major malformation. Only then can correct information be offered to the parents about the risk of recurrence in future pregnancies. This is often reassuringly low. It may also enable parents to be given more accurate knowledge about the handicap's cause and what the future may hold.

MENDELIAN INHERITANCE

Single gene defects may be inherited in an autosomal recessive, autosomal dominant, or X-linked fashion. These conditions make up only about 10 per cent of all congenital disorders, but they are particularly important because they are often severe and involve a high, often avoidable, genetic risk for family members.

The distinction between single gene disorders and chromosomal defects is now blurred. While many single gene defects involve only deletion or alteration of a single DNA base, others lose or gain sufficient genetic material to be visible on careful electron microscopic examination of stained chromosomes. Furthermore, in many single gene defects a similar clinical picture results from many different mutations of specific genes. For example, over 250 different mutations can cause cystic fibrosis.

Autosomal recessive inheritance

Examples include haemoglobin disorders (0–20 births per 1000), cystic fibrosis (0.4–0.5 per 1000), phenylketonuria (0.05–0.13 per 1000) and Tay–Sachs Disease (0.28 per 1000 in Eastern European Jews).

Genes for recessively inherited conditions are very common, but disease only becomes apparent when an individual inherits the mutant gene from both parents. Since this depends on two carriers meeting by chance, there is rarely a family history unless the couple are blood relatives. On average, when both parents carry the same recessive gene, 25 per cent of their offspring have the disorder, 50 per cent are carriers of the gene, and 25 per cent do not have the mutant gene at all.

Because in Britain families are small, a child with a recessive condition will usually be the only affected member of a sibship. Genetic advice after an affected birth will thus have little influence on overall incidence. A practical approach to reducing the number of children born with such a disorder depends on identifying carriers and carrier couples, ideally before reproduction. Their counselling raises important ethical issues (discussed later in the chapter).

In rare instances there may be problems for the heterozygote. For example the carrier of one gene for sickle haemoglobin may develop problems during anaesthesia, or on prolonged swimming under water, or may very rarely develop harmless haematuria. Carriers of β-thalassaemia may mistakenly be thought to be iron-deficient because they have small hypochromic red blood cells and a somewhat low haemoglobin. They may be at risk of iatrogenic iron overload.

Autosomal dominant inheritance

The disease becomes apparent when only one of a pair of chromosomes carries the mutant gene. The children of a person with a dominant disorder have a 50 per cent chance of inheriting the same gene. They usually then develop the disease, though sometimes the gene is not fully expressed. In some affected children the condition arises from a new mutation, and thus the recurrence risk within the family is usually low. New mutations are higher with older parents, especially older fathers. A child whose father is 45 has five times the risk of being born with a new mutation than the child of a father of 30. The rate is very much higher still if the father is over 60 (Modell and Kuliev 1990). There are, broadly speaking, two groups of dominant disorders, sporadic and familial.

Sporadic disorders, such as severe forms of osteogenesis imperfecta, cannot be inherited because they cause death in infancy or prevent reproduction. New cases are due to new mutations.

Familial disorders. Examples of those which have a relatively late onset include Huntington's disease (1 in 3000), adult polycystic disease of the kidney (1 in 250). As they may well cause disease only after reproduction has started, they can be handed on within the family.

X-linked disorders

Important X-linked disorders are: glucose-6-phosphate dehydrogenase deficiencies (there are several types, affecting seven per cent of the world population and they occur, as do haemoglobin disorders, predominantly in areas where malaria was endemic); fragile-X mental retardation (thought to be about 0.5 per 1000 in males and 0.6 per 1000 in females); haemophilia (1 per 10 000 boys); and Duchenne muscular dystrophy (1 per 4000 boys).

In X-linked conditions the abnormal gene is carried on the X chromosome and is thus recessive in the female. A mother who is a carrier can expect that half her sons will have the disorder and that half her daughters will themselves be carriers. The reliable identification of carriers can usually be achieved using DNA methods which allow prenatal diagnosis or, for the 50 per cent of sisters of the index case who are not carriers, reassurance. Usually carrier females show mild biochemical or clinical abnormalities because half their X chromosomes are inactivated in a random fashion (although this is not always so, for example, fragile-X see below). On average, half the remaining X chromosomes will carry the mutant gene. Such individuals will produce half the normal amount of the gene product.

UNIPARENTAL DISOMY

An interesting recent development is the unexpected discovery that for some genes, the effect on the fetus depends on which parent they are inherited from. For example, Prader–Willi syndrome (fat, retarded child with undescended testes and a voracious appetite) and Angelman syndrome (a retarded child with a happy puppet face) both result from the same chromosomal deletion (15q11-3), but in the former both chromosomes come from the father, in the latter from the mother. During the formation of gametes some parts of some chromosomes are handled differently, according to which parent they originally came from, and the genes on those particular bits of the chromosomes function differently thereafter.

GROSS CHROMOSOMAL ABNORMALITIES

About eight per cent of diagnosed pregnancies have a chromosomally abnormal conceptus. Nine-tenths of these die *in utero*, accounting for over half of all spontaneous abortions.

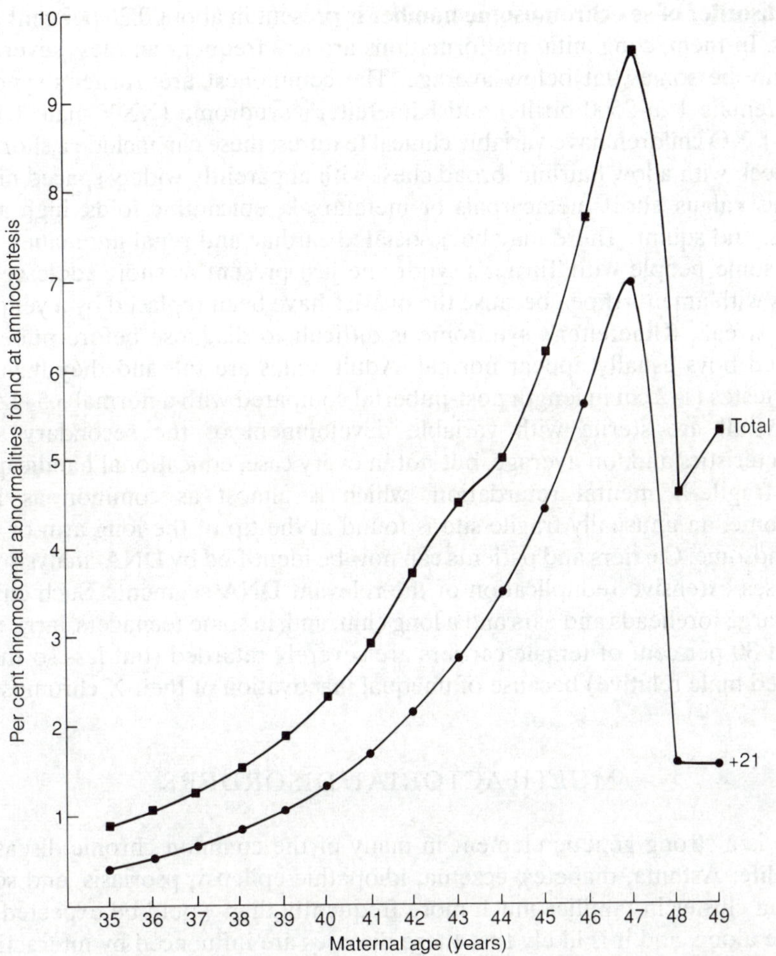

Figure 22.2. The figure shows data for fetuses at amniocentesis. The incidence at birth is about 30% lower, due to late miscarage of chromosomally abnormal fetuses. The apparent fall in incidence of fetuses with trisomy 21 after maternal age 46 may be an artefact due to small sample size,or the result of an increased rate of early miscarriage of chromosomally abmormal fetuses. (From Modell and Modell (1992): based on Ferguson-Smith and Yates 1984.)

Both the incidence of abortion and the chance of the birth of a child with a chromosomal disorder increase with maternal age (Fig. 22.2). The commonest chromosomal disorder at birth is trisomy 21 leading to Down syndrome. Those infants with other disorders of autosomal (non X or Y) chromosome number rarely survive the neonatal period. If they do they usually die in early infancy. Detailed analysis of individual chromosomes can occasionally demonstrate minor abnormalities, allowing the aetiological classification of some other malformed or mentally retarded babies.

A disorder of sex chromosome number is present in about 0.26 per cent of live births. In them, congenital malformations are less frequent and less severe. The IQ may be somewhat below average. The commonest are Turner's syndrome (XO female 1 in 2500 births) and Klinefelter's syndrome (XXY male 1 in 700 births). XO children have variable clinical features; these can include a short webbed neck with a low hairline, broad chest with apparently widely spaced nipples, cubitus valgus, short metacarpals or metatarsals, epicanthic folds, high arched palate, and squint. There may be associated cardiac and renal anomalies. However, some people with Turner's syndrome just present as short adolescents or adults with amenorrhoea because the ovaries have been replaced by a yellowish-white streak. Klinefelter's syndrome is difficult to diagnose before puberty as affected boys usually appear normal. Adult males are tall and they have very small testes (1–2 cm in length post-pubertal compared with a normal 3.5–4.5 cm). Nearly all are sterile with variable development of the secondary sexual characteristics and, on average, but not in every case, educational handicap.

In fragile-X mental retardation, which is almost as common as Down syndrome, an unusually fragile site is found at the tip of the long arm of the X chromosome. Carriers and patients can now be identified by DNA analysis which discloses extensive reduplication of the relevant DNA segments. Such children have large foreheads and ears and a long chin, and, in some teenagers, large testes. About 30 per cent of female carriers are severely retarded (but less so than an affected male relative) because of unequal inactivation of their X chromosomes.

MULTIFACTORIAL DISORDERS

There is a strong genetic element in many of the common chronic diseases of adult life. Asthma, diabetes, eczema, idiopathic epilepsy, psoriasis, and schizophrenia cluster in families much more frequently than would be expected from chance alone, and it is likely that these diseases are influenced by interaction of several genes (polygenic effects) or of genetic and environmental factors (multifactorial effects). Many normal characteristics, such as height, blood pressure, intelligence, and hair colour, are inherited in the same way. Diseases such as diabetes form a heterogenous group, some cases having a larger genetic component than others. Congenital malformations inherited multifactorially include congenital dislocation of the hip; cleft lip and palate; and meningomyelocele. This type of inheritance has several distinctive features.

1. There is an empirical 2–10 per cent rate of recurrence in siblings and offspring of an affected person.

2. The more severe the case the more likely is a positive family history and recurrence in a subsequent pregnancy.

3. The risk of a further affected child is increased if more than one sibling is affected.

4. Incidence falls off rapidly as one passes to more distant relatives.
5. There may be a sex predilection. For example, pyloric stenosis is six times more common in boys than in girls. An affected member of the rarely affected sex is much more likely to have a family history of the condition.

It is often possible to give parents a more exact risk of recurrence by adding other information to empirical data alone; for example, some diseases are associated with particular HLA types (for example, ankylosing spondylitis, diabetes mellitus, and coeliac disease). Offspring of an affected parent who carry the relevant HLA antigen are much more likely to develop the disease in question than those without the antigen.

Both the prenatal and post-natal environment may contribute to the development of certain multifactorial diseases. For example, Barker *et al.* (1993) conclude that babies who are small for gestational age at birth, or fail to gain weight satisfactorily in early infancy, have an increased risk of later cardiovascular disease or non-insulin-dependent diabetes. At present, the mechanism of the association and the possibility of any interventions for future generations are uncertain.

PREGNANCY HAZARDS

Infection

Certain maternal infections during pregnancy can be highly damaging to the fetus and are discussed in Chapter 10.

Drinking and smoking

There is evidence that 30 mL or more of alcohol daily (the amount in two-and-a-half glasses of wine or two pints of beer) affects the fetus to some degree (Vitez *et al.* 1984). The classical fetal alcohol syndrome (mental retardation and poor growth both before and after birth, with a reduced head circumference, a typical facial appearance, and various cardiovascular, renal, and orthopaedic abnormalities) represents the most severe damage. Incidence is about 1.5 per 1000 children. It is more usual to see a poorly-grown child who is somewhat slow mentally and physically and comes from a family where excessive drinking is suspected. It is difficult to prove the connection in an individual case or to separate out congenital from environmental factors.

Darren was discovered to have a loud systolic murmur soon after birth. He developed cardiac failure, and failed to regain his birth-weight by the age of four weeks. After the heart surgery he slowly improved but, by the age of 2½ years, his weight was still way below the third centile. He had a funny face and was only able to say single words. His mother had for many years drunk large quantities of cider in the evenings, partially to help her cope with insomnia.

Maternal smoking in pregnancy is associated with spontaneous abortion, reduced birth-weight, bleeding in pregnancy, an increase in the perinatal death rate, and impaired reading in primary school and educational attainment by adulthood (Fogelman and Manor 1988).

Diabetes

Stillbirths and delivery of sick or overweight infants are more common when the mother suffers from insulin dependent diabetes. There is also a three-fold increase (to about six per cent) in the incidence of congenital malformations, including fatal and multiple ones. Congenital heart disease is particularly common. Careful control of the blood sugar around conception and throughout pregnancy reduces the risk (Ylinen *et al.* 1984).

Drugs

A comprehensive, regularly updated table of the effects of drugs taken in different stages of pregnancy and lactation is included in the British National Formulary and it is always wise to check. Fortunately relatively few drugs in common use appear to cause congenital malformations, the most important exceptions being anticonvulsants, lithium, warfarin, and cytotoxic agents.

Folic acid lack

Folic acid (4 mg daily) after one affected pregnancy reduces the risk of recurrence of a neural tube defect (spina bifida; anencephaly) by 70 per cent. A dose of 0.4 mg daily is recommended for all women hoping to conceive and for the first twelve weeks of pregnancy (Department of Health 1992). It can be taken as a tablet or by eating food rich in folate, such as brussel sprouts, spinach, green beans, and cereals fortified with folic acid.

Irradiation

Mothers-to-be are often concerned that inadvertent diagnostic radiology could have injured their fetus. Though it is advisable to restrict all but the most urgent X-rays to the first few days following the onset of a period (the 10-day rule), the risk of damage appears to be slight. Mole (1979), in a useful review, concluded that if the embryo is exposed to 50 mSV (25 times a chest X-ray and 5 times the usual irradiation of more complex examinations) of radiation there would be 0–2 extra cases of congenital disorders, usually severe learning difficulties, and five extra cases of childhood cancer per 1000 live births. This means that the overall risk of serious damage is probably 0–1 per 1000 women X-rayed in early pregnancy; an opinion that has been confirmed by subsequent studies.

Cancer chemotherapy or organ transplantation involve exposure to high doses of radiation or cytotoxic drugs. Harper (1988) recommends that a couple should wait some months after the man has had such treatment to allow exposed sperm to be shed, before embarking on a pregnancy. Even then, chorionic villus sampling (CVS) or amniocentesis is advised to detect any chromosomal abnormality. It is now becoming commonplace for men to deposit sperm at a sperm bank prior to treatment, so that it can be used for artificial insemination at a later date. Studies of the children of parents who had successful cancer treatment in childhood have not to date shown any increase in abnormalities (Mulvihill *et al.* 1987).

GENETIC RISK

The aim of most genetic screening programmes is to detect individuals who carry a gene for an autosomal recessive condition. This may lead on to the identification of carrier couples who, as mentioned, have a one in four risk of producing an affected child in each pregnancy. They then have a range of options, including taking the risk, not having children, or using prenatal diagnosis with a possibility of aborting an affected fetus. They do, however, lose the option of not knowing, and some may prefer not to be screened for this reason.

Cystic fibrosis (CF) is the commonest genetic disease of Northern Europeans and is carried by about 4 per cent of the population in the UK. The gene for CF was identified in 1989 and it is possible to detect carriers by examining DNA from a mouth wash. Several national pilot screening programmes have demonstrated that screening for CF is acceptable to individuals, but that it is only practicable to detect about 85 per cent of carriers; three-quarters of carrier couples.

Up to 20 per cent or more of some African-Caribbean, African Middle and Far Eastern populations carry sickle cell or thalassaemia. Thus, most non-white and Middle Eastern ethnic groups are at increased risk of carrying a haemoglobin disorder gene. Detection of these carriers by measuring the red cell indices and haemoglobin electrophoresis is simple. There have already been cases of couples who were not screened producing a child with thalassaemia or sickle cell, and then successfully sueing the doctor they felt was responsible (B. Modell, personal communication).

Until recently, individuals and carriers affected by genetic disease have been biochemically identified by direct analysis of the product of the relevant gene (such as haemoglobin in sickle cell anaemia) or by failure of the enzymic step that the product catalyses, as in phenylketonuria, or of the transport function it carries out, as demonstrated by the salty sweat of cystic fibrosis. It is now possible to study abnormal genes directly by analysis of DNA from any nucleated body cell, including the trophoblast surrounding the fetus in early gestation. The applied technology is simple and relatively cheap. In some cases segments of DNA adjacent to the abnormal gene are all that can at present be identified, and family studies are essential in order to be able to decide whether a particular fetus is heterozygous, homozygous, or unaffected. With a fatal inherited disease it may be of critical importance to subsequent pregnancies in family members, to have collected an EDTA blood sample from an affected patient before death, for storage and later DNA analysis.

Chromosomes can be studied—karyotyped—using any cells that can be persuaded to grow in culture. They are examined most easily at mitosis, when the culture is fixed and stained, using methods that give a characteristic pattern of bands specific for each chromosome. Fetal cells from CVS divide more rapidly than those obtained from amniocentesis. This allows a diagnosis of a chromosomal abnormality after only a few days, rather than waiting two or three weeks.

PREGNANCY SCREENING TECHNIQUES

Ultrasound

A gestational sac can be visualized by five to eight weeks, and the fetal heart-beat from about seven weeks onwards. If there has been vaginal bleeding in early pregnancy, then ultrasound examination is helpful in confirming whether a viable conceptus is still present. If no viable fetus is present, then a mother can have an elective D&C rather than waiting until she spontaneously miscarries.

The main indications for ultrasound are confirmation of a viable pregnancy, detection of multiple pregnancies, calculation of gestational age, monitoring of intrauterine growth, the detection of a low-lying placenta or of fetal malformation. It is possible to detect a surprising number of the latter by scanning in early pregnancy. However routine 'fetal anomaly' scanning is usually carried out at about 19 weeks' gestation when the fetal organs are well formed. At this stage an expert can detect over 90 per cent of major malformations with very few false positives (Campbell and Smith 1984). The pick-up rate in a non-expert centre is 50–75 per cent (Ellwood 1995). At present it should be offered to women at an increased risk of producing a child with a congenital malformation, such as those with a raised maternal serum AFP (ultrasound will then identify the vast majority of neural tube defects), a history of a previous malformed child, some familial genetic diseases, exposure to potential environmental teratogens, maternal diabetes and parental consanguinity.

However, most congenital malformations occur in pregnancies in women who are not in known risk groups and so may not currently be identified.

Blood testing

If maternal serum concentrations of human chorionic gonadotrophin, unconjugated oestriol, and AFP are measured at 16–17 weeks of pregnancy and interpreted in relation to maternal age, a figure can be calculated for the risk of carrying a Down syndrome fetus. Amniocentesis is usually offered to women with a risk greater than 1 in 200 but at present 40 per cent of Down fetuses will not be picked up by this approach alone.

Potentially more exciting is the possibility of extracting fetal DNA from small numbers of cells of fetal origin isolated from the maternal circulation.

Chorionic villus sampling

The chorionic villi are of embryonic origin and can be used to study its chromosomes, DNA, and certain enzymes. Occasionally they have a different chromosomal constitution from the fetus—mosaicism—and if findings raise this possibility, confirmation on fetal cells from amniocentesis is advisable. The risk of CVS to the pregnancy is similar to that of amniocentesis, provided the procedure is carried out in an expert centre. Very early CVS might be associated with an increased risk of the birth of a child with limb abnormalities, so CVS should be done after ten weeks gestation; patients who have had the procedure are being offered a detailed scan at 18–20 weeks gestation (Rodeck 1993).

Amniocentesis

Amniotic fluid also contains cells of fetal origin and is collected at about 17 weeks after the last menstrual period. Its cells can be cultured and examined for chromosomal or DNA abnormalities. A DNA diagnosis can often be done directly on amniotic fluid cells so that the results are available much sooner than the approximate two weeks needed for reliable karyotyping. There appears to be an increased fetal loss of about one per cent with this procedure. There is possibly a slightly increased risk of breathing difficulties immediately after delivery and of correctable orthopaedic deformities such as club feet. At present the main indications are:

1. Increased risk of Down syndrome. Some mothers may prefer an earlier CVS.
2. An established risk of bearing a child with certain single genetic defects or chromosomal abnormalities.
3. Failed or doubtful CVS.

Amniocentesis done before 14 weeks appears to have an increased risk of provoking a miscarriage.

ASPECTS OF GENETIC COUNSELLING

The principles of genetic counselling should not differ from those of counselling in general. The counsellor should expect to provide people with accurate, comprehensible information, or to direct them to where such information can be obtained. We share the view that counselling should be non-directive and couples or individuals should be encouraged to make up their own minds on the basis of the best information available, with the doctor backing them up in any decision they make. In general practice, basic counselling is most likely to be given to a

Table 22.3 Issues to raise with parents before and after a genetic screening test

Counselling before a test
You may be a carrier.
Brief description of the condition.
Implications for child bearing.
Limitations of test (for example, 85% of CF mutations only are identified; does not test for other conditions).
Counselling carriers (leaflets usually available)
Carriers are healthy.
More about the disease.
Reproductive risks.
Desirability of testing partners and relatives.

woman who has been offered an antenatal screening test, before screening to detect carriers of a recessive disorder, and to newly identified carriers (Table 22.3). GPs may also be consulted by a carrier couple uncertain whether to accept prenatal diagnosis or not.

Genetic advice to a couple whose baby has been born with a predominantly genetic disorder should not be lightly undertaken because of diagnostic uncertainty in an individual case and the variability of inheritance patterns of apparently similar conditions. There are also a very large number of rare disorders of which neither the GP nor the paediatrician will have had enough experience to allow confident genetic advice, and for all these, referral to a specialist genetic clinic is invaluable. The counsellor needs to bear quite a range of topics in mind. Even if the diagnosis is correct does it explain all the child's problems? Is the condition likely to be equally severe in future affected babies? Is carrier detection or prenatal diagnosis possible? Are the apparent parents really the parents?—and, the obvious question, what is the risk of a further affected pregnancy? A reassessment of contraceptive method may be indicated, or a discussion on sterilization, or abortion, or even of artificial insemination.

Genetic counselling thus requires specific knowledge, training, and adequate time. It is difficult to explain genes and inheritance in a relatively short consultation. Understanding depends on the parents' earlier educational attainment, cultural background and the counsellor's ability to communicate rather complex concepts in a simple manner. It is useful to give patients clearly written leaflets containing the relevant information as a basis for discussion at a second consultation, when the patient has had time to digest the information. Leaflets can often be obtained from the relevant voluntary organization (for example, the Sickle-cell Society and Cystic Fibrosis Research Trust), and will soon be computerized.

TERMINATION FOR GENETIC REASONS

Whatever his personal opinion about termination, the doctor needs to ensure that the parents have access to comprehensive and comprehensible information given in a non-judgemental manner. How do women respond to the offer of prenatal diagnosis? In Italy and Greece systematic carrier screening and prenatal diagnosis for thalassaemia major has proved highly acceptable and the birth incidence of thalassaemic children has fallen dramatically (Modell *et al.* 1991). Most couples who choose prenatal diagnosis will decide on abortion of the fetus if affected and subsequently have another pregnancy in an attempt to achieve the desired family size. In the UK the upper gestation limit for a termination is usually 24 weeks. However, this limit does not apply if the fetus has a lethal condition or there is a serious risk of major handicap. Termination of a wanted pregnancy is always traumatic, but late termination after an abnormality is found in mid-pregnancy poses especial emotional problems for the parents, whose fetus is already more than 14 cm (5.5 in) long and whose movements may already have been felt. As in the case of a stillbirth, the parents may be helped with their inevitable and necessary mourning by handling the dead fetus after termination.

Bibliography

Barker, D. J. P., Gluckman, P. D., Godfrey, K. M., Harding, J. E., Owens, J. A., and Robinson, J. S. (1993). Fetal nutrition and cardiovascular disease in adult life. *Lancet*, **341**, 938–41.

Campbell, S. and Smith, P. (1984). Routine screening for congenital abnormalities by ultrasound. In *Prenatal diagnosis*, (ed. C. H. Rodeck and K. H. Nicolaides). John Wiley, Chichester.

Czeizel, A. E., Intôdy, Z., and Modell, B. (1993). What proportion of congenital abnormalities can be prevented. *British Medical Journal*, **306**, 499–503.

Department of Health. (1992). *Folic acid and the prevention of neural tube defects*. Report from an Expert Advisory Group.

Editorial. (1991a). Chorion villus sampling: valuable addition or dangerous alternative. *Lancet*, **337**, 1513–15.

Editorial. (1991b). Folic acid and neural tube defects. *Lancet*, **338**, 153–4.

Ellwood, D. A. (1995). The role of ultrasound in prenatal diagnosis. In *Handbook of prenatal diagnosis*, (ed. R. J. Trent). Cambridge.

Ferguson-Smith, M. A. and Yates, J. R. W. (1984). Maternal age-specific rates for chromosomal aberrations and factors influencing them: report of a collaborative European study on 52 965 amniocenteses. *Prenatal Diagnosis*, **4**, 5–44.

Fogelman, K. R. and Manor, O. (1988). Smoking in pregnancy and development into early adulthood. *British Medical Journal*, **297**, 1233–6.

Harper, P. S. (1988). *Practical genetic counselling*, (2nd edn). Wright, Bristol.

Medical Research Council Vitamin Study Research Group. (1991). Prevention of neural tube defects: results of the Medical Research Council Vitamin Study. *Lancet*, **338**, 131–7.

Meyer, M. B. and Tonascia, J. A. (1977). Maternal smoking, pregnancy complications, and perinatal mortality. *American Journal of Obstetrics and Gynecology*, **128**, 494–502.

Modell, B. and Kuliev, A. M. (1990). Changing paternal age distribution and the human mutation rate in Europe. *Human Genetics*, **86**, 198–202.

Modell, B., Kuliev, A. M., and Wagner, N. (1991). *Community genetic services in Europe.* WHO Regional Publications, European series No. 38.

Modell, B. and Modell, M. (1992). Towards a healthy baby; congenital disorders and the new genetics in primary health care. Oxford University Press.

Mole, R. H. (1979). Radiation effects on prenatal development and their radiological significance. *British Journal of Radiology,* **52**, 89–101.

Mulvihill, J. J., Myers, M. H., Connelly, R. R., Byrne, J., Austin, D. F., and Bragg, K. (1987). Cancer in offspring of long-term survivors of childhood and adolescent cancer. *Lancet,* **ii**, 813–7.

Robinson, R. J. (1992). Is the child the father of the man? *British Medical Journal*, **304**, 789–80.

Rodeck, C. H. (1993). Prenatal diagnosis—fetal development after chorionic villus sampling. *Lancet*, **341**, 468–9.

Vitez, M., Koranyi, G., Goncy, E., Rudas, T., and Czeizel, A. (1984). A semiquantitative score system for epidemiologic studies of fetal alcohol syndrome. *American Journal of Epidemiology,* **119**, 301–8.

Ylinen, K., Aula, P., and Stenman, U.-H. (1984). Risk of minor and major malformations in diabetes with high haemoglobin A_2 values in early pregnancy. *British Medical Journal,* **289**, 345–6.

23 Chronic disease, malignancy, and death

THE CARE OF THE CHRONICALLY SICK CHILD

Most GPs look after several families with chronically unwell children. The range of sickness is wide and includes severe asthma, epilepsy, diabetes, congenital heart disease, and malignancy. A patient may also suffer from one or another of the vast range of rarer disorders.

There are many important factors common to the care of these children, although details of management will, of course, vary according to the disease they suffer from. Many professionals are involved in their care: nurses, doctors, social workers, health visitors, physiotherapists, and teachers. These families must have medical advisers who are easily available and who will negotiate an approach to management with the family.

The personal doctor

It is important that one doctor is the child's personal physician—the individual who works with the family to establish their *modus vivendi* with the illness. The key to successful management is continued personal support and a two-way flow of information. The parents, and ultimately the child, should be well informed about the disease, its management, and the management of its complications. They need to know what they can do, when to seek help, and from whom. The doctor should understand what the illness means to the family and what they themselves have learnt from living with the condition. To some extent with all chronic disorders, and especially with rare diseases, the parents often become more expert in aspects of management than any professional. It is important that doctor and parents appreciate and accept this. The modern trend towards the team approach has benefits, but patients cannot be looked after by a committee. The personal physician may be the GP but that will not necessarily be the case, and the family doctor should not feel slighted if he is not the most important medical person in his patient's life. The hospital paediatrician or paediatric surgeon may fulfil the role, as long as he recognizes this and does not excessively delegate care to a succession of junior staff.

David suffers from dysautonomia, an autosomal-recessive condition causing severe disturbance of the autonomic nervous system. He has corneal abrasions, recurrent chest infections, scoliosis, and episodes of unexplained fever. Mrs Symon usually consults the paediatrician directly about David's problem, and the GP accepts this and has learnt a lot about the disease and its management from her. The GP's main contact with David is via a request for repeat prescriptions, although he has a good relationship with the family, and is often consulted by its other members.

With children whose chronic illness is subject to acute or life-threatening complications, the family is particularly apt to consider the hospital doctor, or sometimes the sister on a specialized children's unit, or the specialist community nurse, to be the best source of immediate advice in a crisis. This is reasonable, especially if the family doctor knows little about the particular illness the child is suffering from, or feels anxious or insecure when asked to deal with the child when sick, because the treatment includes a high degree of technology. Nevertheless, the GP must continuously keep a finger on the situation in order to help other family members, and to be in a position to pick up management when the child's situation is on a more even keel, or when the child grows out of the paediatric age group. Adult hospital departments are sometimes unable to give the level of personal ongoing care that families come to expect from a paediatric service, and it is often a good move for a GP to become the personal doctor at adolescence, even if he has not assumed that role before. He may have to pick up adolescent issues that have been delayed or which the paediatric department has overlooked: sexual identity and function, and genetic risk to possible offspring, independence from parents, job opportunities.

Occasionally the GP has another important role, that of becoming a bridge between the family and hospital staff, particularly if the latter have not established a reliable system of communication. He can raise issues that a parent is embarrassed to discuss, and explain to the consultant the family's fears, anxieties, and discontents. He may be the most appropriate person to explain to the family the need for compliance with hospital therapy and may be able to persuade them to be more understanding in their demands on the hospital. This negotiating role is easier for an experienced doctor than for the trainee. Conversely, the consultant may feel that the practice could usefully take a more active role in management of the child's condition. All this may take quite a lot of time and effort as it is easy for the GP to lose his grip on the care of the child whose problems are being managed almost entirely by the hospital.

Breaking bad news

When the doctors have decided that a child has definitely got a serious disease the news should, if possible, be given to both parents together, emphasizing at the onset that this is a burden that they will have to carry jointly. If this is done there is less opportunity for misunderstanding between the parents, and between them and the doctor, because if the mother does not ask an important question to clarify a point the doctor has made, the father may do so, and vice versa. Usually several consultations should be arranged so that the doctor can impart facts at a speed which keeps pace with the parents' ability to assimilate the information. The diagnosis may not be accepted at first, especially if the child appeared normal in the early months or years of life. Anger is a natural initial emotion, and may be more marked if the parents sensed for months that there was something seriously amiss with the child in spite of reassurance by the doctors that all was well. It is difficult for them to understand that a delayed diagnosis of a disease that presents with common symptoms is, in the absence of a family history, almost inevitable. Infants often get recurrent respiratory infections; in the vast majority of cases this is not a sign of cystic fibrosis.

Parents feel a varying amount of guilt, usually unjustified, but more difficult to bear if the drug-using mother was HIV positive, or drank very heavily around conception and thus bore at least part of the responsibility for the child's problem. Some parents find it difficult to come to terms with the inevitable negative emotions mixed with positive feelings aroused by their handicapped child. They may, however, feel relieved if the doctor spontaneously tells them that it is normal for parents to feel angry or partly to blame if their child is born with a serious illness. A single mother coping on her own will need even more health visitor, social, and medical support. It may sometimes help to have a relative or friend present when the doctor is breaking bad news or formally reviewing the situation with her.

Parents also need time and support in grieving for the disappearance of their hopes of a strong and healthy child, and in growing to accept the real limitations chronic disease imposes. The GP may need to amplify and clarify what the consultant or registrar has told the family; sometimes a briefing telephone call is required. Good communication within a family is always important, but the stresses upon a sick child's mother may become intolerable if she is not able to share her anxiety with the other parent. The GP should continue to see the parents together from time to time so that he can evaluate their mutual support and try to facilitate it.

Where to refer

One of the most important early decisions a GP has to make is where to refer a chronically sick child, especially if he suffers from an unusual illness. Should it be the local hospital or a specialist unit? It may be difficult to redirect the care of a child elsewhere if treatment has already been started by the paediatric unit in the hospital where the infant was born. However, the best interest of the child must take precedence over a desire not to hurt the feelings of the local consultant. Our preference is for the expert unit. If it is situated some distance away from the family, a shared care scheme is a reasonable compromise, whereby the child attends the local hospital for basic care but visits the specialized unit for an annual assessment.

Consultations with the family

It is useful to go through a mental checklist of areas to be covered when the family consults. They may need help in claiming all the benefits they are entitled to. Grants available include Income Support, Family Credit and payments from the Social Fund. Stable neurological problems and asthma are not contra-indications to any of the routine immunizations. In the presence of a chronic disorder, other disabilities, such as deafness or poor vision, can have a particularly serious impact and should be detected and treated as early as possible.

In the case of a younger, chronically sick child, the GP, or, perhaps even more appropriate, the health visitor or the district nurse, need to be constantly on the lookout for signs that the mother, whether single or supported, is beginning to find the situation impossible. A reassessment of the situation may be needed. Deployment of more resources, temporary fostering, or a brief admission may allow her to recover her strength. The mother may have a high level of anxiety normally kept more or less at bay, but the stress of another family crisis, or of dramatic or unexpected symptoms such as hypoglycaemic coma or haemoptysis, may be intolerable.

Mrs McCarthy has twins aged five. One, Mark, is very severely intellectually and physically handicapped. The other twin, James, was healthy except for recurrent ear infections until he developed intractable epilepsy. His mother then felt she had to watch James so carefully that Mark for the first time had to go into temporary care.

The threshold for hospital admission is often low and this can be a problem as repeated hospital admissions are a blow to the family's self-confidence and self-reliance, and, in hospital, children, like adults, may feel unloved and abandoned.

Parents should also be encouraged to bring to the doctor for discussion the inevitable therapeutic suggestions which will be generated by relatives or by the media. In conjunction with the specialist it is often useful to offer them a second opinion to back up their confidence that the correct course is being followed. Families need the doctor for support but he must not necessarily feel that they expect him to change the course of the disease. Even if he has nothing specific to offer, a positive comment on progress made by the child or good caring by the parents, may be of tremendous value in fuelling their ability to cope with their task. Forethought may enable reassurance to be given about unspoken fears. Sudden death is not seen in most varieties of congenital heart disease; and epilepsy does not cause madness or mental handicap, although it may be associated with the latter. It is sometimes hard to remember all the possible fears. Parents often get tremendous relief and also often practical advice from discussion with parents of other similarly afflicted families. It is therefore usually helpful to put them in touch with the appropriate self-help organization (Chapter 24) at an early stage, unless the parent does not like the idea.

Many of these children require regular medication, or special diets, or physiotherapy, and, paradoxically, as treatment improves, it often becomes tougher for everybody—the doctors, the parents, and the children. However, if the improvement offers an increased hope of a normal life or of longer worthwhile survival it will usually be possible to maintain the family's morale. A generation ago it was technically easy to manage children with lymphoblastic leukaemia—easy, but the disease was fatal within a few months. Now, there is a harrowing treatment regimen with many risks, but also a cure in a majority of cases. The same issues apply with equal or greater force to the many conditions for which major palliation can now be achieved without a complete cure: surgery for neonatal biliary atresia, renal dialysis and transplantation for neonatal renal failure, cystic fibrosis management culminating in cardiothoracic transplantation, and complex surgery for neonatal heart disease. Although therapeutic agents and dietary regimens vary according to the disease, they all have the effect of limiting the family's freedom and creating sources of conflict between parents and child which may be heightened at adolescence. When parents accept the illness without shame or evasion and honestly explain the situation to the child, he seems best able to accept it. He is less likely to comply if there is denial on their part.

Children's questions should be answered honestly at a level appropriate for their age and understanding. This is easier said than done, and may be more a matter of the doctor's tactful and appropriate response to comments by the child or to parental remarks made in front of the child than of a formal educative session. Not only should the sick child be kept informed, but healthy siblings should also not be kept in the dark. If we take cystic fibrosis as an example, at different ages, an affected child must learn the name of his illness, and that it is inherited from both parents. He must accept that it is a lifelong disease which will vary in intensity; sometimes he will be sick, sometimes he will be well, but continuous therapy is necessary. If he is a male he will be sexually competent but infertile; information only to be imparted with great sensitivity, though most will know from patient groups. However, a purely gloomy approach is not justified, the management of cystic fibrosis is continually improving, many patients live into middle life and the gene therapy is being piloted.

If the question arises, it is usually a mistake to inaccurately deny to a child that his life may be shortened. An honest approach is the only realistic policy in these days of open discussion and of frequent TV publicity about serious diseases. The truth can be coped with remarkably well by even young children, and provides a better basis for coping with life than evasion, although hope based on the possibility of therapeutic advance is always justifiable:

John had a Wilms' tumour excised when he was 2, followed by resection of pulmonary secondaries on two subsequent occasions. His parents always warned him that 'the bad bit like the bad bit of banana' might come back again, and that this might mean that he would die and they would have to say goodbye to each other. Fortunately he made a good recovery.

Whereas the doctor must not evade helping the patient accept tragic and unpalatable truths, he should not force this information on the child, but wait until questions arise. The common mistake is to give untruthful off-the-cuff reassurance when the doctor is caught suddenly unawares by a remark of the parent or child. If the doctor can think quickly enough the response to the question 'He is not going to die is he, doctor?' could be, 'Is that what you fear is going to happen?'.

Doctors fail to update the patient's knowledge as a child gets older. As mentioned, the child will, where appropriate, need to be given reassurance about sexual function and about the relatively small chance of his children being similarly affected when this is the case, as it frequently is:

Tim was an intelligent 16-year-old with a severe, but controlled inborn error of metabolism. This was inherited as an autosomal-recessive condition, but, despite having a medical parent, he did not know that his children would not be at significant risk of having the condition.

The GP must also not forget to update his own knowledge of the disease. Has the prognosis changed? Can the child's epilepsy be better controlled with new anticonvulsants? Is antenatal diagnosis now available if the mother becomes pregnant again?

The child and the family

The alteration in hopes for the child's future that chronic disease implies must be very painful for most parents but, even so, the child should be encouraged to live as normal a life as possible and should not be restricted in his activities more than is absolutely necessary. They should be encouraged to develop and expand those skills which are not stunted by disability, in the same way that the child with severe myopia will pursue intellectual rather than sporting pursuits. Most children will have to discover their own limitations, even if this entails taking some risks. This is better than forcing them to operate within a parental straitjacket. Nevertheless, parental discipline is reassuring and is one of the factors enabling a child to feel like other children:

William, a boy with severe asthma, used to say to his mother when she was particularly indulgent: 'Mummy, you are so nice to me, does it mean that I'm going to die?'

Parents who have already lost a child are especially liable to be overprotective and show a marked difference in expectation for the second child affected by a disease. These parents may find it very difficult to maintain the state of optimism which is so helpful to the satisfactory development of the ill child.

Parents will often lead a restricted social life if they consider that one of their children needs constant vigilance. They may be reluctant to leave the child in the care of a baby-sitter whilst they go to the cinema, or to spend a holiday out of reach of a trusted paediatric unit. The presence of a sick child affects the whole family, including well brothers and sisters, who have to come to terms with the situation. In some cultural groups attitudes to illness will be coloured by its effect on the possibility for arranged marriages. Parental preoccupation with the illness may limit their perception of, and their ability to respond to, the physical and emotional needs of the other children. Younger siblings of the patient may have been more likely to miss out on the intense parenting they need in the earlier years. Problems can also occur because of the attitude of the sick child himself, particularly if his demands are given priority over those of his well siblings. Despite the inevitable problems, by no means all the reactions of healthy siblings are negative. Older brothers and sisters often show positive protective feelings towards the younger child, defending him if attacked verbally or physically by others. Worries that they themselves might fall ill must occur at some time to most children in these families.

The NHS is a boon to families with chronically sick children, even in times of financial constraint. Unlike corresponding families in many parts of the world, the disease is not likely to cause serious financial hardship, though it may restrict the family's income in a number of ways, influencing the parent's mobility and their employment possibilities so that they become less affluent than they would otherwise have been.

Chronic disease in adolescence is considered on p. 109.

MALIGNANT DISEASE

Although malignant disease is rare in children and accounts for about one per cent of all cancers, it is nevertheless important as a cause of death. In children of school age it is, after accidents, the most common category. About half the cases are leukaemias and lymphomas; the remainder include brain tumours, the embryonic nephroblastoma of the kidney (Wilms' tumour), neuroblastoma, arising from cells that form the adrenal medulla and sympathetic nervous system, retinoblastoma of the retina, and various sarcomas, such as the rhabdomyosarcoma of muscle, and the osteosarcoma seen more commonly in older children. The common cancers of adult life are almost never seen.

Delays in diagnosis are commonplace. This is not surprising when it is remembered that only 1 in 250 cancer deaths are in children under 15 years; a reassuring figure for the doctor who is continually seeing children who develop a palpable spleen during an acute infection, or who present with prominent cervical lymph nodes. The average GP will see only two new cases of childhood malignancy during his professional career.

Presentation

Leukaemia is almost always acute in childhood. The combination of pallor, bruising, and malaise often leads to a fairly early diagnostic blood test. Anaemia, thrombocytopenia, and either a low, normal, or raised white-cell count will be found. Usually, but not invariably, there are circulating blast cells. Less commonly, acute leukaemia presents with persistent limb or joint pains, or as a pyrexia of unknown origin (PUO). These quasi-rheumatic or quasi-infectious presentations are also sometimes seen with a neuroblastoma.

Lymphomas, such as Hodgkin's disease, usually declare themselves with a mass or a large gland. The typical malignant gland is so large that it is unlikely to be confused with the moderately enlarged, visible glands in the neck that are so commonplace. It is not tender during a cold as they are. In addition, it will usually be in a somewhat unusual site and be larger a few weeks later. Moderate, persistent lymphadenopathy of no pathological importance is also often seen with eczema. It is reasonable, if in doubt, to give a two week course of antibiotics, but close follow-up of gross, unexplained lymphadenopathy is mandatory.

Enlargement of the spleen during acute infections is common, but persistent palpability is also a source of anxiety to the doctor. The soft spleen, only palpable 1–2 cm below the costal margin on inspiration, can usually be ignored. Firmer spleens may be an indication of lymphoma. A search for anaemia, peripheral lymphadenopathy, and hilar gland enlargement on chest X-ray is therefore reasonable. Nevertheless, malignancy presenting as isolated splenomegaly is very uncommon. A large, firm spleen is more likely to be the result of metabolic or hepatic disease, or of haemolytic anaemia.

Central nervous system tumours may present with headache and vomiting, especially in the morning when intracranial pressure will, for postural reasons, be at its highest. Such symptoms suggest the need for a detailed neurological examination, including inspection of the fundi. At first the symptoms are intermittent, but they recur with increasing prominence, later associated with ataxia, head tilt, squint, or other neurological signs.

Nephroblastomas and neuroblastomas tend to present in toddlers as an abdominal mass. The former can also present with haematuria. An unexplained persistent lump on a bone or in a soft tissue may imply the presence of an osteo- or other sarcoma.

Management

It may be difficult for the GP to decide where to refer the child he suspects suffers from cancer. Should the patient be seen by the paediatrician at the local hospital or should he be sent to a paediatric unit which has special experience in the treatment of malignant disease, even though this may mean a journey of many miles for the family? The ideal solution is for the GP and the local paediatrician to have such an easy relationship that the problem of referral can be discussed between them. Failing this, a telephone call for advice to the nearest teaching hospital paediatric oncologist may be helpful. If and when the child is referred to the specialist paediatric oncology unit with a likely diagnosis of childhood malignancy, the GP should tell the family that they will be going to a cancer centre where children already on treatment (some with side-effects such as alopecia) will be visible. First impressions are long lasting.

The addition of prolonged courses of systemic chemotherapy to radiotherapy and, where appropriate, surgery, has had a considerable impact on the prognosis for childhood malignant disease. For example, the long-term remission rate of children suffering from acute lymphoblastic leukaemia has gone up from about

0.5 per cent to 70 per cent over the last 30 years; the latter figure applies to children treated with multiple-agent chemotherapy on intensive nationally organized protocols. Many leukaemic children have now been in remission off all therapy for more than 20 years. Of children in remission three years after treatment for most tumours, the great majority will still be alive at 10 years and relapse after that time is extremely rare.

In addition to the obvious strains on family, patient, and doctor of two or three years' intensive chemotherapy, there are other problems the GP needs to be aware of. During chemotherapy, lymphocyte and other white-cell function is very much impaired. Indeed, in some series deaths from infection because of immunosuppression are almost as common as fatal relapse. A PUO in a child on chemotherapy is an emergency. It may be due to bacterial infection or possible viral or protozoal infection. All unexplained fevers in such children require urgent blood and other cultures and broad-spectrum antibiotic therapy. Untreated they may proceed to death within less than 24 hours. Pneumonia—or, less obviously, dark red, tender, infective skin lesions—may also be the first sign of fulminating infection. Some live viral vaccines, or infection with chickenpox or measles, may be fatal in children immunosuppressed with anti-cancer drugs. This is especially true of those with low lymphocyte counts. Any child on anti-cancer treatment needs to be kept away, as far as possible, from infectious contacts, especially if he has not had chickenpox, measles or measles vaccination before his illness. If exposed they need urgent immunoglobulin within a maximum of three days of contact for measles, and acyclovir, and perhaps immunoglobulin, for chickenpox. The oncologist needs to be contacted promptly.

Once any programme of treatment is complete there remain certain problems, including the risk of tumour recurrence. The latter varies, being less than 10 per cent for a nephroblastoma treated while it is still restricted to the renal capsule, but over 90 per cent for high grade gliomas of the brain-stem. In the case of acute lymphoblastic leukaemia, the prognosis depends on both the host and the malignancy. It is worse, for example, in children under the age of 2 years, or over the age of 10, or who are black, and the prognosis also depends on the number of leukaemic cells present in the body at the time of diagnosis, as well as on their particular sub-type. Doubtless the same sort of factors are involved in the prognosis of other tumours.

Later difficulties in the 'cured' child may be many. They include educational impairment, with, for example, a patchy loss of about 10 IQ points following leukaemia especially in younger children who have had cranial irradiation. They may also have learning problems not reflected in the IQ. Educational difficulties are worsened by the unduly low disciplinary and academic expectations that both parents and teachers may have when faced with cancer. Recovered children also have to learn to cope with their parents' anxiety, which is re-aroused whenever the child becomes unwell. Leukaemia or other tumours, especially sarcomas, may occur as 'second malignancies' years later. These were found in up to eight per cent of children followed up for 20 years (Meadows 1988). Tumours may occur both within and outside the area of body affected by any irradiation. Radiotherapy may also impair subsequent growth, either by direct damage to the spine, or through the effects of cranial irradiation on pituitary growth hormone release. Partial or total infertility, and, sometimes, failure of puberty, requiring hormone replacement, may follow therapeutic damage to the gonads. Finally, there is the possibility that siblings of a child with neurofibromatosis or retinoblastoma, for example, may also subsequently develop a tumour. Genetic advice may be needed on family risk or about the possibility of antenatal diagnosis for future pregnancies. This is a rapidly developing field.

It is becoming apparent that cytotoxic agents themselves can have late effects, such as severe cardiomyopathy, which may result in catastrophic cardiac failure many years after initial treatment, perhaps during pregnancy or following severe physical exertion. Other drugs may have effects on renal function and increase the incidence of secondary tumours. The GP needs to be aware of these possibilities in a young adult with a past history of successfully treated cancer.

If one adds to these problems the tremendous psychological stresses induced by having a child with malignant disease in the family, it is obvious that, even when the patient appears to be being fully managed by a hospital department, the GP, because of his responsibility as a family doctor, will need to help the family cope with this disaster in many ways.

DEATH

The death of any child is considered grossly unfair in the 'civilized' Western society of today; very different from attitudes in the large Victorian families of a century ago and from those in some ethnic minorities. Many deaths in childhood are sudden and unexpected catastrophes. About a third of deaths of children between one and 14 are due to an accident, and parents will have had no time to prepare themselves. Their mourning and grief may be compounded by feelings of guilt; perhaps the accident was partly due to lack of parental supervision or followed a row. A GP who hears of the sudden death of one of his child patients will want to contact the family quickly to open lines of communication. Similar issues also apply to stillbirth. For example, later grieving may be easier if the parents have seen the body (Lewis 1976).

We discuss some of the practical problems of parents faced with sudden death in the section on cot death (p. 16). This section is concerned with deaths that are the last event in a long, drawn-out illness. The decision that further vigorous treatment or surgery is inappropriate, whether the case be one of malignancy, or of a genetic disorder like cystic fibrosis, or of complicated congenital malformation, is often very difficult. Again the GP may need to involve himself in the negotiations, remembering that it may be in the best interests of the child to stop active treatment before the parents are entirely ready to accept this. However, the GP has also to consider the parents' continued well-being, and sometimes treatment is continued longer than one would wish.

One of the decisions facing parents and doctors is of the best location for an expected death of a child. Satisfactory terminal care may often involve co-operation between GP, community services, hospital, and hospice. For a death to be satisfactorily managed at home several essential requirements must be met. It must be accepted by all that, whatever the intention, emotions and practicalities may get out of hand and emergency admission to hospital for terminal care may be needed, even if this was not the original plan. A doctor taking on the management of a dying child at home must ensure that the family have adequate access to 24-hour personal doctoring. This may prove to be one of the occasions where an individual partner should give a family his home telephone number, regardless of what arrangement the practice makes for night cover. In the latter stages daily or even more frequent visiting by him or by another member of the practice team will be necessary. If the doctor is going away, a joint home visit by the child's GP and the doctor who is covering during his absence will help continued smooth management. Intensive support from the district nurse will almost invariably be essential, and in the terminal phase she also may visit several times a day and arrange for nursing equipment, incontinence pads, laundry services, and so forth. Especially for cancer it is often possible to arrange part- or full-time home nursing for a limited period using charitable funds. A social worker can be very helpful in arranging such practical details and in supporting the parents. Many oncology units have liaison nurses especially for this purpose, and many areas have palliative care support teams. The majority of parents of children with terminal malignancy prefer death to occur at home—the preferred option of the children themselves, rather than in hospital. A children's hospice can provide an excellent alternative.

Whenever possible, GP visits to the home should not be hurried. The doctor may sit beside the bed, perhaps looking at the child's books and toys, and giving the family an opportunity to raise any topic they wish to discuss. Open communication between members of the family can be facilitated by the GP. The mother may express an anxiety to the doctor as she shows him to the door, saying 'don't tell my husband', and then be relieved to hear that the father had raised the same issue with the doctor on a previous occasion. Certain issues may need to be specifically discussed with the parents. They include the likely manner of death (discussion of this in very precise practical terms can be very helpful), and what should be said to the sick child who asks what is going to happen to him. It is difficult to be confident of the appropriate response unless the child has been given an opportunity to say what he thinks the future will be. Generally, siblings should be told as much of the truth as is appropriate to their age and maturity; they may of course pass this information on to the dying child.

Confidence in the handling of opiates is essential. Diamorphine is an extremely useful drug, with a starting dose depending on the age and size of the child—approximately 2.5 mg for a 5-year-old made up to 5 mL with honey and flavouring. To maintain an effective analgesic dose it is often necessary to double the concentration every 48 hours and, as the drug is highly soluble, it is easy to do so without making the child swallow increasing volumes of elixir. Some children may reach doses of over 100 mg. Very shortly before death is expected the doctor may sometimes find it helpful to add large regular doses of sedatives, perhaps by injection. Nights are often a problem for families and Vallergan (trimeprazine) oral suspension 4 mg/kg body weight is usually effective. To avoid a distressingly sore mouth, it is useful to encourage a reasonable intake of clear fluids. Bed sores, although uncommon in children, should be prevented by changing the position of the unconscious child.

Throughout the management of the terminal phase the doctor should remain flexible in his attitude and, if the patient rallies unexpectedly, it may be reasonable to reduce the dose of regular analgesics. He will also often be helped by a domiciliary visit with the hospital specialist or by reviewing the situation together with a partner. It is a very stressful situation for the GP and it is useful to feel one has the support of a colleague in the course of action being pursued. Nurses from palliative care teams may be particularly skilled in advising on appropriate drugs regimens, both for analgesia and other distressing symptoms.

Certain tendencies in the parents can be difficult. One is a rather distressing process of parents distancing themselves emotionally from a dying child, almost as if they were getting used to the child's death before it occurs. This is often more obvious in hospital, when the parents begin to visit less and less. Secondly, many parents displace some of their grief into anger directed towards relatives, doctors, or other people in their circle. The doctor has to ride this out without getting caught up in it. However, it is important not to dismiss all parental anger and criticism as groundless.

It may be important on occasion to discuss with parents the possibility of a post-mortem, particularly if the disease may have had a genetic component, or if there appear to be unresolved questions about the nature of the child's condition which might resurface at a later date. If the GP feels it is appropriate, the family often find comfort in his attendance at the child's funeral. As well as giving immediate support, it is usually wise for the doctor to contact the parents some weeks later in order to reopen the relationship with them on a new footing and to help with any problems in their grieving. Often they will wish to recapitulate elements in the child's illness and to discuss matters about which they require further counselling, either of a genetic nature or to do with their understanding of the child's illness and its incorporation into the family's story.

Families often find themselves in a situation some time after the child's death when he or she is never mentioned by neighbours, friends, or relatives. The doctor can play a helpful role by being brave enough to mention the child by name and to discuss him for a minute to two when he happens to see the parents.

Bibliography

Baum, J. D., Dominica, Sister, F., and Woodward, R. N. (1990). *Listen, my child has a lot of living to do*. Oxford University Press.

Burton, L. (1975). *The family life of sick children: a study of families coping with chronic childhood disease*. Routledge & Kegan Paul, London. (A detailed study of the family life of children with cystic fibrosis.)

Lansdown, R. (1980). *More than sympathy—the everyday needs of sick and handicapped children and their families.* Tavistock Publications, London.
Lewis, E. (1976). The management of still birth: coping with an unreality. *Lancet,* **ii**, 619–20.
Meadows, A. T. (1988). Risk factors for second malignant neoplasms: report from the Late Effects Study Group. *Bulletin of Cancer*, **75**, 125–130.
The principles and provision of palliative care. (1992). Joint Report of the Standing Medical Advisory Committee and Standing Nursing and Midwifery Advisory Committee. HMSO, London.
Services outside hospital for children with life-threatening conditions and their families. A national directory. (1993). Produced by M. Tatman, Institute of Child Health, London with the help of the RCN Paediatric Community Nurse's Forum and ACT.

24 Miscellaneous information

HEIGHT, WEIGHT, AND HEAD CIRCUMFERENCE CHARTS

These charts can be obtained from the Child Growth Foundation, 2 Mayfield Avenue, London W4 1PW (Chapter 6).

PEAK EXPIRATORY FLOW RATE (L/MIN) AND HEIGHT

Table 24.1

Height (cm/in)	Median age (years)		Girls PEF	Boys PEF
	Boys	Girls		
100/39.5	3.5	4	40	40
120/52.5	7	7	200	210
140/55	10.5	10.5	310	310
160/63	14	13.5	420	420
180/71			530	550

After Godfrey *et al.* (1970).

BLOOD PRESSURE

The practice needs a couple of sizes of paediatric sphygmomanometer cuffs. The rubber bag inside the cuff should be long enough to go right round the arm and wide enough to cover two-thirds of the arm between shoulder and elbow. Too small a cuff will produce an abnormally high blood pressure reading—the commonest cause for alleged childhood hypertension. Too large a cuff may have the opposite effect.

Table 24.2 Blood pressure in children

Age of child	90th centile
Up to 6 years (higher in crying children)	111/70
At 10 years	117/75
At 15 years	129/79

From Second Task Force on Blood Pressure in Children (1987).

The mean male and female blood pressures are not substantially different until the late teenage years.

RESPIRATORY AND HEART RATE AT REST

Table 24.3

Age of child	Respiratory rate per minute	Heart rate beats per minute
Up to 6 months	30–50	120–140
6–12 months	20–40	95–120
1–5 years	20–30	90–110
6–10 years	18–25	80–100

From Apley (1979).

BLOOD SAMPLING

Ideally gloves should be worn before taking blood. Capillary collection is, with luck, satisfactory for up to 1 mL of blood from babies. The heel is a good place from which to collect capillary blood (or in toddlers the finger-tip). The foot should be warmed by soaking it in a basin of warm water, and dried. A thin film of Vaseline facilitates satisfactory drops of blood. The heel is partially encircled by the doctor's thumb and first finger and compressed. Ideally a spring-loaded lancet device (Autolet, (Owen Mumford)) should be used rather than the manual method for stabbing the heel.

Venous blood can almost always be obtained from the antecubital fossa and back of the hand, if the child is well held and is not too fat. The venepuncture may be easier using a (23-gauge) 'butterfly' needle unconnected to a syringe until blood begins to flow.

INTRADERMAL INJECTION (MANTOUX AND BCG)

Intradermal injection requires skill and prior training. A 25-gauge tuberculin or 26-gauge insulin needle with the bevel upwards is inserted into the superficial layer of skin, stretched between thumb and forefinger. If correctly inserted the needle will be visible under the dermis and the injection will raise a tense white bleb. Incorrectly injected BCG may result in an abscess. In some child health clinics and/or maternity hospitals a percutaneous preparation of BCG administered by a modified Heaf Gun is used instead of intradermal injection in infants. This mode of administration requires less operator skill.

Both subcutaneous and intramuscular injections (for example, for immunization) are usually given into the anterolateral part of the upper arm or thigh. The latter site is recommended for large volume injections, such as penicillin.

GUIDE TO AVERAGE DEVELOPMENTAL PROGRESS

(modified from Illingworth 1980)

Six weeks—Smiles responsively, watches the face of his mother when she talks to him. Follows a light or bright object through about 90 degrees. In ventral suspension the head is held for a few moments in the same plane as the rest of the body. Considerable head lag when pulled to sitting position.

Seven months—Responds to name and imitates simple acts. Turns his head to person talking. Vocalizes with single syllables such as ma, ba, ka. Sits with minimal or no support. Unidextrous approach to objects, which he can transfer. Chews solid food.

Fifteen months—Jargon, with some intelligible single words. Beginning of domestic mimicry and asking for objects by pointing to them. Spoons food into his mouth. Likely to be shy. May build tower of two bricks. Still casting objects. Able to walk but falls frequently.

Two-and-a-half-years—Joins three or four words together and may talk interminably. Can point to whispered parts of body. May help to put things away. Can imitate vertical and horizontal lines with a pencil. Can build tower of 6–8 bricks. Manages his toilet needs except wiping. Runs, climbs, and jumps with both feet.

Four years—Continually asking questions, may count a few numbers and repeat three digits. Can usually be reasoned with, and can give and take somewhat in his play with other children. Will draw 4–6 basic parts of a man. Can button up clothes, and go down stairs one foot per step.

NORMAL BIOCHEMISTRY

(haematological values are on p. 249)

Table 24.4

Variable	Range	Comments	Blood container
Urea (mmol/L)	2.5–6.7		Lithium heparin
Sodium (mmol/L)	135–144		Lithium heparin
Potassium (mmol/L)	3.3–5.6	Upper limit often exceeded if specimen haemolysed	Lithium heparin
Chloride (mmol/L)	98–106		Lithium heparin
Bicarbonate (mmol/L)	22–29		Lithium heparin
Alanine transaminase (U/L)	Infants 10–80 Children 10–40		Lithium heparin
Alkaline phosphatase (U/L)	100–850	High values (e.g. 500–800 IU/L) occur during peak puberty. Normal range depends on methodology and therefore consult with the local laboratory.	Lithium heparin
Creatinine (μmol/L)	20–80		Lithium heparin
Bilirubin (μmol/L)		90% or more unconjugated up to the age of 1 month	Lithium heparin
in cord blood	up to 50		
first 24 hours	up to 103		
2–5 days	up to 205		
after 1 month	1.7–26		
Calcium (mmol/L)	2.2–2.7		Clotted or lithium heparin
Glucose (mmol/L)	3.3–5.5	Fasting	Fluoride-oxalate
Cholesterol (mmol/L)	3–6	Fasting	Clotted
Ferritin (ng/mL)			Clotted
1 year	16–100		
5–15 years	10–100		
Thyroxine (nmol/L)		Higher in newborn	Clotted
1 month–1 year	90–195		
1–10 years	70–180		
TSH (mU/L)	<5		

Modified from Forfar and Arneil (1992).

PRESCRIBING AND DRUG USAGE

The British National Formulary (BNF) provides much more useful information than does *Mims*. It includes sections on drug interactions, and on prescribing for children and for pregnant and lactating women. The BNF, if occasionally amplified by the *Data Sheet Compendium*'s list of side-effects, contains all the drug information needed. Large sections of the pharmacopoeia should ideally remain closed in paediatric practice, and a limited list of drugs only, need to be prescribed. Most paediatric prescribing for systemic use initiated in general practice, could be met from the following list: amoxycillin, erythromycin, flucloxacillin, penicillin, co-amoxiclav, trimethoprim, and nystatin; paracetamol, ibuprofen; promethazine, trimeprazine, and a less sedative antihistamine such as terfenadine; salbutamol/terbutaline, sodium cromoglycate, beclomethasone/budesonide and prednisolone; oral rehydration solution, such as Dioralyte; rectal diazepam as an emergency anticonvulsant.

We would not include in such a list symptomatic drugs for diarrhoea and vomiting, pharmacologically active cough suppressants, day-time sedatives and tranquillizers and third-generation cephalosporins.

The perfect prescriber needs a mental checklist over his prescription pad of points he wishes to make to himself or to the mother:

1. A prescription is often used to reduce the level of maternal anxiety and to preserve the doctor–patient relationship rather than for its direct pharmacological effect. Keep such prescriptions simple. It is better to use harmless linctus simplex for a cough rather than a proprietary cough mixture containing two or three drugs, or kaolin mixture (BNF) for diarrhoea and vomiting, rather than unnecessarily toxic agents such as prochlorperazine (Stemetil). Better still to use neither, although some parents, children of our culture, require a bottle of medicine to give them the confidence to cope. Recurrent requests for symptomatic relief for minor illnesses should be cause for re-evaluation of the reason for consulting. A registrar will often find it more difficult to avoid prescribing a medicine than a doctor whom the mother has known for many years. It is partly a question of finding the right phrase to sell observation alone—'resting the gut' rather than 'irritating it with drugs'.

2. Is there a safer alternative to the drug proposed, one that has been established for longer or with few known side-effects? Does a warning need to be given of potential toxicity?

3. Has the family been given clear instructions? For example, penicillin is best absorbed when taken on an empty stomach (may not be practical in frequently fed breast-fed babies). Complicated instructions need to be written down.

4. Self-medication is almost universal. The question 'What have you tried already?' often results in useful information, not only about medicines bought over-the-counter, but also about non-drug approaches. Complementary medicine is in fashion. A non-judgemental reception of this information helps negotiation of a mutually agreed treatment plan.

5. Many parents, including medical ones, find it difficult to give medicines to babies and recalcitrant toddlers. Infants under a year may accept liquid if it

is squirted slowly onto the tongue in small doses from a syringe. This will be automatically supplied by the chemist if doses of less than 5 mL are prescribed. With most medicines the mother can be told that a second incomplete spoonful can be given to make up for losses, without risk of overdose.

6. Syrups cause problems that tablets do not, although they are easier to administer. Long-term use is bad for the teeth, unless a sugar-free formulation is available, a drink after the dose may help. Prolonged storage is not usually possible because the active ingredient often degrades.

7. Computer issued prescriptions need to be carefully checked; micrograms may have inadvertently become milligrams.

8. Keep all drugs (especially the deadly ones: aspirin, paracetamol, iron, and antidepressants) away from toddlers.

9. Drugs are rarely given by parents exactly as prescribed by the doctor.

Dosage

The doses need to be altered in any child with renal impairment, liver disease, or other serious organ failure. As the BNF points out, special care with dosage needs to be taken in the first 30 days of life. 'The risk of toxicity is increased by inefficient renal filtration, relative enzyme deficiencies, differing target organ sensitivity, and inadequate detoxifying systems causing delayed excretion'.

Table 24.5 Drug doses for infants and children

Age of the child	Percentage of adult dose
1 month	15
4 months	20
1 year	25
3 years	33
7 years	50
12 years	75

After Catzel and Olver (1981).

SELF-HELP ORGANIZATIONS

Some of the most severely handicapped children are ones with diseases for which management is burdensome and difficult, or for which, perhaps, there is no useful therapy at all. One of the successful developments has been the founding of many self-help groups. While not all parents welcome this sort of group activity, many find it a tremendous help to be able to share their problems, not with professionals, but with somebody who has been through the same experiences. It may on occasions be important to warn parents that members attending the local branch meeting, may include young people with more severe forms of the disorder that affects their child.

The list of associations is too long to give here in full, but some examples are:

Association for Children with Life Threatening Conditions

Institute of Child Health, Royal Hospital for Sick Children, St Michael's Hill, Bristol BS2 8BJ, tel. 01179 221556
ACT provides a resource for parents and professionals caring for children with life threatening and terminal conditions.

Bacup

3 Bath Place, Rivington Street, London EC2 3JR, tel. 0171 613 2121
National telephone information service staffed by cancer nurses offering advice, information, and emotional support on any aspect of cancer. London based counselling service available.

British Diabetic Association

10 Queen Anne Street, London W1M OBD, tel. 0171 323 1531
The British Diabetic Association (BDA) aims to give practical help and advice to all diabetics, to create greater public understanding, and to support diabetic research. The Association organizes educational and activity holidays for diabetics of all age groups, and produces a wide range of literature covering all aspects of the disease.

British Epilepsy Association

Anstey House, 40 Hanover Square, Leeds LS3 1BE, tel. 01132 439393
Services include a National Information Centre providing advice and information to lay and professional people. Supplies a wide range of leaflets, books, and video packages to purchase or hire.

Child Growth Foundation

2 Mayfield Avenue, Chiswick, London W4 1PW, tel. 0181 994 7625/995 0257
Provides counselling and information for parents of any child suffering from a disorder which leads to abnormal growth.

Contact a Family

170 Tottenham Court Road, London W1P 0HA, tel. 0171 383 3555
This service networks parents of children with rare disabling or life threatening conditions, usually through established self-help and voluntary groups. These are

available on an information database of over 1100 national and local groups via the contact line.

Department of Social Security Benefits Enquiry Line, tel. 0800 882200
Ring between 9.00 and 16.30, Monday to Friday. For information about Disability Living Allowance. Leaflets on benefits and help with NHS costs are available at post offices or from Health Publications Unit, HMSO, Oldham, Broadway Business Park, Broadgate, Chadderton, Oldham OL9 0JA.

The Eating Disorders Association

Sackville Place, 44 Magdalen Street, Norwich, Norfolk NR3 1JU. Helpline, tel. 01603 6214141. Young people's helpline, tel. 01603 621414
Provides help for young people with anorexia nervosa and bulimia.

Foundation for the Study of Infant Deaths

14 Halkin Street, London SW1X 7DP, tel. 0171 235 0965
Cot death helpline, tel. 0171 235 1721
This help line is available 24 hours a day for bereaved families.

The Genetic Interest Group (GIG)

Farringdon Point, 29–35 Farringdon Road, London EC1M 3JB, tel. 0171 430 0090
The Genetic Interest Group is the national umbrella body for voluntary organizations and support groups for people affected by genetic disorders. Part of their remit is to raise public and health professional awareness of the services and support available for those affected by these conditions.

Hospice Information Service

St Christopher's Hospice, 51 Lawrie Park Road, Sydenham, London SE26 6DZ, tel. 0181 778 9252
Resource for the public and health professionals seeking information on the work of the hospice movement.

MENCAP: Royal Society for Mentally Handicapped Children and Adults

Mencap National Centre, 123 Golden Lane, London EC1Y 0RT, tel. 0171 454 0454
Mencap is exclusively concerned with people with learning disabilities and their families. Mencap runs residential, training, employment, and leisure services. It campaigns to improve public awareness of services for people with learning disabilities.

National Asthma Campaign

Providence House, Providence Place, London N1 0NT, tel. 0171 226 2260; 0345 010203
The Campaign funds research into all aspects of asthma and related allergy. It produces a wide range of patient education materials, including self-management plans and a schools pack.

National Eczema Society

163 Eversholt Street, London NW1 1BU, tel. 0171 388 4097
It promotes quality care through the provision of information, support, and education and by funding research. A range of literature is available.

The Royal National Institute for the Blind

224 Great Portland Street, London W1N 6AA, tel. 0171 388 1266
Supports visually impaired children both in mainstream and special schools. Produces books and trains readers in Braille; talking book service; promotes research; monitors legislation; advisory service for parents; family case-work; information service for professionals.

The Royal National Institute For Deaf People

105 Gower Street, London WC1E 6AH, tel. 0171 387 8033 (voice)
The main objective of the RNID is to improve services and opportunities for deaf, deaf-blind and hard of hearing people. It also aims to increase public and professional awareness of the difficulties encountered by the deaf. Amongst the services provided are: residential care, specialist telephone services, the sale of assistive devices, training, communication support units, and information.

SCOPE (previously the Spastics Society)

12 Park Crescent, London W1 N4EQ, tel. 0171 636 5020
Freephone helpline: tel. 0800 626 216
Offers educational assessment, social, and information services for children and adults with cerebral palsy.

There are many associations for the numerous very rare conditions such as the Angelman's Syndrome Support Group and the Lowe's Syndrome Association. These associations can be particularly helpful when the family has to cope with an unusual disease that fellow parents and local doctors know little about; remembering that occasionally a parent running such a group may have a rather idiosyncratic view of the disorder or of the caring professions.

Bibliography

Apley, J. (1979). *Paediatrics*, (2nd edn). Baillière Tindall, London.

British National Formulary. (1995). No. 28. British Medical Association and the Pharmaceutical Society of Great Britain, London. (Essential if rather purist.)

Catzel, P. and Olver, R. (1981). *The paediatric prescriber,* (5th edn). Blackwell Scientific Publications, Oxford.

Data Sheet Compendium. (1995–96). Together with the Code of Practice for the Pharmaceutical Industry. Datapharm Publications Limited. (Useful for a quick check on side-effects or dosage.)

Forfar and Arneil's textbook of paediatrics. (1992). 4th edn, (ed. A. G. M. Campbell and N. McIntosh). Churchill Livingstone, London.

Godfrey, S., Kamburoff, P. L., Nairn, J. R., Connolly, N. M. C., Davis, J., Packham, E., and Samuels, L. S. (1970). Spirometry: lung volumes and airways resistance in normal children aged 5-18 years. *British Journal of Diseases of the Chest,* **64**, 15–23.

Illingworth, R. S. (1980). *The development of the infant and young child, normal and abnormal*, (7th edn). Churchill Livingstone, London.

Second Task Force on Blood Pressure Control in Children. (1987). Report. *Paediatrics,* **79**, 1–20.

Index